Bonney's Gynaecological Surgery

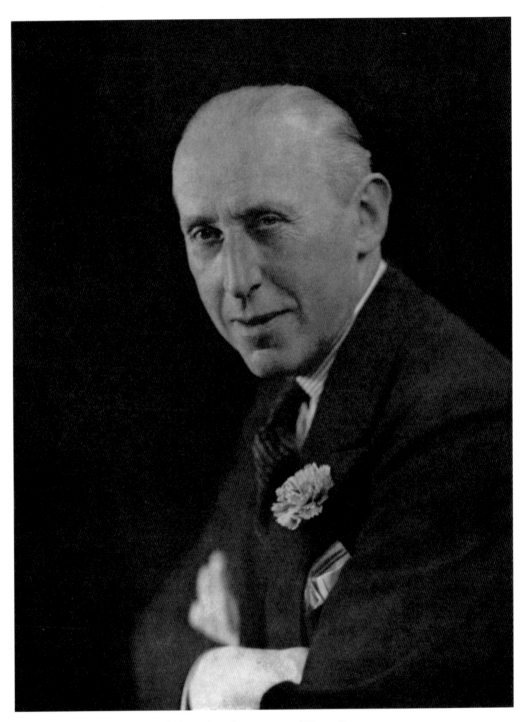

This book is dedicated to the memory of Victor Bonney.
It is also dedicated to Jane, Vicki, Roopal and Maggie for their support, understanding, patience and love, which they have shown us in our lives together.

Bonney's Gynaecological Surgery

Tito Lopes

MBChB, FRCOG
Consultant Gynaecological Oncologist
Royal Cornwall Hospital
Truro
UK

Nick M. Spirtos

MD
Professor and Vice-Chairman, Department of Obstetrics and Gynecology
Director, Division of Gynecologic Oncology, University of Nevada School of
Medicine, Reno, and the Women's Cancer Center of Nevada, Las Vegas
NV, USA

Raj Naik

MD, FRCOG
Consultant Gynaecological Oncologist and Surgeon
Clinical Director of the Northern Gynaecological Oncology Centre
Queen Elizabeth Hospital
Gateshead
UK

John M. Monaghan

MB, FRCS (Ed), FRCOG
Retired Senior Lecturer in Gynaecological Oncology, University
of Newcastle Upon Tyne
Retired Gynaecological Oncologist, Regional Department of
Gynaecological Oncology
Queen Elizabeth Hospital
Gateshead
UK

ELEVENTH EDITION

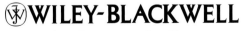

A John Wiley & Sons, Ltd., Publication

Blackwell Publishing was acquired by John Wiley & Sons in February 2007. Blackwell's publishing program has been merged with Wiley's global Scientific, Technical and Medical business to form Wiley-Blackwell.

Registered office: John Wiley & Sons Ltd, The Atrium, Southern Gate, Chichester, West Sussex, PO19 8SQ, UK

Editorial offices: 9600 Garsington Road, Oxford, OX4 2DQ, UK
The Atrium, Southern Gate, Chichester, West Sussex, PO19 8SQ, UK
111 River Street, Hoboken, NJ 07030-5774, USA

For details of our global editorial offices, for customer services and for information about how to apply for permission to reuse the copyright material in this book please see our website at www.wiley.com/wiley-blackwell

Library of Congress Cataloging-in-Publication Data
Bonney's gynaecological surgery. – 11th ed. / Tito Lopes ... [et al.].
    p. ; cm.
  Other title: Gynaecological surgery
  Includes bibliographical references and index.
  ISBN 978-1-4051-9565-2
  1. Generative organs, Female–Surgery. I. Lopes, Tito. II. Bonney, Victor, 1872–1953. Gynaecological surgery. III. Title: Gynaecological surgery.
  [DNLM: 1. Gynecologic Surgical Procedures. 2. Genitalia, Female–surgery. WP 660 B7171 2010]
RG104.B65 2010
618.1–dc22
                        2010015117

ISBN: 9781405195652

A catalogue record for this book is available from the British Library.

This book is published in the following electronic format: ePDF 9781444325232; Wiley Online Library 9781444325225

Set in 9/11.5 pt Sabon by Toppan Best-set Premedia Limited

Printed and bound in Singapore by Markono Print Media Pte Ltd

01 2011

Contents

Preface to the eleventh edition

Next year, *Bonney's Gynaecological Surgery* celebrates its 100th birthday, the first edition having been published in 1911 by Comyns Berkeley and Victor Bonney. In those 100 years, major advances in anaesthetics, transfusion services, antibiotics and instrument development have not only resulted in safer surgery for the patient but also have allowed increasing innovation in surgical procedures.

In gynaecology this is exemplified by the almost routine use of minimal access techniques in everyday practice, as well as the increasing surgical options in the urological and oncological subspecialties.

Despite these advances, many of the basic surgical principles remain unchanged, and this is highlighted by the retention in this edition of some of Bonney's original drawings 100 years on.

Three of the current editors have worked in the department of gynaecological oncology in Gateshead started by Stanley Way in 1948. It is therefore not surprising that this 11th edition reflects an evolution rather than a revolution from the 9th edition edited by John Monaghan in 1986, the preface of which follows this current preface.

As with previous editors, I have taken the liberty of removing elements from the last edition which are no longer relevant to current practice. The format has also changed and the current edition is divided into three sections. The first section, covering general principles and basic techniques, lays the foundation for any trainee wishing to develop into a competent gynaecological surgeon. The second section, presented by anatomical site, covers the common procedures undertaken in day-to-day benign gynaecology. The last section recognizes the two surgical subspecialties of urogynaecology and gynaecological oncology. Although several of the procedures described are currently undertaken by the experienced generalist as well as the specialist, this is becoming less common, especially in cancer surgery. This section also covers surgery for other sites that may arise during gynaecological surgery, either as a planned procedure or as the result of an unexpected finding or complication. Although rarely encountered in general gynaecology, and usually within the remit of one's surgical colleagues, it is important to understand the principles of the procedures involved.

As the senior editor I am indebted to John Monaghan and Raj Naik for their continued support and I am extremely grateful to Nick Spirtos for agreeing to join us in editing this current edition. His skills in both laparoscopic and radical open surgery are recognized internationally and his methodical approach to these procedures is reflected in his contributions to the book. I also wish to thank David Richmond and Gillian Fowler for their contributions to the section on urogynaecology.

Lastly, my thanks to Wiley-Blackwell and especially to publisher Martin Sugden for inviting me to lead on this edition of *Bonney's Gynaecological Surgery*. The support and encouragement of their team along with that of Lindsey Williams has made the whole process a pleasure.

Tito Lopes
Truro, Cornwall
September 2010

Preface to the ninth edition

The influence of Victor Bonney and his pupils upon gynaecological surgery has developed from the publication of the first edition of *A Textbook of Gynaecological Surgery* in 1911. The first to the fourth editions were the results of the collaboration of Bonney with Sir Comynus Berkeley. Following the death of the latter, Victor Bonney produced the fifth and sixth editions alone. Bonney's pupils Howkins and Macleod then produced the seventh edition. The death of Macleod signalled virtually the end of those practising surgeons who had been trained by Victor Bonney. The very successful eighth edition was prepared by John Howkins and Sir John Stallworthy. These two great figures of Commonwealth Gynaecology had worked together as junior colleagues during the last years of Bonney's clinical career.

When the eighth edition was published in 1974 many changes were incorporated into the text. However, in the next 10 years, an enormous number of new developments have occurred, possibly the greatest being a resurgence of interest in gynaecological surgery and the growth and establishment of gynaecological oncology as a recognized subspecialty. The present editor has only a tenuous link with Victor Bonney in that he has been greatly influenced in his career by the late Dr A.F. Anderson of Edinburgh and by Mr Stanley Way, both of whom spoke frequently with great affection and reverence of the master surgeon. Indeed it was Way who introduced me to the Bonney scissors, which instruments the reader will see referred to throughout this edition.

When asked by the medical editor of Baillière Tindall for my opinion of the eighth edition of *Bonney's Gynaecological Surgery* some 2 years ago, I replied that I thought that it was undoubtedly the leading textbook of gynaecological surgery in the world, but would nevertheless benefit from a major revision. I also jokingly said 'Give me five years and I will do it for you'. The prompt rejoinder was 'We will give you two years if you will take it on'. Little did I know at the time that I had been 'set up', as the Americans say. I felt hesitant at the prospect of making major changes to such a well-established book but realized that large-scale changes were necessary and also that if modern materials and instruments were to be incorporated, most of the drawings would require reworking.

It was also clear that no single surgeon could encompass all the skills of modern gynaecological surgery and that I would need assistance with three major sections. I have been delighted with the response and the quality of the contributions from Sir Rustam Feroze, Stuart L. Stanton and Professor John R. Newton. I am indebted to them.

Victor Bonney had skills far beyond those of mere mortals; to be able to operate to the highest level and then to be capable of transferring those ideas to paper as the most clear and concise drawings was an amazing talent. I have been especially fortunate in obtaining the services of Mr Douglas Hammersley, once head of graphics at the University of Newcastle upon Tyne, to illustrate all the chapters which have been rewritten. Doug has now moved to Norfolk to be a little closer to his chief interest, that of observing and drawing butterflies. I am sure that the reader will appreciate the outstanding quality of the drawings in this new edition, in particular the way in which they have captured the movement and dynamism of surgery. I am totally indebted to Doug for bringing to life my attempts at surgery.

This book is very much my own; the philosophy of the surgery is entirely mine and the responsibility for making such drastic alterations to this classic text are also mine. I do not make apologies as I feel that Bonney would have approved because I have attempted to keep his beloved gynaecological surgery moving forward. Indeed, even between the beginning and end of the 2-year writing period, new developments have occurred which have had to be incorporated into the text.

I have attempted to show that by adopting an economy of movement in surgery as well as in the text, operations can be performed cleanly and neatly, without ritual. Operations should flow with a style and a natural pace, rather like a well-choreographed dance. There should be no great crises and the procedure should not be performed to the point of total exhaustion for the surgeon and his staff. I have tried to show the enormous enthusiasm which I have for gynaecological surgery and the way in which I feel that it can become a source of great satisfaction and pride. I hope that a little of this enthusiasm is transmitted to the reader and that this book will bring forth new energies for the development of our fascinating subject.

The updating of this text has been for me an enormous honour and a great pleasure. I have had to clarify my thoughts on many aspects of surgery and take bold decisions to cut out large quantities of the previous edition, particularly the results and compli-cations sections, which although historically interesting are not relevant to modern-day practice except as records of the past. Their repetition would simply occupy space.

This ninth edition hopefully reflects the most modern aspects of gynaecological surgery as well as retaining all that is still valuable and relevant from past editions. It also emphasizes the continuing role of gynaecological surgery in the management of a multitude of gynaeco-logical conditions, particularly highlighting the place of surgery in cancer care and the newer surgical technique relating to the infertile woman. The place of new tools such as the laser and staples has been added to the more standard instrumentation.

I would like to thank Baillière Tindall and in particular Dr Geoffrey Smaldon for his constant support. To all those who have assisted, guided and encouraged me during my career, occasionally allowing this stubborn, single-minded Yorkshireman to have his way, I am grateful.

Very special thanks must go to Mr Alan Evans who, as my senior registrar, painstakingly read all my first drafts and attempted to bring a Welsh view of the English language to bear upon my efforts.

I stand in great awe at the end of a long line of illustrious names in gynaecological surgery. I hope that I have done them justice in this the ninth edition of *Bonney's Gynaecological Surgery*.

John M. Monaghan
Newcastle upon Tyne
April 1986

Part 1: General

1

Introduction and prologue

Surgery remains only as safe as those wielding the scalpel.

Tito Lopes

Introduction

Surgical training

Surgical training in gynaecology has seen dramatic changes in both the UK and the USA over the last 20 years.

When the current editors were in training, there were no restrictions to the number of hours that they could be asked to work. It was common to be resident on call every third night in addition to daytime work, which often resulted in a working week in excess of 110 hours. In the UK, adoption of the European Union Working Time Directive will mean that trainees will legally be allowed to work only 48 hours per week. In the USA, the working week for residents is limited to 80 hours.

Although the reduction in working hours is important for one's work–life balance, it has inevitably had a major impact on surgical training. The concept of the surgical team or firm to which a trainee was attached has all but disappeared. The introduction of shift systems has made it difficult, and in some cases

impossible, for trainees to attend the surgical and clinical sessions of their team.

At the same time, there has been a marked reduction in the number of hysterectomies performed as a result of more conservative management options for dysfunctional uterine bleeding. In the 9-year period from 1995 to 2004, there was a 46% reduction in the number of hysterectomy operations performed in NHS hospitals in England (Hospital Episode Statistics). In 2003, at the 'Fellows' ceremony at the Royal College of Gynaecologists, the then President stated that not every specialist gynaecologist would be expected to be able to perform a hysterectomy.

With the increasing use of laparoscopic surgery in elective gynaecology, including for hysterectomy, the 'open' approach to gynaecological surgery, the surgical 'bread and butter' for trainees, is also on the decline. Equally, a large number of ectopic pregnancies are now managed conservatively so that trainees are lacking exposure to emergency laparoscopic surgery for tubal pregnancies.

Gynaecology training

Current training in the UK is a competency-based process and it is envisaged that the majority of trainees will take 7 years to complete the programme. As part of the training, the trainee must be competent in opening and closing a transverse incision before commencing his or her third year but need only be assessed for opening and closing a vertical abdominal incision in the advanced module for benign surgery in years 6 and 7. In these last two years the trainees are obliged to complete a minimum of two of 21 available advanced training skills modules, which include separate modules for benign abdominal, vaginal, laparoscopic and hysteroscopic surgery.

Basic skills and training opportunities

Trainees wishing to develop as gynaecological surgeons should attend appropriate courses including cadaver and live animal workshops. However, they are no substitute for learning the basic surgical skills, and picking up good habits, early in training; bad habits are difficult to lose at a later stage. As assistants, they should question any variations in technique among the surgeons. As surgeons, they should review every operation they perform to assess how they could have done better.

In relation to laparoscopic surgery, there is no excuse for trainees not practising with laparoscopic simulators that are often readily available or easy to construct. It is readily apparent to trainers which trainees have spent adequate time on simulators.

Sadly, a consequence of the new training is an inevitable lack of knowledge and experience of the 'unusual', with the all too frequent result of difficulties for both the patient and the surgeon. These difficulties are often manifest in an almost complete failure to appreciate the wide range of possibilities for management. Previous editors of this text have advocated that any surgery should be tailored to the specific needs of the patient and her condition. Unfortunately, when modern patients are managed they are in real danger of being treated by surgeons with a limited experience and a narrow range of skills which may be applied in a 'one-size-fits-all' pattern. In this text, we have attempted to provide a wide range of options for management which we would encourage all trainees to practise assiduously in order to give their patients the very best possible chances of a successful outcome.

Despite the recent changes in gynaecological training, the essence of surgery remains essentially unchanged. The editors have felt it appropriate in this 11th edition to retain the prologue written for the 9th and 10th editions by JM Monaghan based on that of the 1st edition of this series, *A Textbook of Gynaecological Surgery*, published in 1911 by Comyns Berkeley and Victor Bonney. It remains just as relevant today as it was a century ago.

Prologue: after Comyns Berkeley and Victor Bonney

The bearing of the surgeon

A surgeon when operating should always remember that the character of the work of his subordinates will be largely influenced by his own bearing. Whilst it is impossible to lay down definite rules suitable for all temperaments, nevertheless there are certain considerations which will prove useful to those embarking on a gynaecological career. Anyone who has taken the trouble to study the work of other operators cannot fail to have observed how variously the stress and strain of operating is borne by different minds and will deduce from a consideration of the strong and weak points of each operator some conception of the ideal.

The thoughtful surgeon, influenced by this study, will endeavour so to discipline himself so that he will strive constantly to achieve the ideal. By so doing, he will encourage all who work in the wards and theatres with him – young colleagues in training, anaesthetists, nurses, theatre assistants and orderlies – to appreciate the privileges and responsibilities of their common task. Expert co-ordinated teamwork is essential to the success of modern surgery. This teamwork has resulted in a significant lowering of operative morbidity and mortality.

However, it is important to recognize the enormous contribution to the safety of modern surgery made by other disciplines, especially anaesthesiology. The preoperative assessment and the postoperative care carried out by the anaesthetist has rendered surgery safer and has also allowed patients who would not in the past have been considered eligible for surgery to have their procedures performed successfully. The role of specialties such as haematology, biochemistry, microbiology, radiology, pathology and physiotherapy are also well recognized.

Bonney maintained that the keystone of a surgeon's bearing should be his self-control; and whilst it is his duty to keep a general eye on all that takes place in the operating theatre and without hesitation correct mistakes, he should guard against becoming irritable or losing temper. The surgeon who when faced with difficulties loses control has mistaken his vocation, however dextrous he may be, or however learned in the technical details of the art. The habit of abusing the assistants, the instruments or the anaesthetist, so easy to acquire and so hard to lose, is not one to be commended; the lack of personal confidence from which such behaviour stems will inevitably spread to other members of staff, so that at the very time the surgeon needs effective help it is likely to be found wanting. However, the converse of accepting poor standards of care and behaviour is not to be condoned. The continual presentation of inadequately prepared instrumentation should not be accepted. There is little excuse for staff or equipment to arrive in theatre in a state ill prepared for the task ahead.

The whole team should look forward to a theatre session as a period of pleasure, stimulation and achievement, not as a chore and a period of misery to be suffered. The surgeon should also remember that he is on 'display' and his ability to cope with adversity as well as his manner when the surgery is going well will be keenly observed. The surgeon should teach continuously, pointing out to assistants and observers the small points of technique as well as related facts to the case in hand.

Bonney enjoined that the surgeon should not gossip; the present editors feel that day-to-day chit-chat is not out of place in the operating theatre and is to be preferred to the media view of an operating theatre as a place of knife-like tension fraught with grave interpersonal relationships. However, the mark of the good surgeon and his team is that, at the time of stress, the noise level in theatre should fall rather than rise, as each member of the team goes about his or her task with speed and efficiency.

It is inevitable that at some point the surgeon will come face to face with imminent disaster; even the most stalwart individual will feel his heart sink at such a moment. The operator should always remember that at such moments if basic surgical principles are applied quickly and accurately the situation will be rapidly rescued. Hesitation and uncertainty will all too often terminate in disaster. A sturdy belief in his own powers and a refusal to accept defeat are the best assets of a calling which pre-eminently demands moral courage.

Before operating the surgeon should prepare by going over in his own mind the various possibilities in the projected procedure, so that there may be no surprises and he may all the better meet any eventuality. Likewise following the procedure it is valuable to go over in one's mind every step in the operation in

order to analyse any deficiencies and difficulties experienced; it is only by this continuous self-assessment and analysis that the surgeon can from his own efforts improve his practice.

It is of increasing importance that the surgeon understands the need for meticulous record-keeping in order to build a comprehensive database for future analysis. The modern surgeon has to continually examine his and others' work in order to practise to the highest possible standards. More and more guidelines are being generated; the surgeon has to be sure that his work meets the quality requirements of modern practice. Patients, purchasers and professional bodies wish to be able to access the best possible practices. Transparency of standards is essential to modern medical practice. The high-quality surgeon has little to fear from the implementation of guidelines and should look upon these times as opportunities for developing the highest quality of care.

Surgery is physically and mentally tiring. The surgeon should be sure to be adequately equipped in both these areas to meet the demands of theatre. It is important to remember that driving the staff on for long, tiring sessions is counterproductive; there is little merit in performing long procedures with an already exhausted staff. The surgeon's hands and mind become less steady, his assistants less attentive and the nurses tired and disillusioned. It is under these circumstances that mistakes occur. It is important, however, not to be dogmatic about the ideal length either of individual operations or of operating lists. A full day in the operating theatre may suit one surgical team but be anathema to another.

Speed in operating

Speed, as an indication of perfect operative technique, is the characteristic of a fine surgeon, as striving for after-effect is the stock-in-trade of the charlatan. An operation rapidly yet correctly performed has many advantages over one as technically correct yet laboriously and tediously accomplished. The period over which haemorrhage may occur is shortened, the tissues are handled less and are therefore less bruised, the time the peritoneum is open and exposed is shortened, the amount and length of anaesthesia is shortened and the impact of the operative shock, which is an accumulation of all these factors, is lessened. Moreover, less strain is put upon the temper and legs

5

of the operator and his assistants with the result that the interest of the latter and the onlookers is maintained at the highest level.

However, this speed must be tempered with attention to detail, particularly of haemostasis, and by a conscious effort not to unnecessarily handle tissue.

Operative manipulation

The surgeon should continually endeavour to reduce the number of manipulations involved in a procedure to the absolute minimum consistent with sound performance. If an operation is observed critically, one is struck by the vast number of unnecessary movements performed, the majority of which are due to the uncertainty and inexperience of the operator. In older surgeons, unless care is taken to analyse these movements and eliminate them they will become part of the habits and ritual of the procedure.

Minimizing trauma is of fundamental importance for uncomplicated wound healing. *The art of gentle surgery must be developed* (Moynihan). Sadly, many surgeons achieve speed by being rough with tissue, particularly by direct handling. This must be avoided at all costs, and the temptation to tear tissue with the hands rather than to delicately incise and dissect with instruments is to be eschewed. All operative manipulations should be gentle; force is occasionally essential but should be applied with accuracy, only to the tissue to be removed and for limited periods of time. The surgeon who tears and traumatizes tissue will see the error of his ways in the long recovery periods that his patients require and in the high complication rate.

Moynihan spoke in 1920 at the inaugural meeting of the British Association of Surgeons on 'The Ritual of a Surgical Operation', stating that 'he [the surgeon] must set endeavour in continual motion, and seek always and earnestly for simpler methods and a better way. In the craft of surgery the master word is *simplicity*.'

Further reading

Berkeley C, Bonney V. *A Text-book of Gynaecological Surgery*. London: Gassell and Company, 1911. See www.archive.org/details/textbookofgynaec00berkuoft

Hospital Episode Statistics. See www.hesonline.nhs.uk/

Moynihan BGA. The ritual of a surgical operation. *Br J Surg* 1920;8:27–35.

2 Preparation for surgery

Before major surgery,

> Submit yourself to your God, your love to
> your beloved and friends and your trust in
> your doctor.
>
> *Lord Gowrie (1999)*

Most gynaecological surgery is elective. Consequently, for most patients, there is no excuse for preoperative assessment and preparation for surgery not to be comprehensive. There should be a departmental protocol in place so that all staff involved with the care of the patient provide consistent high-quality care. A medical history, examination and relevant investigations are undertaken as part of preoperative assessment. The patient is provided with appropriate information, often in conjunction with support from a nurse specialist, and an informed consent is taken. A review of all available information, including preoperative scans and laboratory tests, should be performed prior to surgery. In theatre, patient safety may be increased by use of the World Health Organization (WHO) Surgical Safety Checklist.

Initial visit

Most patients will be first seen in the outpatient department, where a preliminary assessment and provisional diagnosis will be made. At this first visit, the clinician should obtain a comprehensive history, fully examine the patient including the pelvis and abdomen and organize the next series of steps in the diagnostic process. Once this information is collated, admission dates for surgery, if appropriate, are organized, or referral made to the appropriate specialist. In the UK, there is increasing pressure on clinicians to see patients rapidly, come to a definitive diagnosis and arrange appropriate management as quickly as possible. Although this pressure is most acute in the diagnosis and management of cancer, it is being extended in a more limited fashion to the management of benign conditions.

In order to attain targets, clinics have to be structured so that referral can be made by telephone, fax or online if necessary, and appropriate diagnostic facilities such as endometrial sampling, ultrasound and colposcopy are available at the one visit. This requires considerable collaboration with supporting services including radiology and pathology.

History-taking and documentation

As the clinician progresses through training, every effort should be made to concentrate on developing a style of clear and concise history-taking. Initially, this process of meticulous systematic questioning may seem cumbersome. However, with constant practice, an abbreviated technique will develop which concentrates on the major fields of interest but also allows for peripheral areas of relevance to be included.

Documentation of the history is vital for medico-legal purposes, for transmission of information to colleagues and for analysis in clinical research and

Bonney's Gynaecological Surgery, 11th edition.
© Tito Lopes, Nick Spirtos, Raj Naik, John Monaghan.
Published 2011 by Blackwell Publishing Ltd.

audit. The editors have over many years organized standardized questionnaires for all patients, the details of which build up a complete picture of the patient, her cancer and her progress through therapy. This huge database allows rapid access for office administration, audit, research and analysis.

In an increasingly litigious world, the careful but not necessarily cautious doctor who keeps good records and takes the time to communicate and document all meetings will to a significant extent protect him- or herself from the very distressing circumstances of litigation.

Patient information

Gynaecological patients require considerable support and assistance when making decisions about treatment, particularly surgery. The most important factor is the manner in which the patient conceives the impact of the operation upon herself, particularly her sexuality. The surgeon must be prepared to spend a considerable amount of time discussing and explaining the content of any surgical procedure. This important process is frequently aided by the use of literature and drawings, copies of which should be included in the medical record. Departmental websites and contact numbers are a great assistance.

It is at this point that the clinician may feel the need to involve other areas of expertise, including a nurse specialist, psychologist, stoma therapist and dietician. A factor that is often of enormous reassurance to the patient is to meet other patients who have been treated for a similar problem and experienced similar procedures.

Clearly, such a detailed approach is not practical for all procedures, especially minor ones; however, it is important not to trivialize minor procedures, especially those involving anaesthesia, as complications can and will occur and warning of the possibility and appropriate consenting is vital for all operations, even those of a diagnostic nature carried out in the outpatient department under local anaesthetic. It is important not to 'talk down' to patients; always use accurate terminology with appropriate explanation and resist the temptation to use gross inaccuracies, which become perpetuated in the mythology of the subject, such as the vaginal hysterectomy being described as a 'suction' hysterectomy.

The offer to the patient to attend with her partner, a close family member or a friend is also of vital importance in providing support and reassurance to the patient and often contributes to the essential dialogue and communication which is necessary. Patients take in and understand information at very varying rates; some are comfortable with a brief once-only visit, whereas others may need repeat visits or telephone calls to answer questions and seek reassurance. This wide range must be accommodated within a successful practice.

Clinic information

If at all possible, information in written form should be sent to patients prior to the first visit. This should not only include details of appointments, parking facilities, transport access, etc. but also as many broad details as can be envisaged. This should include warnings about examination, time involved and the advisability of having a partner or companion present. For many specialist clinics, such as those for colposcopy, specific details of procedures can be outlined. A list of contact telephone numbers and departmental websites should be included.

Information sheets and documents

At the end of the clinic visit, it is of inestimable value to be able to give the patient and her accompanying person a sheet of information with an outline summary of what has been said and discussed in the clinic. The type of document will usually have space for drawings and handwritten notes. If the sheet can be of a 'carbon copy' type, the patient will be able to take home the original and an exact copy is stored within the clinical record. Locally or nationally produced leaflets or booklets regarding the specific condition and operation should also be given to the patient to take home and read.

Drawings

Drawings of procedures indicating tissues to be removed with small annotations alluding to potential complications and future difficulties are of enormous value. The drawings should be made in the clinical record or included in the information sheet mentioned above and the copy kept in the records. Such drawings, however crude and simplistic, are often critical when complaints or legal proceedings occur.

Consent for surgery

In recent years considerable effort has been expended in trying to improve the whole process of consent. The main reason for this is the extensive publicity given when operations are allegedly performed without 'proper' consent.

Patients must give consent for operation in the light of full knowledge of the procedure, the nature of the condition for which it is being proposed, any serious or frequent complications of the surgery, as well as any reasonable or accepted alternative treatments, including no treatment. In the UK, four standard consent forms have been created for all categories of patients including for those with parental responsibility and use where the patient is an adult unable to consent. In gynaecology, most patients who are undergoing surgical treatments are able to give consent on their own behalf.

Current legal principles and philosophies require that patients are informed of all potential complications associated with the planned surgical procedure irrespective of the likelihood of their occurrence or rarity. Although many surgeons may oppose such practice because they do not want to burden the patient with fearful information to the point of seriously complicating the patient–doctor relationship and the loss of the patient's trust in the surgeon, it is important to address during the consultation how much information the patient is willing and able to receive through direct questioning and to document clearly in the notes if she demands an abbreviated list of risks and complications. When the patient prefers a full and thorough discussion then it is important that the surgeon presents the risks of surgery that relate to his/her own individual and personal practice rather than reference to accepted or published rates, which may differ considerably and will serve only to misguide the patient and surgeon.

Concept of risk

For the majority of patients an understanding of risk is not clear. Journalistic increases of risk of 50% may sound alarming, but explaining that this change involves a move from 0.5% to 0.75% will be immensely reassuring. All populations are bombarded with 'statistics' which require careful analysis and explanation. It is incumbent upon all surgeons preparing patients for operation to be able to translate risk into understandable and meaningful terms. Although it is vital to be scrupulously honest with the patient about all potential risks, putting the risks into perspective is a skill to be developed by all trainees.

Consent to surgical trials

Recruitment to surgical trials often adds further complexities to the consent process. It requires an understanding of our current knowledge 'or lack of it' in relation to the disease process or treatment procedure being researched, and the ability to explain to patients the vital need for research to improve the quality of care for future patients by providing good quality evidence relating to new or currently available treatments. Such consultations can be testing to junior surgeons, and it is only through good consultative technique that they are able to translate commonly used terms and research principles for the patient, including 'randomization' and 'blinding'. Although good levels of recruitment are often a proxy of a good consultation, it is crucial not to coerce patients into a trial that they clearly have no understanding of. The employment of a trials nurse, although not diminishing the important need for an enthusiastic approach by the surgeon, can be invaluable in achieving adequate recruitment to available trials while ensuring that the patient has given consent to enter the trial based on sound moral and ethical grounds.

Timing of consent

There has been considerable discussion but no firm conclusions about the best time for consent for an operation to be obtained.

The taking of consent as part of the clinic visit has been viewed by supporters as enabling the patient to take this important step away from the stress of admission to hospital and an imminent operation. The contrary view is that, at the time of the clinic visit, there is far too much information to be taken in and that the patient is suffering from information 'overload' and will have problems in making a sensible, balanced decision.

The taking of consent at the time of admission for surgery has been viewed as incorrect because of the stresses already mentioned. This problem may be exacerbated as we move more and more to admission times very close to the time of surgery. The positive side of this approach is that the patient has had time to weigh the points of management that have been put to her at the original clinic visit. Contact may have been made in the interim and further concerns dealt with. This approach also reflects the principles of obtaining patient consent as a 'continual process' rather than as a 'discrete event'.

Preoperative assessment

In many centres, preoperative assessment clinics have been set up and run by nursing staff at which all preoperative investigations and admission procedures can be performed. This is excellent when patients live close to the hospital; however, making an extra journey to the hospital is either inconvenient or impossible when patients have to travel any distance, as is found in association with centralized services. In this situation pre-assessment may be undertaken by the referring hospital or centres may organize the pre-assessment to be undertaken as part of the initial visit.

Pre-assessment clinics have the added advantage of ensuring that all investigations and information can be obtained well in advance of the intended surgery so that unexpected results can be addressed and the patient optimized without resorting to postponement of surgery, as may be the case when the investigations are performed just prior to the date of surgery. The clinic is becoming increasingly valuable as more patients require specific investigations such as echocardiograms and pulmonary function tests prior to surgery. It also avoids the embarrassing scenario of the surgeon having overlooked the need to discontinue/ modify or schedule vital medications at the appropriate times, including clopidogrel and warfarin.

Assessment of medical conditions such as cardiovascular disease, hypertension, diabetes, pulmonary disease and mental state may all require input from an expert in the field. It is important to allow adequate time for appropriate consultation and correction of problems prior to surgery. Often, the expert

anaesthetist will be able to give a clear opinion on the physical state of the patient. It is the editors' opinion that the decision to anaesthetize is taken by the anaesthetist and the decision to operate by the surgeon following on.

Early admission may be necessary on occasions for patients who have specific problems which may need to be corrected prior to surgery. However, the majority can be admitted on the day of, or the day prior to, surgery.

Preoperative investigations

It is not the place of a surgical text to exhaustively detail all preoperative investigations. The guidelines on *The Use of Routine Preoperative Tests for Elective Surgery*, produced by the National Institute for Health and Clinical Excellence (NICE), provide a useful assessment of the investigations advised based on American Society of Anesthesiologists (ASA) status and type of surgery. Specific tests will be outlined in relevant chapters; only a general outline will be provided here.

1 *Haematological investigations.* Every patient should have a full blood screen performed to include haemoglobin, haematocrit, white cell count and differential, platelets, and a blood film when indicated.

2 *For all procedures in which there is a significant risk of requiring a blood transfusion,* typing of serum should be performed so that blood and blood products can be obtained at short notice. In recent times, acceptance of lower haemoglobin levels, especially postoperatively, coupled with a nervousness about blood and blood products and the use of intraoperative cell salvage have led to a marked reduction in the use of transfusion. A postoperative haemoglobin level of 7 g/dL is often treated with oral iron.

3 *Biochemical investigations.* In most centres it is customary to use computerized assessment of blood, which allows a large range of investigations to be performed rapidly on a small volume of blood. For the majority of procedures, the assessment of the blood electrolytes and liver function test are appropriate.

4 *Tumour markers.* When malignancy is suspected, it is essential that a range of tumour markers is performed to assist in the diagnostic process. This may

include one or a number of the following: CA125, CEA, CA19-9, CA15-3, AFP, HCG, LDH, SCC, inhibin and/or a hormonal profile.

5 *Urinalysis.* Using simple 'stick' tests, a range of analyses can be performed accurately and rapidly on the urine obtained on admission. These are usually screening tests leading the clinician on to more detailed tests when necessary.

6 *Radiological investigations.* Chest radiograph, abdominal and transvaginal ultrasound, computed tomography (CT) scan, magnetic resonance imaging (MRI), positron emission tomography (PET)-CT and other contrast radiology may all be helpful in making a preoperative diagnosis. Their specific indications and value will be discussed in the individual chapters.

7 *Meticillin-resistant* Staphylococcus aureus *(MRSA) screen and decolonization.* As of March 2009, the majority of patients admitted for elective surgery in the UK undergo MRSA screening. Swabs are taken from the patient's nose and one further site, and all positive patients receive a 'decolonization pack' to use prior to admission.

Preoperative meeting

One valuable introduction that the editors have included into their practice in recent years is the weekly 'preoperative meeting'. At this meeting, all patients listed for surgery the following week are presented and discussed in the presence of the preoperative assessment nurse who has collated all the notes and investigation results, including reports following anaesthetic, cardiology, respiratory or haematological assessment. The meeting provides a further 'failsafe' in the process of patient assessment and preparation by ensuring that nothing has been overlooked. It provides the opportunity to reassess the proposed surgery and whether this requires modification based on review of the case and the results of investigations.

It also contributes to the education of the trainee surgeon, who develops the habit of working as part of a team, learns the importance of careful assessment of patients submitting themselves to surgery, and who may also on occasion have to justify clinical decisions on cases they have listed.

Preoperative discussion of the scope of surgery

This discussion should be a continuation of the information given at the first clinic visit. Many of the details outlined at the first visit may have been forgotten or misunderstood; therefore, it is recommended that the clinician repeats the whole explanation of the need for the operation as well as the expected findings and outcome. In particular, this should include all that the patient should expect to happen in the postoperative period. The presence of drips, suction drains, catheters and patient-controlled analgesia devices must be described. The likely timing of their removal is often reassuring, especially if the proposed timetable is adhered to.

Complex postoperative needs such as the possibility of stomas or prolonged application of devices is often best described by experts such as a stoma therapist.

Preoperative visit by the anaesthetist

For most patients the major fear associated with surgery is related to the anaesthetic. Consequently, a sympathetic, reassuring and confident anaesthetist will help to allay most phobias; some patients have fears about needles, some about masks. The skilled anaesthetist will be able to ensure that a particular technique will or will not be used. Clearly, it is important that the person visiting the patient is the clinician who will be present at the anaesthetic.

Preoperative medication may be prescribed at this visit and its timing carefully organized to fit in with the timing of surgery. The advantages of the surgeon and anaesthetist working together as a team can clearly be seen. The drugs to be prescribed are recorded on the anaesthetic record so that the actual time of administration can be checked by the anaesthetist in theatre.

Thromboprophylaxis

Since the 1970s, there has been general agreement that efforts to reduce the incidence of thromboembolism must be made for virtually all patients undergoing major surgery. There is considerable debate as to the relative benefits of mechanical methods both intra- and postoperatively compared with the use of heparin prophylaxis beginning preoperatively and continuing into the postoperative period until the patient is fully mobilized.

Current recommendations are that women with no patient-related risk factors use compression stockings whereas those with risk factors have a combination of mechanical prophylaxis and low-molecular-weight heparin.

The editors' preference for high-risk patients is to use a combination of compression stockings, low-molecular-weight heparin as well as intermittent pneumatic compression during surgery.

Patient-related risk factors should be identified in the pre-assessment clinic and include:

- age over 60 years
- obesity
- use of oral contraceptives or hormone-replacement therapy (HRT)
- pregnancy and puerperium
- cancer and other thrombotic states
- anticipated colorectal surgery (recommended in the USA)
- personal or family history of venous thromboembolism
- thrombophilias
- immobility
- prolonged travel.

Oral contraception and hormone use

Controversy remains as to whether or not to stop the combined oral contraceptive pill (COC) before major surgery. The small increase in risk of postoperative thromboembolic disease (0.5–1%) needs to be balanced against the possibility of an unwanted pregnancy as a result of stopping the pill 4–6 weeks before surgery.

When considering stopping the COC prior to elective surgery, one should discuss the balance of risks and benefits with the patient. Alternative contraception must be provided if the COC is discontinued. If continued, appropriate thromboprophylaxis must be administered based on risk factors.

Venous thromboprophylaxis should be given routinely in women taking the COC who undergo emergency surgery.

Women on high-dose progestogen, HRT and raloxifene are also at an increased risk of thromboembolic disease.

Mechanical prophylaxis

Graduated compression stockings exert graded circumferential pressure from distal to proximal regions of the leg, increasing blood velocity and promoting venous return. These should be worn on admission and the patients encouraged to wear them until they return to their usual levels of mobility. Ideally, the stockings should be thigh length, but if this is not appropriate for reasons of fit or compliance then knee-length stockings may be used instead.

Intermittent pneumatic compression devices involve the use of inflatable garments wrapped around the legs which are intermittently inflated by a pneumatic pump. This enhances venous return and prevents venous stasis.

Pharmacological prophylaxis

Patients at increased risk of thromboembolic disease should have low-molecular-weight heparin in addition to mechanical prophylaxis. This should be continued for at least 5 days or until the time of discharge.

Other strategies

For major surgical procedures, one should encourage the use of regional anaesthesia as it reduces the risk of thrombosis compared with general anaesthesia.

Vena caval filters should be inserted if the patient has existing or a recent venous thrombosis.

Patients must be encouraged to mobilize as soon as possible after surgery.

Do not allow patients to become dehydrated during their stay in hospital.

Bowel preparation

Bowel preparation is used in gynaecological surgery for a variety of reasons.

- *Mechanical.* In both laparoscopic and open procedures, an empty bowel improves access to the pelvis by facilitating bowel retraction away from the pelvis and by producing an empty sigmoid colon and rectum.

• *Vulval soiling.* In vulval and vaginal surgery to reduce the risk of perineal soiling by faecal incontinence resulting in infection of the wounds.

• *Bowel surgery.* In complex operations where bowel surgery is likely to be involved to reduce infectious complications and anastomotic leaks.

Although a Cochrane review of mechanical bowel preparation in elective colorectal surgery showed no evidence of reduced infectious complications and anastomotic leaks, this cannot be translated to complex gynaecological surgery. Bowel surgery in these situations is often the result of an inflammatory or malignant process in which the bowel serosa will not be pristine. In exenterative surgery, bowel will often have been irradiated, compromising healing of any anastomosis while formation of an ileal conduit requires as 'sterile' a segment of bowel as possible to avoid a pyelonephritis.

Minor to intermediate procedures do not usually require significant bowel preparation; at the most, two suppositories on the morning of surgery will suffice. Major procedures during which it is envisaged that bowel will not be resected may benefit from an oral aperient on the day prior to surgery.

Major procedures in which bowel is to be resected will require that the bowel content be reduced to a minimum and sterilized. This is best achieved by putting the patient on a low-residue diet for 2 days prior to operation and giving strong aperients. A non-absorbable antibiotic such as neomycin may be given for 48 hours prior to surgery. Ultimately, the degree and type of bowel preparation used depends on the surgeon's preference and ongoing published evidence.

Dehydration can commonly be associated with preoperative bowel preparation and some patients will require preoperative intravenous hydration to ensure that they are in optimal condition when presented to the surgeon.

In the operating theatre

Prophylactic antibiotics

Prophylactic antibiotics should be used for all major gynaecological operations as they fall under the cat-

egory of clean–contaminated surgery or contaminated surgery. The choice of antibiotics is often based on the local antibiotic formulary, which will be based on prevalent infective organisms and their antibiotic resistance. A single dose of antibiotic prophylaxis should be administered intravenously on starting anaesthesia.

Hair removal

Traditionally, all patients undergoing gynaecological surgery were given a full abdominal and vulval/pudendal shave to reduce the risk of wound infection. It is now felt that there is no need to remove the hair routinely to reduce the risk of infection, although it may still be appropriate if the incision in is a hair-bearing area if only to ease opening and closing of the wound.

If hair has to be removed, this is best done with electric clippers with a disposable head immediately prior to surgery. Razors should not be used as they increase the risk of surgical site infection.

Bladder catheterization

The need for catheterization will depend on the surgical procedure being performed and the personal experience and preference of the surgeon. If catheterization is to be avoided, it is important that the patient empties her bladder immediately before going to theatre.

As with most minor procedures, catheterization using an aseptic technique is rarely taught and often badly performed. The vagina should be prepared at the same time as performing the catheterization. This is the ideal time for the surgeon to perform a bimanual pelvic examination if not recently done to assess the pelvic organs and guide him as to the most appropriate approach.

Skin preparation

Prepare the skin at the surgical site using an antiseptic (aqueous or alcohol based) preparation such as povidone–iodine or chlorhexidine. This should be performed in a methodical fashion starting over the intended site of the incision and radiating out to the edges of the intended area of skin exposure.

Preparation of the vagina should be considered as part of the general skin preparation for abdominal procedures when a hysterectomy is being performed. It is best undertaken at the time of bladder catheterization.

Draping

Drapes should be applied in such a way that the site of the incision and any appropriate landmarks are visible. They must be placed accurately, as they offer lines which the surgeon will use to orientate himself. The use of self-adhesive paper drapes is a vast improvement on the old cloth ones. The adhesion to the skin is firm and complete and does not allow soiling beyond the adhesive area.

WHO Surgical Safety Checklist

In June 2008, the WHO launched a second Global Patient Safety Challenge, 'Safe Surgery Saves Lives' to reduce the number of surgical deaths across the world. A core set of safety checks was identified in the form of a WHO Surgical Safety Checklist for use in any operating theatre environment. A study of the checklist in nearly 8000 surgical patients showed a significant reduction in deaths and complications (Haynes et al. 2009). In January 2009, the NHS announced that an adapted WHO Surgical Safety Checklist must be in place in all hospitals in England and Wales.

The operation note

The operation note is often used in medico-legal cases, and maintaining a proper and legible record is the professional responsibility of the surgeon. The Royal College of Surgeons of England, in its document *Good Surgical Practice*, recommends that every operation note should record:
- date and time
- elective/emergency procedure
- the names of the operating surgeon and assistant
- the operative procedure carried out
- the incision
- the operative diagnosis
- the operative findings
- any problems/complications

- any extra procedure performed and the reason why it was performed
- details of tissue removed, added or altered
- identification of any prosthesis used, including the serial numbers of prostheses and other implanted materials
- details of closure technique
- postoperative care instructions
- a signature.

Further reading

In the UK, we are fortunate to have NICE, an independent organization responsible for providing national guidance on the promotion of good health and the prevention and treatment of ill-health. It produces numerous guidelines each year around public health, health technology and clinical practice. A full list of its guidelines can be found through its website (www.nice.org.uk), but specific guidelines related to this chapter are listed below along with other relevant reading material.

General Medical Council. *Consent: Patients and Doctors Making Decisions Together*. London: GMC, 2008. See http://www.gmc-uk.org/static/documents/content/Consent_2008.pdf.

Haynes AB, Weiser TG, Berry WR, et al. and the Safe Surgery Saves Lives Study Group. A surgical safety checklist to reduce morbidity and mortality in a global population. *N Engl J Med* 2009;360:491–499.

National Institute for Health and Clinical Excellence. *The Use of Routine Preoperative Tests for Elective Surgery*. NICE guideline no. 3. London: NICE, 2003. See http://www.nice.org.uk/CG003.

National Institute for Health and Clinical Excellence. Reducing the Risk of Venous Thromboembolism (Deep Vein Thrombosis and Pulmonary Embolism) in Inpatients Undergoing Surgery. NICE guideline no. 46. London: NICE, 2007. See http://www.nice.org.uk/CG046.

Royal College of Obstetricians and Gynaecologists. *Obtaining Valid Consent*. RCOG Clinical Governance Advice no. 6. London: RCOG, 2008. See http://www.rcog.org.uk/womens-health/clinical-guidance/obtaining-valid-consent.

Royal College of Surgeons. *Good Clinical Practice*. London: RCS, 2008. See www.scts.org/documents/PDF/GoodSurgicalPractice2008.pdf.

World Health Organization. *Safe Surgery Saves Lives*. The Second Global Patient Safety Challenge. Geneva: WHO, 2009. See www.who.int/patientsafety/safesurgery.

3

Instruments, operative materials and basic surgical techniques

The choice of instruments used by a surgeon is influenced by his mentors during the formative years of training. Surgical trainees should develop the habit of questioning their superiors as to why a certain piece of equipment is used in preference to another. They should experiment with the various instruments available to them and critically assess their strengths and weaknesses. Attending surgical procedures in other specialties exposes one to a further plethora of instruments often developed for specific situations but which can be transferrable to gynaecological surgery. With each new training appointment they should scrutinize the instruments available in the basic trays, recognizing old favourites and rapidly evaluating new ones.

This critical evaluation of instruments should continue throughout a surgeon's professional practice, recognizing that no instrument is ideal for every situation. Currently, the generic tray system remains the central plank of instrument provision for the majority of gynaecological procedures and it is imperative that the surgeon dictates the content of the trays to represent the actual requirements of the surgeons involved. However, it is essential that a surgeon does not develop a reputation for desiring every minor new development seen at surgical meetings, but should insist on a broad but concise range of high-quality functioning equipment that does not continually irritate by failing to work, whether this be a simple

pair of scissors or the most sophisticated laparoscopic piece of equipment.

The 'generic' tray should be assessed every so often, removing instruments that are rarely used and introducing new instruments that the surgeon is using increasingly.

With the increasing incidence of morbid obesity, it has become common for many departments to have a 'deep' tray available with extra long instruments.

As with all things, the need for specialized instrumentation has resulted in two major developments. The first is that emerging technologies have produced a number of new instruments aimed at achieving haemostasis during both open and laparoscopic procedures. These include vascular staples and coagulation devices such as the argon beam coagulator, Ligasure (Covidien Inc., Boulder, CO, USA), Harmonic Scalpel (Ethicon Endo-Surgery Inc., Cincinnati, OH, USA), PlasmaKinetic seal system (Gyrus ACMI, Southborough, MA, USA) and Transcollation technologies (Salient Surgical Technologies, Portsmouth, NH, USA).

The second is the wide range of disposable instruments developed specifically for laparoscopic surgery.

Instruments for major gynaecological procedures

The instruments used by the editors in their general operating set vary based on their preferences and years of experience. As surgeons develop their special interests, they may regularly use instruments not required by the generalist. Tables 3.1 and 3.2 give

Bonney's Gynaecological Surgery, 11th edition.
© Tito Lopes, Nick Spirtos, Raj Naik, John Monaghan.
Published 2011 by Blackwell Publishing Ltd.

Table 3.1 Basic gynaecological abdominal set

4 Rampley sponge handle forceps	2 Meigs (Navratil) artery forceps, long
2 Blade handles, no. 4	5 Littlewood tissue forceps
1 DeBakey dissecting forceps, 200 mm	6 'Zeppelin' slight curved hysterectomy clamps, 220 mm
1 Dissecting forceps, toothed, 175 mm	1 Vulsellum, toothed, 250 mm
1 Dissecting forceps, non-toothed	2 Morris retractors, 1 medium, 1 large
1 Scissors, straight, 155 mm	2 Langenbeck retractors
1 Scissors, straight, 200 mm	1 Cushing vessel retractor
1 Monaghan dissecting scissors	1 Raytec intra-abdominal pack
2 Needle holders, 200 mm	1 Receiver
1 Needle holder, 250 mm	2 Gallipots
10 Spencer Wells forceps, straight, 200 mm	1 Ligature tray

Table 3.2 Basic minor procedure set

1 Sims vaginal speculum	1 Blade handle, no. 3
2 Sponge handle forceps	2 Spencer Wells forceps, straight, 200 mm
1 Endometrial polyp forceps	3 Sharp curettes, small, medium and large
1 Vulsellum, toothed	1 Toothed dissecting forceps, 175 mm
1 Uterine sound	1 Scissors, straight, 155 mm
1 Set of cervical dilators	1 Needle holder, 200 mm

examples of a basic major and minor tray suitable for everyday gynaecological surgery.

Editors' picks

The majority of the instruments are standard, but this section is dedicated to the editors' favourites that they felt warranted special comment.

Scissors

Bonney dissecting scissors (Fig. 3.1) are often marketed as Mayo scissors. They are heavy but have a sureness about them that allows for accurate gentle dissection, particularly of the 'separate and cut' type. The ends of the scissors are relatively blunt and will do little damage when separating tissue, whereas the blades are powerful enough when coupled with the long levers of the 25-cm handles to cope with the toughest of scar tissue. This latter characteristic is especially important in cancer work when operating on tissues previously treated with radiotherapy.

Monaghan dissecting scissors (Fig. 3.2) were developed out of a need for a lighter pair of dissecting scissors which retained the wonderful 'feel' of the Bonney scissor without the weight. This instrument has allowed the scissor dissection technique taught by the editors to reach the level of anatomical dissection required to meet the most stringent standards of cancer surgery. The tips of the instrument remain relatively blunt but do allow for accurate point dissection without the risk of trauma to tissues to be preserved.

Tissue clamps

On many occasions in gynaecological surgery, it is necessary to clamp discrete blocks of tissue firmly and then suture the block to occlude the vessels contained with it. It is important that these clamps are strong, that the jaws appose accurately and that tissue does not slide out from between the jaws. Many different varieties have been designed and produced, which is probably a reflection that the requirements above are difficult to achieve. As a general principle, it appears

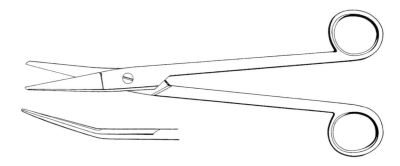

Figure 3.1 Bonney gynaecological scissors.

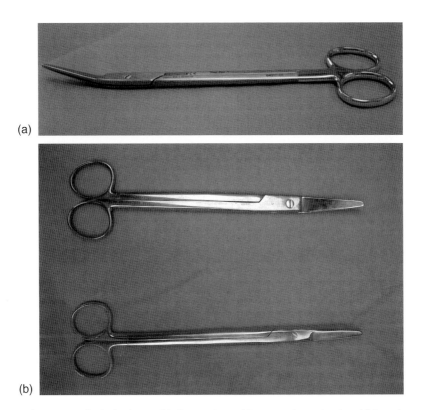

(a)

(b)

Figure 3.2 (a) Monaghan gynaecological scissors. (b) Comparison of Bonney scissors (top) and Monaghan scissors (bottom).

that those designs with longitudinal ridging of the jaws have an advantage over those with transverse ridging.

Downs hysterectomy clamps (220 mm) with a slight curve and 2/3 atraumatic jaws are shown in Fig. 3.3. Three of the editors initially used Zeppelin clamps but changed to using the Downs clamps now as they meet the requirements mentioned above. The markedly angled clamps are useful when incision of a pedicle is required at right angles to the line of application of the clamps (e.g. when clamping the paracolpos during a Wertheim hysterectomy).

Dissecting forceps

Singley forceps (Fig. 3.4) are used to grasp the nodal tissue during pelvic and para-aortic node dissection.

17

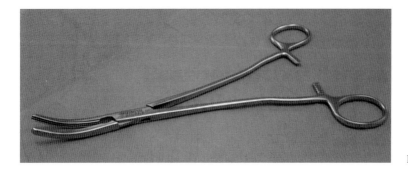

Figure 3.3 Hysterectomy clamps.

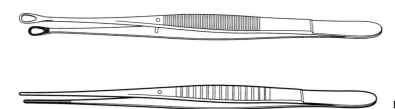

Figure 3.4 Singley forceps.

Figure 3.5 DeBakey forceps.

These instruments are similar to Russian forceps except they are somewhat lighter as the central defect removes unnecessary weight and, with concentric transverse ridges, allows for an improved ability to grasp and place countertraction on the nodal tissue.

DeBakey forceps (Fig. 3.5) were developed by the famed cardiovascular surgeon for use during cardiothoracic surgery. They provide a fine, delicate and atraumatic surface allowing for the handling of delicate tissues.

Artery forceps

These can be straight or curved based on the surgeon's personal preference and include the *Meigs–Navratil forceps* (Fig. 3.6). The use of right-angled forceps such as these is of great value in dealing with vessels deep in the pelvis; the right angle of the small head of the instrument allows ties to be accurately placed. The throw of the suture material or tie can be placed around either the points or the heel of the forceps and, if the assistant then rotates the forceps, the opposite end automatically loops around the tie, allowing the surgeon to deal with vessels surely and confidently. As with many instruments in the set, the Meigs–Navratil forceps are long, reaching easily into the depths of the pelvis.

Retractors

Self-retaining retractors
• The *Balfour self-retaining retractor* (see Fig. 4.6), designed by the gastrointestinal surgeon Donald Balfour, is the standard retractor used by most gynaecologists. The central blade is adequate for standard procedures, but in complex cases the editors prefer to use a hand-held retractor or the Martin arm retractor to allow adjustments during the operation.
• *Ronald Edwards* and *Finochietto retractors* have a rack and pinion mechanism and were originally developed as rib spreaders in thoracic surgery. They have been modified for abdominal procedures and are excellent for retraction when a large midline incision has been used.
• *Martin arm retractors* have two joints that allow for 360° movement and a locking mechanism that allows the placement of any retractor into its jaws, this is an ideal instrument to hold in place retractors that would normally require multiple assistants. This retractor is particularly effective in performing upper abdominal surgery, providing excellent elevation and retraction of the rib cage and gaining exposure to the retroperitoneal lymph nodes.
• The *Bookwalter retractor* is a self-retained retractor system which attaches to the operating table, from

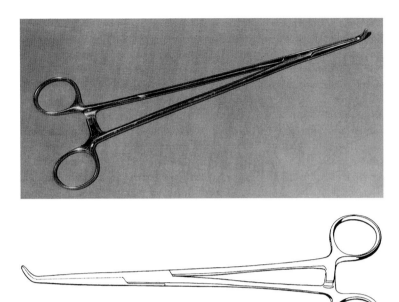

Figure 3.6 Meigs–Navratil forceps.

which rings of different sizes are attached. A variety of adjustable retracting blades can be placed at any desired location around the suspended ring and the angle of that blade be individualized at the point of fixation on the ring.

Hand-held retractors
• The *Morris retractor* has a lip which aids the elevation of the wound edge. The shallower blade of the retractor is less likely to endanger the delicate internal structures, as may occur with deeper retractors.
• The *Cushing vessel retractor* is an ideal retractor for displacing the iliac vessels during pelvic lymphadenectomy.

Sutures

Suture materials

It is important to understand that there is no ideal, universal, suture material. The purpose of a suture material is to hold tissue in apposition until such time that the tissues have achieved enough tensile strength to maintain the apposition. Successful repair requires not only proper surgical techniques but also knowledge of the physical characteristics and properties of the suture and needle.

Ideal suture characteristics

These will include good knot security, inertness, adequate tensile strength, flexibility, ease of handling, non-allergenic nature, resistance to infection, smooth passage through the tissues and absorbability. Sutures are classified as natural or synthetic, monofilament or multifilament, absorbable or nonabsorbable. Synthetic materials have all but replaced natural materials such as catgut and silk. The smooth surface of monofilament sutures causes less tissue trauma and prevents harbouring of microorganisms unlike multifilament sutures. However, multifilament sutures have greater strength and are soft and pliable, making handling and knotting easier.

Absorbable sutures provide temporary wound support; with synthetic materials absorption is by hydrolysis, causing less tissue reaction than natural sutures such as catgut. It is important to recognize that loss of tensile strength and rate of absorption are not related. Table 3.3 lists the absorbable synthetic

19

Table 3.3 Absorbable suture materials

Suture, trade name (year developed)	Construction	Time to complete loss of tensile strength (days)	Absorption profile (days)	Uses
Polyglycolic acid, Dexon II (1968–70)	Multifilament	28	60–90	
Polyglactin 910, Vicryl (1974)	Multifilament	28	56–70	Pedicles
Polyglactin 910, Vicryl Rapide (1987)	Multifilament	14	42	Ileal conduit T-tube fixation stitch
Polydioxanone, PDS II (1981)	Monofilament	63	183–238	Rectus sheath; intestine
Polyglyconate, Maxon (1984)	Monofilament	56	180	
Poliglecaprone 25, Monocryl (1992)	Monofilament	21	91–119	Intestine; urinary tract; subcuticular stitch

suture materials used by the editors with their strength retention and absorption profiles. Antibacterial forms of some of these sutures have been produced to try and reduce the risk of infection.

Non-absorbable suture material such as nylon or polypropylene is used for permanent wound support in slowly healing tissues, such as for closure of the rectus sheath. Care must be exercised in their use as their permanent nature always runs a small risk of sinus formation to skin or other structures.

Suture selection

As with surgical instruments, once the various characteristics of the available suture materials are understood, the choice depends on the surgeon's training and preference, as numerous suture materials are available for each location and structure. The surgeon should select the finest suture that adequately holds the healing wound edges and the tensile strength of the suture should never exceed the tensile strength of the tissue. Sutures are needed only long enough for a wound to reach maximum strength. Therefore, one should consider non-absorbable sutures in skin and fascia (slowly healing tissues), whereas mucosal wounds (rapidly healing tissues) may be repaired with absorbable sutures.

In the presence of contaminated tissue, monofilament sutures should be used as multifilament materials are more likely to harbour microorganisms and degrade more rapidly.

Common errors of suture use are:
• too many throws, which increases foreign body size and can cause stitch abscesses
• intracuticular rather than subcuticular sutures, which can cause hypertrophic scars
• holding monofilament sutures with instruments reduces tensile strength by over 50%
• holding the butt of the needle causes needle and suture breakage.

Suture needles

Virtually all needles used today are swaged (eyeless) needles in which the needle is drilled and the suture is inserted into the base of the needle, creating a continuous unit. They have obvious advantages over the old eyed needles. A modification of the standard permanent swaged suture is the controlled release or 'pop-off' suture in which the needle and suture are easily separated by means of a light tug. These sutures facilitate rapid interrupted suturing techniques and are favoured by some surgeons.

Needles have three basic components: the swage as discussed above, the body and the point. The body of the needle is the part grasped by the needle holder and its curvature can vary, giving different characteristics. The curvature may be a 1/4, 3/8, 1/2 or 5/8 circle, with the 1/2 circle probably being the commonest used in gynaecology.

In a deep narrow pelvis or other area with limited space, there is some advantage to using a smaller

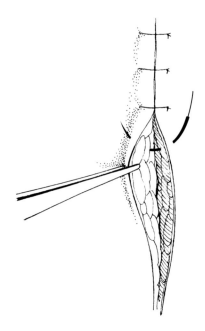

Figure 3.7 Simple interrupted suture.

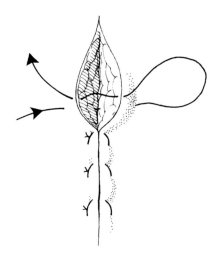

Figure 3.8 Vertical mattress suture.

needle and an increased curve to allow easy passage of the needle.

There are basically three types of points: cutting, taper and blunt. The cutting needle is designed for cutting through dense tissue such as fascia and skin. The reverse cutting needle has its third cutting edge on the outer convex curvature, reducing the risk of tissue cut-out. The taper point has no cutting edge and the needle pierces and spreads the tissue without cutting it, making it ideal for easily penetrated tissue such as bowel, bladder and peritoneum. Blunt point needles dissect rather than cut tissue; they are usually used to avoid needle-stick injuries, especially in high-risk patients.

Editors' picks

The editors' favourite sutures include the following.
• *General.* W9421 – Ethicon polyglactin 910 (coated Vicryl) 1 gauge; 90 cm long with a 40 mm 1/2 circle reverse cutting needle. A general purpose suture, including for hysterectomy pedicles and vaginal vault.
• *Rectus sheath.* W9262 – Ethicon polydioxanone (PDS II) 1 gauge loop; 150 cm long with a 48 mm 1/2 circle round-bodied needle. For a continuous suture.

• *Skin.* W3650 – Ethicon poliglecaprone 25 (Monocryl) undyed 3/0 gauge; 70 cm long with a 60 mm straight needle. For a subcuticular suture.
• *Bowel.* W3664 – Ethicon poliglecaprone 25 (Monocryl) 3/0 gauge; 70 cm long with a 26 mm 1/2 circle JB Visi-black taper point plus needle.

Suture techniques

In previous editions of this book, a large variety of suture techniques were shown. The current editors have selected those that are of most value to the gynaecologist and, where possible, retained some of Bonney's original drawings.

Interrupted sutures
Interrupted sutures use a number of strands to close the wound, with each strand tied and cut separately. This provides a more secure repair than the continuous suture because, if one suture breaks, the remaining sutures will hold the wound edges together. They are used where there is infection present and suture viability might be compromised.

The interrupted suture may be simple (Fig. 3.7) or a vertical mattress (Fig. 3.8). The mattress suture has the added advantage that haemostasis will be further improved by an increased area of local pressure on fine bleeding points. A horizontal mattress suture spreads tension along a wound and is used for pulling

21

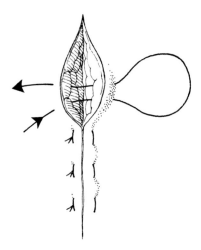

Figure 3.9 Horizontal mattress suture.

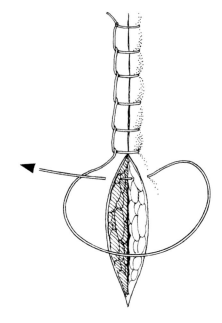

Figure 3.10 Locked or blanket sutures.

wound edges together over a distance, or as the initial suture to anchor two wound edges (holding sutures) (Fig. 3.9). With both mattress techniques, it is important to note that the suture should be used to *appose* the tissues not to *necrose* them; excessive force must not be used. Following all surgery the tissue thickness will initially increase, so the suture can be placed relatively lightly to achieve apposition and haemostasis.

Continuous sutures
Continuous sutures can produce a near perfect closure and apposition of two surfaces with excellent haemostasis. This technique is more rapidly performed than interrupted sutures and obviously requires fewer knots. It derives its strength from tension being distributed evenly along the full length of the suture. In the presence of infection, a monofilament suture should be used to avoid infection being transmitted along its full length.

Locked or blanket stitches (Fig. 3.10) are of great value in achieving haemostasis; the editors use this stitch to oversew the vaginal edge at the completion of the hysterectomy procedure.

Subcuticular sutures
These are popular for skin closure as they give an immediate attractive cosmetic effect. They can be performed as a continuous suture or interrupted. A fine absorbable monofilament suture such as Monocryl is ideal for large incisions as it results in minimal

scarring and can be left *in situ* while the wound strength increases.

Other sutures
Puckering sutures are used for shortening tissues and where there are a series of small vessels in a tissue edge which cannot be easily dealt with individually (Fig. 3.11).

Purse-string sutures (Fig. 3.12) are continuous sutures placed around a lumen and tightened like a drawstring to invert the opening. They can be used prior to inserting a tube such as for drainage of a large benign ovarian cyst, and to repair small defects in the bladder or bowel. Although traditionally used for burying the stump of the appendix (Fig. 3.13), this is now thought to be unnecessary.

Surgical knots and methods of tying

Facility in tying knots is an important part of the surgical technique in which all young surgeons should attempt to excel. They must also remember that it is not adequate to be competent to tie one knot – they should practise a wide variety, learning the indication

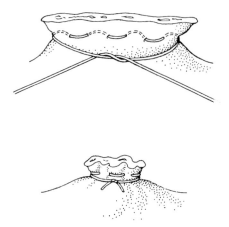

Figure 3.11 Puckering sutures.

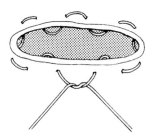

Figure 3.12 Purse-string suture.

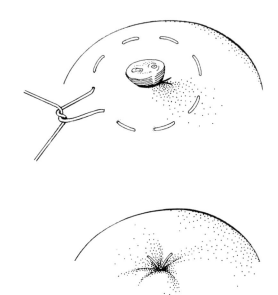

Figure 3.13 Purse-string inverting sutures.

more suture. This mode of presentation is also more economical in the long term.

The granny knot

This is the simplest and quickest knot to make, consisting of two identical hitches. It has the advantage that the first hitch is easily held tight while the second is being made and that should the first tie slip the second will tighten it up again. This applies only to monofilament suture materials which slide. If surgeons use multifilament sutures, they must learn to tie all knots as they wish them to end up – the tension on the first knot must be exactly as it is wished to be, as there is no possibility of 'snugging' down the second throw. Granny knots are not recommended as they have a tendency to slip when subjected to increased stress. For this reason, when the granny knot is used, a third opposite throw is an important safety feature.

The reef (square) knot

This knot consists of two hitches, one tied with one end of the ligature and one tied with the other

for their uses as skills improve. As an assistant, the young surgeon learns to cut the tails of sutures accurately and quickly, taking care to leave a short but adequate length. The cut should be made with the scissors stationary and with due regard to the position of the tips of the blades at the end of the cutting stroke. The assistant must become proficient in cutting sutures with the non-dominant hand so as not to be continually transferring instruments between hands. Equally, the surgeon should present the suture in such a way that the assistant can easily see and safely cut without causing any hazard to adjacent tissues or organs.

It is often tempting to try to use very short lengths of suture material in difficult places; this practice must be eschewed. The suture material for knot tying must be presented to the surgeon in at least 'half lengths', and, ideally, on the reel so that the surgeon can efficiently continue to tie without continually asking for

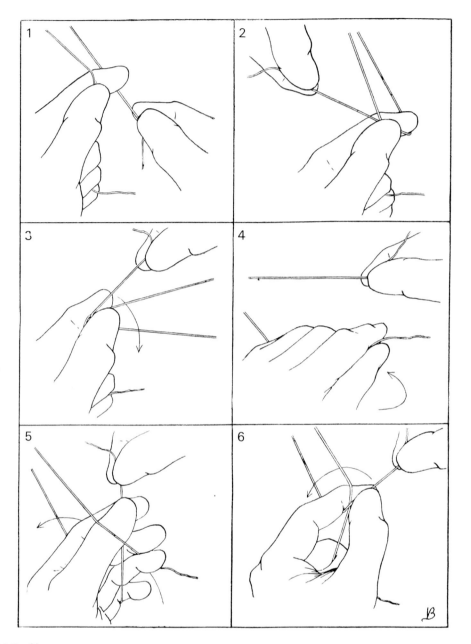

Figure 3.14 Reef knot.

end. Figure 3.14 shows the technique of tying as described by Bonney. This two-handed technique produces a firm knot, but it is possible by crossing the hands to perform a reef knot using the one-handed technique.

The surgeon's (friction) knot

The surgeon's knot is a simple modification to the reef knot. It adds an extra twist when tying the first throw, forming a double overhand knot, thus adding friction which makes the knot more secure.

It is important to remember that any suture with a knot in it is significantly weaker than one without. Do not, therefore, be surprised to find suture material breaking at the knot when excess tension is applied.

The single-handed knot

This fast, elegant and simple technique of single-handed tying with the left hand allows the surgeon to operate dexterously and rapidly without putting down the instruments or requiring special tools for tying knots. The technique is shown in Fig. 3.15(1–4).

The instrument tie

This elegant method of tying is shown in Fig. 3.15(5,6). It is particularly useful when there is only a short piece of suture material available.

Knot tying in deep holes

It has been recommended that the lasso technique be used when a bleeding point occurs in a deep or inaccessible spot. The editors would instead recommend the use of a long, angled clamp such as the Meigs–Navratil. This type of clamp, which has the attributes of gallbladder forceps, will allow the tie to be hooked around either the heel or the tip of the clamp so that it is firmly held while the knot is being made (Fig. 3.16). If the bleeding point is extremely difficult to reach, the use of preloaded small metal artery clips such as the Ligaclip MCA (Ethicon Endo-Surgery Inc.) is of enormous value (Fig. 3.17).

Tying pedicles

In their original textbook, Berkeley and Bonney described nine different ways in which pedicles may be tied, but, other than the simple pedicle tie, the others were variations on the transfixion stitch. The material to be ligated is held in a clamp, which is placed so that a small part of the tip projects beyond the tissue to be tied. This allows the suture material to be firmly held by hooking it around the projecting tip while the knot is tied.

Simple pedicle ties

The ligature may be simple, carrying the entire throw around the mass of tissue to be ligated (Fig. 3.18a).

The major drawback of this method is the potential for slipping; this risk is reduced if the tension is adequate and if the tissue beyond the tie is of a reasonable amount.

It is important to remember not to be too ambitious and try to include so large a mass that the edges slip out and produce haemorrhage, which may be difficult to control. Remember that the simple loop pedicle ligature should never be used if there is tension on the pedicle. Double tying of pedicles should not be used as the tissue distal to the proximal tie is considerable, resulting in a large amount of necrotic material that can become infected.

Transfixion stitches

The mass of material to be ligated can be transfixed at one or both ends (Fig. 3.18b,c) so that the ligature will not slip and material escape. The transfixion stitch should be used with great care in pedicles, which are known to contain significant blood vessels. The risk of damage to vessels is greatest when suturing the ovarian or uterine pedicles during a total hysterectomy. The ovarian vessels in the infundibulo-pelvic ligament are thin and wide. It is the editors' practice to use a simple tie and not to put any tension upon the pedicle. The uterine artery or a large vein may be pierced when stitch ligaturing the lower pedicles alongside the uterus during a hysterectomy. When this occurs, a rapidly developing haematoma grows into the soft tissues of the broad ligament behind the pedicle, discolouring the tissues and making identification of bleeding points extremely difficult. It is not usually safe to simply reclamp the bleeding area as the vein or artery often retracts once it is cut.

There is also considerable danger in blindly clamping alongside the uterus and cervix, as the ureter is not far away. It is better to open up the pelvic side-wall, identify the uterine artery at its origin, tie it and then follow it through to the uterus over the top of the ureter. This simple demonstration of the ureter in its lower course is immensely reassuring.

Staples

The use of staples in surgery began in Hungary in the early part of the twentieth century when Hultl

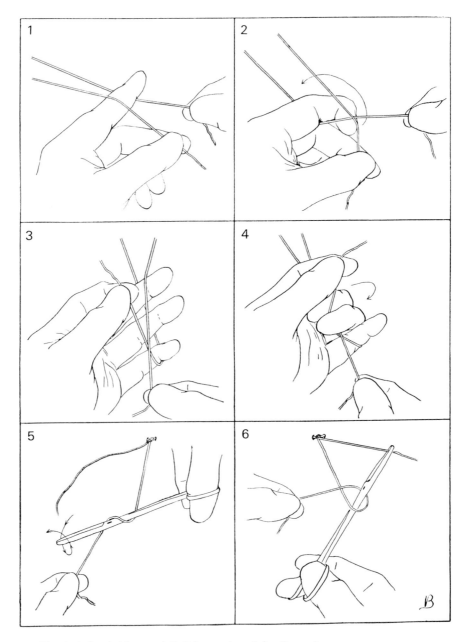

Figure 3.15 (1–4) The single-handed knot and (5,6) forceps knot (after Bonney).

designed staples that closed into a 'B' shape, setting the standard pattern for the remainder of the century.

In general, gynaecology stapling has not enjoyed a significant role except for skin closure. However, in recent times, the increased interest in laparoscopic surgery and the growth of the subspecialty of gynaecological oncology has resulted in a massive expansion of the use of stapling devices. The most common staplers used in gynaecology are linear cutting, endoscopic linear cutting and skin staplers, with circular staplers also used in oncology procedures. The linear cutting staple places two double or triple staggered rows of titanium staples and a knife simultaneously divides the tissue in between. They can be used for taking the pedicles at laparoscopic hysterectomy, open hysterectomy in obese women as well as at radical hysterectomy and exenterative surgery.

Skin staples compare favourably as regards wound complications and cosmetic appearance and result in significant time-saving compared with suture closure, especially with large wounds.

Electrosurgery

Electrosurgery utilizes AC current over a wide spectrum of frequencies (the number of times a current changes directions per second equals the frequency of that current). Briefly stated, AC can be measured by the peak-to-peak voltage, understanding that the effective power is diminished as the current goes to zero upon reversing direction. Average effective power for a sine waveform associated with 'pure'

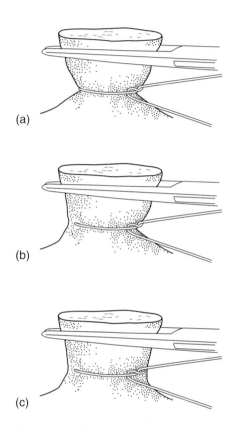

(a)

(b)

(c)

Figure 3.18 (a) Simple pedicle tie. (b) Single-end transfixion tie. (c) Double-ended transfixion tie.

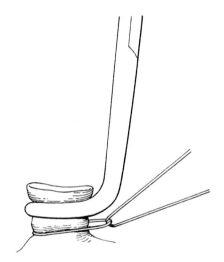

Figure 3.16 Tying a pedicle around Meigs forceps.

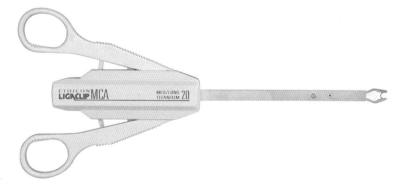

Figure 3.17 A disposable multiple clip applicator. Reproduced with permission from Johnson & Johnson.

27

cutting is 0.7 of the peak voltage. This is referred to as the root mean square (RMS). It is important to remember that the patient is actually part of the circuit as energy flows into the body, but at frequencies high enough (radiofrequencies) that the body does not recognize or respond to them.

Tissue effects include fulguration, cutting and desiccation.

Fulguration is achieved with either minimal or no contact with the tissues and requires the use of much higher voltages than does a cutting current to achieve a similar average effective power, as represented by a higher RMS. This application results in protein denaturation and charred tissue. Essentially, to achieve this effect, the surgeon needs intermittent high voltage with low RMS to prevent tissue vaporization. As current flows for only approximately 5% of the duty cycle, the average effective power of this waveform (current) is less than that of an unmodulated cutting current. Clinically, this requires the surgeon to use a very high-power setting with corresponding high voltage to overcome the reduced duty cycle associated with the 'coagulation' setting on the electrosurgical unit.

The *cutting* phenomenon, associated with an unabated sine wave-shaped current of relative low voltage, occurs as the tissue is heated so rapidly as to cause vaporization of cells. It is best achieved by holding the tip of the pencil ever so slightly above the tissue. The current crosses the high impedance of air and produces heat to the degree that cells are vaporized. It is imperative to understand that the temperatures associated with this technology can reach 700°C, whereas tissue dies at 44°C. This imposes a great deal of responsibility upon the whole surgical team to understand the implications of a stray current or a momentary act of carelessness.

Desiccation results from the direct contact of the electrode and tissue. Current passes through the tissue with resultant dehydration and, ultimately, coagulation. This can be modulated by the temperature and area of contact because, when the electrode contacts the tissues, they do not vaporize as the concentration of the current is markedly reduced.

Even though there have been great advances in generator technology, particularly the development of return electrode technology, there still can be burns associated with the use of monopolar current, most frequently at the return pad site. Return pad site injuries can be minimized by ensuring that it is placed over low-resistance sites such as the lateral thigh, where there is minimal fat, hair or bony prominence. The pad should be large, with a full-surface adhesive present and the area cleaned and dried before applying it to the patient's skin.

Electrical injuries can occur at sites of inadvertent contact with other instruments. This occurs during laparoscopic procedures as well, wherein the electrical instrument is not entirely visualized throughout the procedure. Also, insulation failures can lead to unrecognized visceral or vascular injury, and, rarely, capacitance coupling can occur if metal trocars are still in use.

An important clinical application of this brief and basic review of electrosurgery is the application of 'cutting' and 'coagulation' current to the intraoperative setting. When applying monopolar current to tissue held in a clamp of any type it is best to apply the 'cutting' current since the low continuous voltage allows the current to reach the core of the tissues clamped without producing an eschar and high outer tissue resistance that occurs when using the interval high-voltage 'coagulation', thus preventing the current from reaching the core within the instrument. When using the current directly to an area of bleeding, it is best to use the high-voltage intermittent current 'coagulation' to cause haemostasis.

Another monopolar energy source is the argon beam coagulator, in which argon gas is typically integrated with the electrical current resulting in a relatively non-penetrating current (1 mm) with little lateral spread (1 mm). This can be used to haemostatically divide tissues and achieve excellent haemostasis particularly when working on the liver or spleen or undertaking lymph node dissections. The lateral spread associated with standard monopolar cautery is approximately 3 mm, and care should be used around any nearby tissue at risk.

Bipolar instruments pass current between two plates that act as the active and return electrodes. Theoretically, this should result in virtually no lateral spread and the associated collateral damage of tissue, but that is not the case practically speaking. All bipolar energy sources, including the Gyrus PK device (Gyrus ACMI, Southborough, MA, USA), Ligasure and the Harmonic Scalpel have associated lateral spread and the potential to damage nearby tissue. They do, however, eliminate the risk of injury associated with the grounding pad. The initiating energy source of these instruments may be different, as is the exact mechanism resulting in haemostasis, but the underlying physics of passing that energy between two electrodes remains the same. It is the responsibility of the surgeon to learn about each and every instrument used in the operating theatre, particularly the individual mechanisms of action and the risks associated with the use of that instrument.

Haemostatic agents

Commonly used haemostatic agents require a basic understanding of the intrinsic, extrinsic and common coagulation pathway. Three mechanisms result in haemostasis: (1) vasoconstriction, (2) platelet aggregation due to ADP and thromboxane A2 and (3) the activation of the extrinsic pathway by the release of factor III and intrinsic pathway by the release of factor XII.

Materials and agents commonly used in the operating theatre today include the following.
• *Thrombin factor IIa (the common pathway)*: induces the conversion of fibrinogen to fibrin. There are both human and bovine products available to be applied topically directly to the area of concern or applied to Surgicel (Johnson and Johnson Inc., New Brunswick, NJ, USA) or Gelfoam (Pfizer Inc., New York, NY, USA) and then placed against the bleeding surface.
• *Tisseel (Baxter Inc., Deerfield, IL, USA)*: a combination of factor XIII, calcium chloride and human thrombin. Approved as both a haemostatic agent and a sealant, sometimes used at the site of anastomosis and for distal resection of the pancreas. Applied by spray or drip technique.
• *Evicel (Johnson and Johnson Inc.)*: a combination of human fibrinogen, thrombin and calcium chloride. Approved for haemostasis, but not as a sealant. Applied by spray or drip technique.
• *FloSeal (Baxter Inc.)*: gelatin matrix, thrombin and calcium chloride. Direct application.
• *Arista (Medafor Inc., Minneapolis, MN, USA)*: microporous polysaccharide hemospheres made from corn starch. This material is applied to areas of generalized oozing and absorbs serum while the individual beads expand up to 15 times their original size. This results in the concentration of blood solids to

form a gel matrix that slows blood flow and enhances both platelet function and fibrin formation. As it is absorbed rapidly (under 48 h), its use is not associated with infection/abscess.
• *Surgicel (Johnson and Johnson Inc.)*: made of oxidized cellulose polymer(polyanhydroglucuronic acid). The sheet of absorbable cellulose reacts with blood, forming a pseudoclot which stops bleeding. It also has an antibacterial effect against more than 20 species of both Gram-negative and -positive bacteria.
• *Gelfoam (Pfizer Inc.)*: absorbable sheet of purified porcine skin gelatin. The mechanism of action is not completely understood, but it appears to acts as a physical matrix that promotes coagulation. It is usually absorbed completely within 4–6 weeks. Often, it is soaked in thrombin, and many surgeons use it in this manner.

It should be noted that these haemostatic agents are not replacements for good surgical technique, with isolation and ligation or cauterization of bleeding sites.

Adhesion prevention

There are no randomized prospective studies in major gynaecological or gynaecological oncology surgery demonstrating efficacy of adhesion-preventing agents. There is some evidence suggesting a benefit of using Interceed (Johnson and Johnson Inc.), an oxidized regenerated cellulose, in patients undergoing distal tubal surgery. There has been a large randomized prospective study (Fazio *et al.* 2006) in patients undergoing low anterior resection for colon cancer that has demonstrated a small but significant benefit associated with the use of Seprafilm (Genzyme Inc., Cambridge, MA, USA), a sheet of sodium hyaluronate carboxymethylcellulose (HA-CMC), in the prevention of adhesions. Seprafilm acts as a barrier during the critical first 7 postoperative days, soon after which it is absorbed completely. In addition to preventing adhesions, there was a slight increase in pelvic abscess and anastomotic leaks associated with its placement near or over bowel anastomoses. It is currently recommended when using Seprafilm to make sure it is not placed over the site of anastomosis. Many gynaecological oncologists have extrapolated the general surgery literature to their field of interest and routinely place one or two sheets of Seprafilm in the pelvis and beneath the abdominal wall incision.

There are non-randomized data in obstetrics suggesting a reduction in adhesions following caesarean section; as a result, as the number of repeat caesarean sections has increased dramatically, so has the use of Seprafilm in this clinical setting.

Drainage

In modern gynaecological practice, the indications for drainage of the pelvis/abdomen are very few. The widespread use of intraoperative antibiotics has probably contributed to this situation, and has reduced the indications to the following:
• any procedure in which it has been impossible to achieve perfect haemostasis and the surgeon wishes to monitor potential blood loss
• where there is a danger of urine leakage, such as following repair to a damaged bladder or ureter or following elective surgery on these structures
• where there has been widespread contamination of the peritoneal cavity with infected material.

The routine use of drains following pelvic or para-aortic lymphadenectomy has been shown not to reduce the risk of lymphocysts and should not be used. However, they continue to be used following inguinal node dissection. Retrospective data from the (American) Society of Gynecologic Oncologists suggested that any value in draining the groin is lost after 7 days, and, after this point, the drain may be the inciting agent in causing the accumulation of lymphatic fluid. A small prospective study from Gateshead suggested no benefit in leaving the drains *in situ* for more than 3 days (McAuley *et al.* 2003).

Drain types

The use of suction drains is efficient for drainage of lymph fluid or assessing potential urine leakage and leaves little scarring at the drainage exit site. However, if one is concerned about blood loss or if there has been gross soiling of the peritoneal cavity, such as following bowel opening, a larger bore drain is necessary, such as a Jackson–Pratt or Robinson drain.

Management of drains

Drains should be removed when they have ceased to function or drainage has stabilized at a low level. It is important that they be anchored carefully by adequate fixation in theatre.

The presence and type of drain must be accurately recorded in the operation note, and clear instructions for drain care included in the postoperative instructions. Decisions for removal are usually made and recorded during the postoperative ward rounds.

Further reading

The suture manufacturers have produced manuals on knot tying and wound closure which are readily available on the Internet. Although produced by commercial companies, they are written by surgeons and are useful teaching guides. They include:

Ethicon Wound Closure Manual. See www.pilonidal.org/pdfs/wound_closure.pdf

Ethicon Knot Tying Manual. See www.medisave.co.uk/pdf/Knot_Tying_Manual.pdf

Covidien Surgical Knot Tying Manual, 3rd edn. See www.covidien.com/imageServer.aspx?contentID=11850&contenttype=application/pdf.

References

Fazio VW, Cohen Z, Fleshman JW, *et al.* Reduction in adhesive small-bowel obstruction by Seprafilm adhesion barrier after intestinal resection. *Dis Colon Rectum* 2006;49:1–11.

McAuley WJ, Nordin AJ, Naik R, *et al.* A randomised controlled trial of groin wound suction drainage after radical vulvectomy and bilateral groin node dissection. *Int J Gynecol Cancer* 2003;13:5.

4

Opening and closing the abdominal cavity

Opening and closing the abdomen should be one continuous movement.

J.M. Monaghan

The length and position of the abdominal incision will depend on the purpose of the operation and on the physical state of the patient. Complicated and time-consuming incisions are inappropriate for emergency surgery, and small, cosmetic incisions are of little use for the removal of large masses; conversely, it is wrong to produce large unsightly scars when performing simple pelvic procedures. Just as the operation is planned, the incision must allow the surgeon to carry out the procedure with ease and full access to the operative field. The incision must allow an adequate exploration of the abdomen, especially if there is any possibility of other pathology than that expected.

The patient should be left with a scar that is neat and, like the memory of the surgical intervention, fades with time. An unsightly scar will continuously remind the patient of the procedure, bringing back memories of the worst aspects of the operation.

Most gynaecological procedures are best performed through one of two incisions – the low transverse incision (Pfannenstiel) or the subumbilical midline incision. The Cherney and Maylard incisions may

prove useful in the obese patient with a pannus when optimal exposure to the pelvis is needed. In this situation, they can be combined with a panniculectomy to further ease access. Paramedian incisions have a limited place.

Gynaecologists practising benign gynaecology invariably use a transverse incision and some consider a midline incision disfiguring or mutilating. The result is that the Pfannenstiel incision is occasionally used inappropriately, thereby compromising the surgery. In reality, the majority of women prefer the incision that will result in a safe procedure with minimal complications.

Operative stance

Surgeons must be comfortable when they are operating; young surgeons will realize very quickly that they have a preferred side to stand. The editors stand on the patient's right, as did Bonney; this allows the dominant right hand to perform all the dissecting, cutting and suturing procedures while the left hand is used for tying, applying tension to tissues and displaying the operative field. The tyro can frequently be seen leaning and contorting as though glued to the spot. He or she should remember that the feet can be moved to obtain a more comfortable operating position and, if a part of the procedure is more easily performed from the opposite side of the table, the surgeon and his or her assistant should not hesitate in changing places.

The table should be adjusted for the surgeon's requirements to provide a comfortable operating

Bonney's Gynaecological Surgery, 11th edition.
© Tito Lopes, Nick Spirtos, Raj Naik, John Monaghan.
Published 2011 by Blackwell Publishing Ltd.

position and the very best access to the operative field. The editors' use varying degrees of head-down tilt for most abdominal procedures; this allows the bowel to be easily packed out of the pelvic field and ensures minimal blood pooling in the lower limbs. However, it does make for poor visibility for the scrub nurse and second assistant and means that special care has to be taken to ensure that the patient does not slide off the operating table.

When laparoscopic surgery is being performed, a steep Trendelenburg may be required to move the bowel contents from the pelvis and to obtain a clear operative field. Rarely, special positions of the patient may be required in order to obtain access to specific areas of the pelvis and upper abdomen.

Draping the patient

Drapes should be applied to the abdomen in such a way that the bony landmarks are visible and accessible. For the midline and Pfannenstiel incisions these are the anterior superior iliac spines and the symphysis pubis. The umbilicus should also be visible for the midline incision. Some surgeons use plastic adhesive drapes for skin cover and cut through the surface; the editors feel that these are unnecessary for most procedures and reserve their use for covering over and sequestering potential sources of wound infection, such as stomas and sinuses.

In modern practice, the use of self-adhesive paper drapes is becoming increasingly common. They can be placed very accurately, assisting the surgeon's orientation prior to the incision.

The drapes must be placed accurately, as they offer lines which the surgeon will use to orientate himself. An untidily draped abdomen will all too frequently result in a squint ugly scar. If disposable paper drapes are not used, it is of paramount importance that drape clips should not be put into the patient's skin; these small wounds will often cause more discomfort than the incision itself. The incision should also lie within the drapes; the cut must not reach into the towels and, if extension is necessary and there is not enough room available, the patient should be redraped. Consequently, a very wide area of the abdomen should be prepared for this eventuality.

Instruments

The basic instruments required are those described in Chapter 3, Instruments for major gynaecological procedures.

Subumbilical midline incision

This is adequate for most gynaecological operations; it should extend from the skin fold below the umbilicus down as far as the hair line or one finger's breadth above the symphysis pubis. The incision can be easily extended for removal of very large intra-abdominal masses or for better operative access. This extension should be carried out upwards either through or around the umbilicus.

The incision

Once the patient has been draped and the scrub nurse and the anaesthetist are ready, the incision can be performed. The surgeon places the left hand across the upper part of the incision site with the fingers and thumb outstretched; the knife is grasped firmly in the palm of the right hand with the index finger along the length of the handle. A bold stroke is now made accurately down the midline, the full length of the required incision (Fig. 4.1). The first cut should extend well down into the fatty layers; these are then separated with the knife down to the rectus sheath, which is incised for a short distance in the same line. Small vessels in the fatty layer bleed and may be clipped and tied or diathermied. In the interests of speed some surgeons ignore these small bleeding vessels and simply pick them up at their leisure on the way back out of the abdomen. This technique, used by some of the editors, avoids tying or diathermy of every single bleeding point, with only significant bleeding points tied on the way into the abdomen.

The use of electrocautery to open the abdomen is common practice. The surgeon should use the cutting mode, as use of the coagulation current is associated with increased tissue damage and reduction in tensile strength. This should be reserved for its intended role, that of coagulation of small vessels.

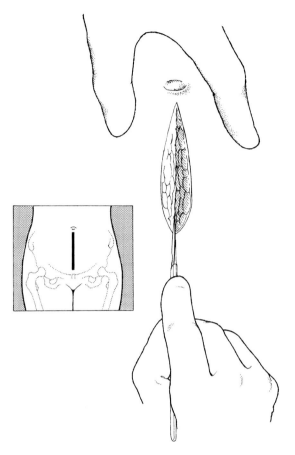

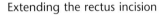

Figure 4.1 The subumbilical midline incision, incising the skin.

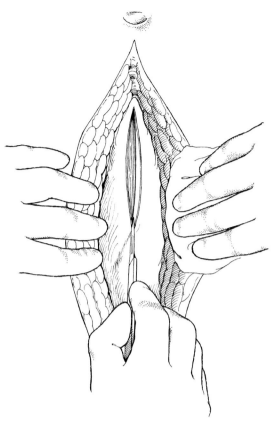

Figure 4.2 Incising the rectus sheath.

Extending the rectus incision

The small incision in the rectus sheath is now extended the full length of the skin incision using the scalpel (Fig. 4.2), dissecting scissors or diathermy. The scissors allow easy and bloodless separation of the rectus sheath prior to cutting by the simple expedient of running the scissors under the sheath in the fascial plane and opening the blades.

Separation of the recti

The midline is identified and the recti separated by using either a knife or the scissors to cut down through the fascia to the posterior layer of the rectus sheath. The incision is now extended the full length of the wound by inserting the index finger of each hand and drawing the hands apart (Fig. 4.3). The fingers run easily along the plane, completely separating the muscle and bringing the posterior rectus sheath and the peritoneum into view.

In the slim patient, separating the recti and extending the incision along its full length can be easily performed with the scalpel without the need for digital separation.

It is important not to deviate from the midline as it is easy to traumatize vessels that run along the posterior surface of the rectus sheath, causing troublesome bleeding and haematoma formation. Similarly, division of the muscle longitudinally should be avoided.

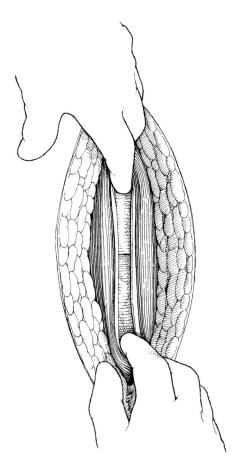

Figure 4.3 Separating the rectus muscles.

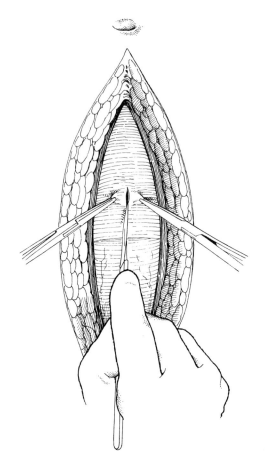

Figure 4.4 Incising the peritoneum.

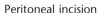

Peritoneal incision

The peritoneum is now in full view excepting in obese patients, in whom a layer of fat of variable thickness may be present. This fat should be separated gently by the fingers or the dissecting scissors. The peritoneum is now picked up at the junction of the mid- and upper third of the wound using two artery forceps. The midline can often be readily identified by the presence of the median umbilical ligament (the remnant of the embryonic urachus) and the medial umbilical ligaments (remnants of the fetal umbilical arteries) shining through the peritoneum. If the urachus is grasped the abdomen can be entered confidently without fear of damage to underlying bowel or bladder. The surgeon and first assistant now slightly elevate the forceps, and the surgeon palpates

the fold of peritoneum between finger and thumb to make sure there is no bowel included and then makes a short incision in the peritoneum (Fig. 4.4). As air enters the cavity of the abdomen the bowel falls away from the abdominal wall and the surgeon can now lengthen the incision under direct vision. If it is clear that there are extensive adhesions beneath the peritoneum then it is prudent to move to another part of the incision and enter the abdominal cavity away from the adhesions.

Alternatively, the surgeon and assistant can lift up the anterior abdominal wall by firmly grasping each side of the incision and then cutting the peritoneal layer using the scalpel with the underlying tissues under tension as entry into the peritoneal cavity is achieved. The upward traction of the anterior abdominal wall places any underlying adherent bowel under

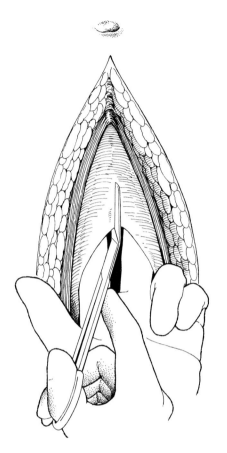

Figure 4.5 Cutting the peritoneum along the full length of the wound.

traction, which can be seen and avoided as the peritoneal layer is cut.

The edges of the incision are now picked up either by the surgeon and assistant hooking their index fingers under the peritoneum or by the surgeon elevating the peritoneum with two fingers of the left hand (Fig. 4.5). The opening is extended longitudinally using the scissors for the full length of the wound. Care is taken at the lower end of the wound to be sure that the bladder is not damaged; this can be avoided by transilluminating the peritoneum to demarcate the bladder edge or by palpating and elevating the catheter balloon in the bladder to the upper limit of the bladder. Occasionally, small vessels are cut in this area and require special attention and ligation.

Exploration of the abdomen and retraction

The editors advocate a combination of manual and visual exploration to be carried out before and after introducing the self-retaining retractor. The habit of routinely exploring the entire abdomen is one that should be adopted early in the surgeon's career; the process takes a very brief time and can be extremely rewarding. It is of particular importance in cancer surgery, in which, for many tumours, the process is part of the surgical staging. If there is any suggestion of malignancy, biopsies and peritoneal washings should also be taken at this time. The development of this habit will allow the surgeon to build up a comprehensive knowledge of normal abdominal and retroperitoneal organs so that any minor variations will register as his or her experience increases.

The choice of retractor is very much a personal decision; the editors preferring a Balfour self-retaining retractor (Fig. 4.6) for most routine gynaecological procedures, dispensing with the lower blade and replacing it with a Morris retractor held by the second assistant (Fig. 4.7). This second option allows the bladder to be moved and protected, producing the tissue tension in the parametrial and paravesical areas which is so valuable during dissection of the ureters. Great care should be taken if the self-retaining retractor is kept in position for an extended period of time, as bruising and even necrosis of the rectus muscles may occur (this is reduced if the patient is fully relaxed). It is interesting that Bonney and Wertheim both preferred manual retraction of the abdominal incision edges by the surgical assistant. This dynamic manual retraction is said to be less traumatic than the use of self-retaining retractors.

Packing away the intestines

In order to facilitate access to the pelvis, all small bowel, omentum and redundant loops of the sigmoid colon must be removed from the pelvis. This is achieved by a combination of Trendelenburg or head-down positioning and packing away of the intestines. The bowel is removed from the pelvis by the left hand with the fingers spread, a large pack is then spread over the fingers and, by sliding out the left hand, the right hand can then gently lift the bowel above the pelvic brim. Packing is best performed using one very large pack rather than a number of small ones. The pack must have a Raytec radio-opaque marker sewn

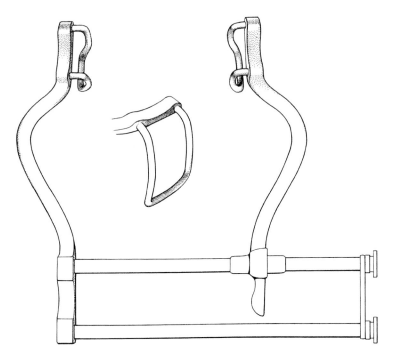

Figure 4.6 The Balfour self-retaining retractor.

into it and a long tape attached, which is brought out of the abdomen and can be marked with a clip. It is very important to use wet packs dampened by saline or water; the packs must not be hot – blood heat is all that is required. This wetting and normal body temperature is important in order to reduce damage to the bowel and the subsequent increased risk of adhesions.

Special circumstances

Previous scar

The surgeon should not feel constrained to utilize a previous scar if that route is inappropriate for the planned procedure. For example, it is folly to attempt to remove a large tumour or cyst through a low transverse incision simply for cosmetic effect. However, if it is necessary to make a different incision, it is frequently found that healing may be impaired at the junction of the two scars.

If it is decided to enter the abdomen through the previous scar, the surgeon must decide whether to remove it or to simply incise through it. As a general rule, if the scar is thin it is easier and quicker to simply cut through it; if it is broad or there has been keloid

formation, the old scar should be excised. Excision is most easily performed by picking up the ends of the scar in tissue forceps, such as Littlewood forceps. With the assistant holding the scar up, the surgeon can cut accurately down either side of it.

Adhesions to the old scar

Previous surgery markedly increases the risk of the development of adhesions, particularly to the back of the scar. Entry into the abdomen must, therefore, be carried out in a circumspect way. If bowel is adherent to the anterior abdominal wall it should not be separated by pulling or rubbing with a swab. If there is no obvious plane of separation, the 'postage stamp' technique should be used. This involves removal of a 'stamp' of peritoneum with the bowel so that there is no danger of damage to the bowel wall.

Extension of the wound

This applies only to the midline and paramedian incisions. For the midline incision a lot has been written about how to handle the umbilicus, varying from cutting straight through to circumnavigation and even a curious oblique incision. Extension can be easily and accurately performed if the surgeon and

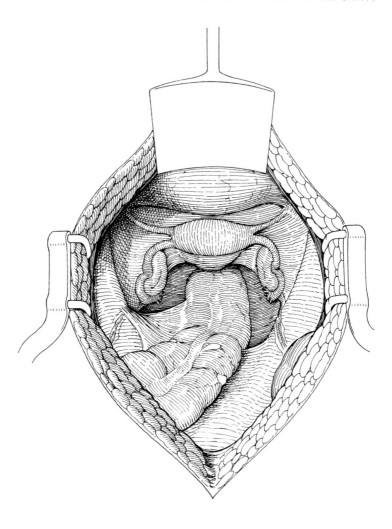

Figure 4.7 The incision retracted using the Balfour and Morris retractors.

the assistant elevate the upper part of the wound using the index fingers, and the surgeon cuts through all layers with a knife, keeping the abdominal contents in full view. The umbilicus is therefore easily circumnavigated using this technique.

Closure of the abdomen

At the end of the surgical procedure, having made certain that there is no untoward bleeding, the abdominal pack is removed; the swab, instrument and needle count is carried out and reported and confirmed to be satisfactory. There is no great advantage in bringing down the omentum to lie in the pelvis unless there is a wide defect in the peritoneum. The

abdominal wall can now be closed; this is facilitated by maintaining the patient in the Trendelenburg position, keeping the bowel out of the surgical field.

Discussion as to whether the abdominal peritoneum should be closed continues among some gynaecologists, but the majority have abandoned the procedure for lack of evidence to its benefit and have adopted mass closure. This has been shown to have a lower incidence of dehiscence and incisional hernia than layered closure. Avoiding closure of the peritoneum has also been shown to reduce adhesion formation.

Mass closure technique
Mass closure incorporates all the layers of the abdominal wall except for the skin and, ideally, the

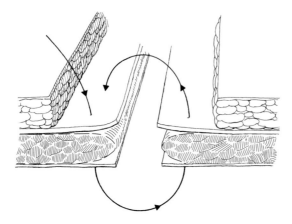

Figure 4.8 The mass closure technique.

peritoneum. A continuous running suture has been shown to be equivalent to interrupted sutures with regards to dehiscence and hernia formation. An absorbable monofilament suture material such as polydioxanone (PDS) is superior to non-absorbable monofilament sutures as there is less wound pain, sinus formation and buttonhole hernias (a hernia that develops lateral to the main incision in association with progressive enlargement of the needle hole through which the permanent suture material passes). The senior editor's preference is to use a no. 1 looped PDS suture, thus avoiding the need for a knot at the start of the closure.

The suture length–wound length ratio should not be less than 4:1 and excessive tension should not be applied. Two of the editors recall being taught to 'appose and not necrose' when closing the abdomen.

The surgeon begins to appose the fascia at the uppermost part of the incision, taking suture bites 1–2 cm from the incision edge and the same distance apart (Fig. 4.8). Each edge should be taken separately using the full curve of the needle to avoid compromising the strength of the closure. The peritoneum should be avoided when possible.

The knot at the end of the closure can be buried by using the remaining length of suture to approximate the fat above the knot.

Fat stitch
There is no evidence that suturing the subcutaneous fat tissue has any benefit and the editors do not perform this routinely. However, as mentioned above,

the editors will often bury the 'sheath knot' using the sheath suture or will apply one or two Vicryl sutures within the fat layer above the knot.

Wound drains
There is no evidence that the use of parietal wound drains has any benefit and they are rarely used by the editors.

Skin closure

There are various techniques of skin closure. The editors' preference is to use stainless steel staples in a preloaded stapling device (Fig. 4.9). However, one of the editors is increasingly using subcuticular 3/0 poliglecaprone 25 (Monocryl), an absorbable monofilament suture which results in excellent wound healing.

If an epidural has not been used, infiltrating the wound with local anaesthetic either as a bolus dose or using a continuous infusion device such as the ON-Q PainBuster catheter can reduce postoperative pain.

Transverse incisions

There are several transverse abdominal incisions available to the gynaecologist, and this is the preferred incision for the obstetrician and gynaecologist dealing with benign pathology. The Pfannenstiel incision is the transverse incision of choice, but the Cherney and Maylard incisions provide excellent exposure to the pelvic sidewall. The advantages include better cosmesis and less pain. However, they limit access to the upper abdomen and are associated with greater blood loss and haematoma formation. Nerve injury resulting in paraesthesia of the overlying skin is also more frequent.

Pfannenstiel incision

The single most important value of this incision is cosmetic. It is important for many women that their abdomens should remain apparently untouched by the surgeon's knife, and, using this technique, the illusion can be maintained. The incision follows Langer's lines, a short distance above the symphysis pubis, usually just within the pubic hair line. Most

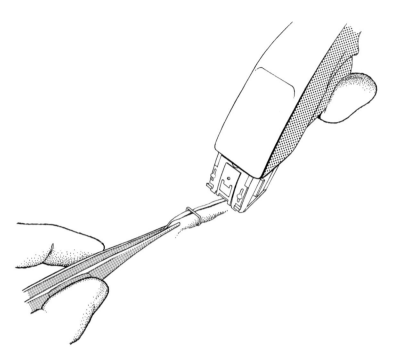

Figure 4.9 Stapling the abdominal skin.

minor pelvic surgery can be easily performed through this incision, and, as surgeons develop their skills, they will find that most hysterectomies and benign ovarian surgery come within the compass of this route of access. In the editors' view, the use of this incision for more radical surgery, particularly Wertheim hysterectomy, should be eschewed, although some clinicians do utilize it in these circumstances.

This incision is also of value when operating on the extremely obese patient with a large pannus, for the area a short distance above the symphysis pubis is often the thinnest part of the abdominal wall; if the massive abdominal pannus is lifted up and held out of the way by large Lane's forceps, access to the abdomen is often amazingly easy. Both the Pfannenstiel and Cherney incision can be combined with a panniculectomy for the very obese patient with a large pannus.

The incision is not advocated for extreme emergency situations as it takes significantly longer to enter the abdomen using this technique. The incision is also more vascular and is, therefore, more prone to haematoma formation than the midline alternative.

The incision

It is extremely important that the initial skin incision is level and symmetrical. A skewed scar after this incision is less acceptable than after any other. The landmarks of the symphysis and the anterior superior iliac spines must be accessible and not covered by drapes. The drapes must be accurately and evenly placed so as not to mislead the surgeon. The incision should be approximately 12 cm long for a hysterectomy; shorter for more minor procedures. The initial cut is made cleanly through the skin, slightly convex towards the pubis (Fig. 4.10). The fat is incised down to the rectus sheath and the aponeurosis of the external oblique muscle. As the incision is completed, the surgeon should make an incision into the sheath on either side of the midline. Small vessels in the fat are more numerous than in the midline incision and must be clipped and tied or diathermied. In particular, a large vein at the lateral edges of the incision is often seen and should be tied and cut unless it can be gently pushed laterally. The techniques of tearing the fatty layers have been advocated and, although functionally satisfactory, they are not aesthetically so.

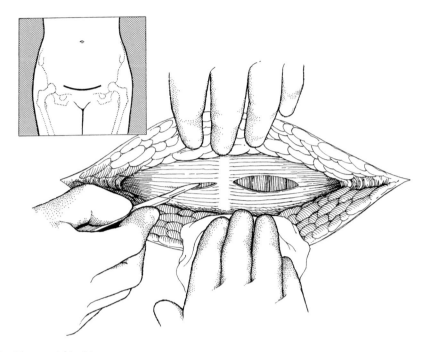

Figure 4.10 The Pfannenstiel incision.

Incision of the aponeurosis

The short incisions in the rectus sheath are now extended for the full length of the skin incision using a scalpel, scissors or diathermy. The upper and then the lower edges of the incision are now grasped in turn by artery forceps, elevated, and the underlying muscle separated from the sheath by a combination of blunt (swab) and sharp (scissors or diathermy) dissection (Fig. 4.11). Small vessels running parallel to the midline are tied or diathermied. The rectus muscles are now separated vertically and the peritoneum visualized.

Opening the peritoneum

This is performed in the same manner as for the midline incision, keeping a watchful eye on the upper limits of the bladder. It is usually easy to see the upper limit of the bladder by identifying the urachus as it appears as a narrow fibrous band in the midline. Grasping the urachus and incising it is a simple way of entering the peritoneal cavity.

Closure of the abdomen

This is carried out as in the midline incision. There is no need to close the peritoneum unless the bowel is protruding above the rectus muscle, which is uncommon. Meticulous attention should be paid to checking for any bleeding from perforating vessels on the rectus muscle and undersurface of the rectus sheath to prevent subfascial haematoma formation. The sheath is closed with a delayed absorbable suture such as PDS. A fat stitch and drains are not routinely used and the skin is approximated with staples or a subcuticular Monocryl suture.

Cherney incision

Cherney described a transverse incision that allows excellent exposure to the pelvic sidewalls. The editors use it rarely in obese woman with a large pannus requiring a radial hysterectomy.

The skin and fascia are entered as in the Pfannenstiel incision. The tendinous insertions of the recti (and

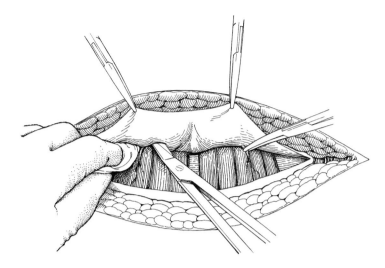

Figure 4.11 Dissecting the rectus sheath.

pyramidalis) are divided from the symphysis pubis using diathermy, allowing the recti to be reflected upwards. The peritoneum is opened transversely above the bladder and laterally to the inferior epigastric vessels. These should be preserved if possible as myonecrosis of the rectus muscle has been described.

Closing the abdomen

The peritoneum can be closed if thought appropriate to prevent the bowel protruding. The free tendinous ends of the rectus muscles can be left free and should not to be resutured to the symphysis pubis as this can cause osteomyelitis. The sheath and skin are closed as for the Pfannenstiel incision.

Maylard incision

As with the Cherney incision, Maylard proposed a transverse muscle-splitting incision to provide exposure to the pelvic sidewalls. The incision usually refers to a subumbilical transverse incision made 3–8 cm superior to the pubic symphysis at about the interspinous level. The anterior rectus sheath is cut trans-

versely and the inferior epigastric vessels are identified under the lateral edge of each rectus muscle and ligated prior to transversely cutting the rectus muscle. As with the Cherney incision, some patients may experience myonecrosis of the rectus muscle.

Closing the abdomen is similar to the Cherney incision, with the anterior rectus sheath closed with a monofilament absorbable suture.

Further reading

Ceydeli A, Rucinski J, Wise L. Finding the best abdominal closure: an evidence-based review of the literature. *Curr Surg* 2005;62:220–225.

Cherney LS. New transverse low abdominal incision. *Cal West Med* 1943;59(4):215–218.

Joel-Cohen S. *Abdominal and Vaginal Hysterectomy*, 2nd edn. London: William Heinemann, 1977. This covers the various techniques in full and is a mine of useful information. It illustrates how the use of time-and-motion studies radically changed Joel-Cohen's approach to surgery.

Maylard A. Direction of abdominal incisions. *BMJ* 1907;2:895–901.

The laparoscopic approach in gynaecology

Since the mid-1960s laparoscopy has grown from very simplistic beginnings to become one of the most commonly performed and most valuable of gynaecological procedures. The procedure is used extensively in the assessment of infertility, in the diagnosis of pelvic infection, ectopic pregnancies and endometriosis, and for sterilization procedures. During the late 1980s and 1990s laparoscopic surgery began to develop into what is now generally called 'minimal access surgery', being applied to a wide variety of conditions and gynaecological problems, changing from a mere observational process into one which has become the mainstay of effective management and treatment of a wide variety of conditions including a number of cancers. Minimal access surgery (MAS) is now used by virtually every surgical specialist and is widely established throughout gynaecological surgery, particularly in gynaecological oncology. The major change allowing this progress has been the continued improvement in instrumentation, particularly the generation of high-quality cameras and monitors. Trocar development, including improvements in both bladed and non-bladed instruments, has reduced the number of injuries associated with initial entry into the peritoneal cavity as well as that associated with the placement of accessory trocars. Similar advances in the quality and variety of laparoscopic graspers, scissors and other accessories has made it possible to safely perform an increasing number of procedures.

The continued development of MAS has meant patients with significant pelvic inflammatory disease, endometriosis and oncological problems can not only have their diagnoses made but also effective treatment carried out using techniques which allow for rapid recovery and return to normal activity.

In the last 10 years robotic surgery has been developed to the point that many prostatectomies are performed using the DaVinci system, and recent publications suggest that many gynaecological and gynaecological oncology procedures can be performed using this new technology, although there seems to be prolonged surgical times associated with its use. We would be remiss if we did not mention that no prospective randomized trial has yet to be conducted comparing standard MAS with that performed robotically. This remains the gold standard in medicine and, until such a trial is carried out demonstrating superior outcomes, given the high cost associated with its use, robotic surgery cannot be considered the standard of care. It should also be noted that, although there have been recent publications from the Gynecologic Oncology Group (GOG) in the USA demonstrating some advantages using MAS in the treatment of endometrial cancer, particularly as it pertains to shortened hospital stay and improved body image, there has been no demonstration of any survival advantage to the patients undergoing MAS.

Positioning of the patient

The patient initially should be positioned in the supine position on a table that allows for maximum

Bonney's Gynaecological Surgery, 11th edition.
© Tito Lopes, Nick Spirtos, Raj Naik, John Monaghan.
Published 2011 by Blackwell Publishing Ltd.

Trendelenburg as well as the use of a C-arm for intra-operative fluoroscopy. The patient's arms should be tucked at the sides and the legs placed in stirrups that allow for both maximum flexure of the knee and maximum rotation of the hip. The stirrup should provide padded support for the calf and foot. To maximize instrument range of motion, the anterior thigh should be parallel to the abdomen and the knee flexed at 90° in the stirrup. This not only reduces the pressure on the popliteal fossa but also helps to maintain the patient's position on the table when the patient is placed into the steep Trendelenburg position. Additional consideration should be given to using shoulder supports in order to keep the patient from sliding towards the head of the table. These supports should be padded with gel to minimize the risk of nerve injury, as should all pads placed against the patient.

Access to the abdomen

Generally speaking there has been no randomized prospective study or meta-analysis demonstrating the superiority of one method of entry over any other and, as a result, the editors would recommend continued use of the method with which each surgeon has developed familiarity and comfort within the context of the guideline produced by the Royal College of Obstetricians and Gynaecologists (RCOG) entitled *Preventing Entry-Related Gynaecological Laparoscopic Injuries*. The only variance with these recommendations one should consider is the placement of the initial trocar 2–3 cm above the umbilicus, so as to maximize the distance between the entry points of the primary 'umbilical' trocar and a potential secondary trocar placed just above the symphysis, in order to facilitate working in the pelvis, as the uterus is elevated during hysterectomy, and in the upper abdomen and in particular performing aortic lymphadenectomy, omentectomy, splenectomy and transverse colostomy. It should also be noted that, despite best efforts to keep the trocar placement at 90° to the skin, most often the angle of insertion varies as much as 20–45°, making the entry point into the peritoneal cavity quite close to the reproductive organs. This issue becomes more important when undertaking radical hysterectomy or the removal of large, complex pelvis masses.

Highlights of the RCOG recommendations include the following.

1 Regardless of the entry method used (within the limits of these recommendations, there is not one technique proven to be superior to another), the patient should remain flat prior to placing the primary trocar.

2 Entry instruments should be used at 90° to the skin.

3 If a Veres needle (disposable) is used to insufflate the abdomen prior to trocar placement, high intra-abdominal pressures of 20–25 mmHg should be achieved prior to placing the primary and secondary trocars.

4 Special care is warranted in patients with a history of previous surgery and in very thin and very obese patients. In these cases, the use of Palmer's point (3 cm below the left costal margin in the midclavicular line) to insert the Veres needle and primary trocar or the use of an open technique is thought to be beneficial.

5 Once the peritoneal cavity is entered, 360° inspection of the abdomen is mandatory to identify bowel or vascular injury, including retroperitoneal bleeding.

6 After completing the procedure, all midline and lateral trocar sites greater than 10 and 7 mm in diameter, respectively, should be sutured closed at the fascial level.

Equipment

Insufflators

It is recommended that high-flow insufflators be used with maximum flow rates of 20–40 litres of carbon dioxide per minute. Most insufflators can be set at any flow rate from 0 to 40 litres per minute with pre-set 'low-flow' rates at 3–4 litres per minute and 20–40 litres per minute for the pre-set 'high-flow' rate. This equipment has both high and low flow rates which allow initial safe low-pressure insufflation that can then be accelerated during the initial phases of the procedure. Virtually all of these are self-regulated with the ability to stop the in-flow of gas when the pre-set pressure limit is set. Most authorities recommend that the intra-abdominal pressure should not exceed 14–15 mmHg pressure.

The gas used for insufflation remains carbon dioxide because of its ability to be rapidly absorbed into the patient's bloodstream and excreted through the lungs and the kidneys. Continued monitoring of the pCO_2 is required and particular attention paid to patients with morbid obesity or any chronic pulmonary disease. If the pCO_2 elevates to 50 mmHg or greater and cannot be reduced with hyperventilation, consideration must be given to either reversing the Trendelenburg position temporarily or possibly aborting the laparoscopic procedure completely.

Trocars

Blunt, bladed and non-bladed radially expanded trocars are regularly used by multiple authorities on this subject, as are trocars that allow for visual entry to the peritoneal cavity. Use of these are all based on the surgeon's preference, making specific recommendations difficult.

Other instruments

There are a variety of instruments for manipulation of the uterus during the procedure, and a wide range of graspers, scissors and cutting devices have been developed. At a minimum, a pair of wavy graspers to grasp the round ligaments in order to retract the uterus are needed, as well as a Maryland dissector to grasp sutures or more delicate structures such as the bowel and ureters. It is the opinion of the editors that endoscopic shears must be quite sharp, and one is best served by using disposable instruments in this setting. The editors have not found the value in using uterine manipulators and, in cases involving endometrial or cervical cancer, would prefer to minimize disruption of the endocervix or endometrium. In that regard, the editors prefer the use of the McCartney tube (Covidien Inc., Boulder, CO, USA) or the Gyne Tube (Paragon Imex Co., Menlo Park, CA, USA).

Energy sources

Although monopolar diathermy remains a mainstay of most minimal access surgical procedures, some clinicians prefer bipolar energy. There are a number of bipolar energy sources in addition to the standard electricity provided using a bipolar platform. The Harmonic Scalpel (Ethicon Endosurgery Inc., Cincinnati, OH, USA), which is a form of ultrasound initiated by vibration in an instrument, provides a similar effect along with the ability to seal vessels up to 5 mm in diameter. The Ligasure device (Covidien Inc.) utilizes radiofrequency resulting in the melting of the collagen and elastin in vessel walls, causing them to be sealed with minimal peripheral damage (less than 2 mm). Essentially, all bipolar energy sources have limited lateral tissue damage of less than 2 mm, and all of the instruments are of excellent calibre; use is left to individual preference. Others clinicians prefer the use of the argon beam coagulator and it should be noted this technology is based on monopolar current integration with a stream of argon gas. Its use is associated with minimal penetration, approximately 1 mm lateral extension and excellent haemostasis. It has been used extensively in achieving haemostasis in laparoscopic liver resection and can be a valuable tool in controlling bleeding from the splenic hilum as well as in performing retroperitoneal lymph node dissection.

There is little indication at this point for the intraperitoneal use of lasers of any sort.

Light source

Modern fibreoptic light sources provide tremendous intra-abdominal illumination so long as their fibres remain intact. Cables should be checked regularly to make sure that there is no loss of fibres and a consequent reduction in light availability.

Cameras and monitors

Over the last few years, significant advances have been made in the cameras and monitors used during MAS. Most centres now have available high-definition (HD) monitors and cameras. The quality of the images associated with this technology is superb to the point that the image almost appears to have a third dimension (3D) to it. Much effort has gone into the development of 3D technology for MAS, yet, to date, there is no system that is widely marketed or commonly in use. That is not to say that the experienced surgeon is without a sense of depth when performing MAS. In the same way one-eyed individuals develop a sense of depth perception with subconscious micro-movements of the eye providing two images centrally, so does the experienced surgeon performing MAS. It is the merging of the two images (binocular vision) that usually provides one with a sense of depth.

In the best of settings it facilitates MAS if four monitors are available: one placed on each side of the patient towards her head and one on each side of the patient near her knees. This allows maximum flexibility and minimizes the unnecessary movement of the equipment, which both wastes time during surgery and can result in damage to the equipment over the long haul. Many MAS surgical suites now have the monitors and equipment installed on mobile arms in cabinetry suspended from the ceiling, achieving both of these endpoints.

Preparation

Patients do not require special preparation for diagnostic procedures. Many of the simple diagnostic tests are performed as day cases and even a number of small MAS procedures will be performed as day cases. More complicated procedures are best preceded by an adequate bowel preparation. This will allow for easier displacement of the intestine into the upper abdomen as well as minimizing bacterial contamination in the case of direct bowel injury.

Anaesthesia

Laparoscopic surgery should be performed under general anaesthesia with the patient intubated and fully relaxed. For extended procedures nitrous oxide gas should not be used, as it is retained intraluminally in the intestine, thereby minimizing visualization of the operative field. It is also helpful to use a combined anaesthetic technique utilizing both general and regional anaesthesia. The regional anaesthesia provides a sympathetic block that constricts the bowel and reduces the lumen size, again facilitating its displacement into the upper abdomen. Similar effects can be achieved with either a spinal or epidural anaesthesia, and it matters not whether an opioid or a member of the amide group (lidocaine, marcaine) of local anaesthetic agents is used. This strategy provides the additional advantage as the regional anaesthesia can then be used in the postoperative period, reducing the need for parenteral narcotics. The use of laryngeal masks has become popular and for short procedures can be used. The use of local anaesthetic techniques is difficult and renders operations more complex and potentially dangerous.

Diagnostic laparoscopy

Operation

Positioning and preparation
The patient should be positioned on the operating table as described earlier in this chapter. The vulva and the vagina are swabbed and the bladder meticulously emptied using a disposable catheter. It is important to observe and record the amount of urine removed from the bladder as some patients undergoing surgery for simple but large central pelvic masses have nothing more than overdistended bladders from a variety of causes. At the same time, the lower abdomen is swabbed and the patient draped. It is recommended that, in draping the patient, one makes sure that the anterior superior iliac spine is within the field so lateral trocar placement can be successfully carried out in the proper field.

Grasping the uterus
The pelvis must be examined prior to the procedure to determine the size, position and mobility of the uterus as well as the presence or absence of adnexal masses and, in the case of cancers of the reproductive tract, local extension of the disease into the parametrial tissues. If one is going to use a uterine manipulator, the cervix is visualized by inserting a Sims speculum into the vagina and grasped by placing a single-toothed tenaculum transversely across the anterior lip of the cervix and attaching it to a simple intrauterine device, such as that used for injecting methylene blue into the uterus, or the Hulka tenaculum, which combines a tenaculum and a sound. These and other devices can allow the assistant to manipulate the uterus to different positions to improve access and visibility for the surgeon.

Producing the pneumoperitoneum
The surgeon grasps the skin of the relaxed lower abdomen with the left hand and elevates the abdominal wall. The right hand firmly introduces the disposable Veres needle directly through the centre of the umbilicus or through a small vertical cut in the fold of skin at the lower part of the umbilicus (Fig. 5.1). Resistance is felt at the level of the rectus sheath causing the blunt obturator in the needle to be forced back, allowing the needle's cutting edge to pass through the sheath into the abdomen. At this point,

45

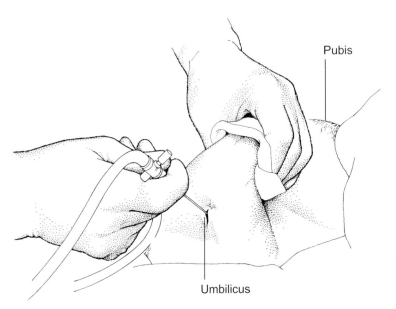

Pubis

Umbilicus

Figure 5.1 Veres needle insertion into the abdominal cavity to produce a pneumoperitoneum.

the spring-loaded obturator moves forward, protecting the abdominal contents from the sharp cutting edge. Utilizing a modern disposable Veres needles, a double click may be heard as the needle passes through the layers of the abdominal wall. The most reliable indicator of proper placement and location of the Veres needle is the recording of intra-abdominal pressures of 7 mmHg or less.

Variations in technique

Although the umbilical site is the commonest site used for straightforward laparoscopic procedures, in patients in whom there has been any evidence of previous surgery or intra-abdominal or pelvic infection it is prudent to utilize an alternative site of entry. Statistically, the left hypochondrium is the site in the abdomen where the surgeon is at least risk of hitting an intra-abdominal structure, unless there is a history of splenectomy or other upper abdominal surgery. The site normally chosen is the point 3 cm below the costal margin in the midclavicular line. This technique is that described by Palmer, and the point chosen is that of Palmer's point. At this point, a small incision some 3 mm wide is made in the skin. The Veres needle is now inserted vertically through the abdominal wall. It is prudent to grasp the needle in the right hand with the fingers of the right hand lying along the shaft of the needle so as to act as a buffer as the needle is

inserted through the skin. Once more, the abdominal wall is elevated with the left hand and the needle passed through the wall; two clicks of the disposable needle are heard as it passes through the rectus sheath and then the peritoneum into the abdominal cavity. By allowing the gas to flow maximally at the time of insertion, the surgeon can watch and use the change in pressures as the Veres needle passes through the abdominal wall as an indicator of proper placement. Generally speaking, the pressures will spike to approximately 30–45 mmHg as the gas line is occluded and then fall to approximately 6–7 mmHg once the peritoneal cavity is entered. In the very obese patient, the intraperitoneal pressure may be slightly higher and the surgeon should not be alarmed if the pressure upon entry is in the range of 9–10 mmHg. Many clinicians do not utilize this technique and adopt a series of small tests including the water test, which consists of attaching a syringe full of sterile water to the Veres needle opening and observing the gentle change in pressure associated with respiration. This technique has not proven itself to be reliable enough to count on as evidence of entry into the peritoneal cavity.

Initially, the gas is allowed to flow in at low rates of approximately 3–4 litres per minute. Once flowing freely with clear signs of wide distribution throughout the abdominal cavity, as can be demonstrated by percussion of the expanding abdomen, the pace of

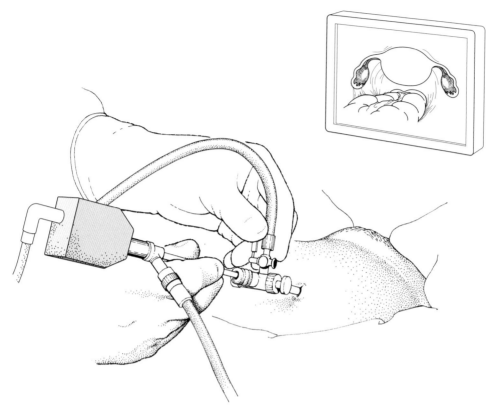

Figure 5.2 Insertion of the laparoscope via the trocar.

insufflation can be raised to a high flow. Care should be taken to ensure that high intra-abdominal pressures are not allowed to exist for prolonged periods of time and, to this end, most insufflators automatically sound an alarm if pressures exceed 15 mmHg. Short-term elevations in intra-abdominal pressures such as those occurring during initial trocar placement do not seem to cause concern to the anaesthetic process.

Insertion of the laparoscope

For most diagnostic procedures a 5 mm trocar and a 5 mm laparoscope will be used in order to minimize trauma. Just prior to insertion of the primary trocar the intra-abdominal pressure should be raised to 20–25 mmHg as suggested earlier in this chapter. At this point, the importance of an adequate skin incision cannot be overemphasized. Skin dystocia should be eliminated at the time of trocar placement and the subcutaneous tissues should be separated so the blade

of the trocar device is essentially touching the anterior abdominal fascia prior to its insertion. The trocar is grasped in the surgeon's right hand with the index finger passing along the length of the trocar. Once more, the index finger will act as a buffer so that the trocar is not inserted any further than the depth of the abdominal wall. At this point, the abdominal wall will be firm from the insufflating gas, and one can boldly insert the trocar with the right hand directing the trocar down towards the pelvis. The modern disposable trocars are very sharp with safety devices built into them which immediately spring to cover the sharp blade as soon as the trocar passes through the abdominal wall. The trocar can be felt passing through the various layers of the abdominal wall and, as soon as this is achieved, the laparoscope can be inserted, the gas attached to the trocar and observation of the intra-abdominal structures begun (Fig. 5.2). It is often useful to apply de-misting solutions to the laparoscope tip prior to insertion and the laparoscope kept in a warmer until just prior to its connection to the camera and insertion into the abdomen. In many centres, the gas is warmed as it is instilled into the abdomen. As it is the gas cooling the laparoscope which causes misting, applying hot water to the laparoscope can minimize this problem as well. A fibreoptic light and camera are attached to the laparoscope, and the pelvis and abdomen can then be visualized. If the laparoscope mists while inside the abdomen (this often occurs in the initial phases of a laparoscopy), it is usually not necessary to remove it from the abdomen. All that is needed is to gently touch the laparoscope onto a clean peritoneal surface or the uterine fundus.

In most procedures, other instruments are inserted into the abdominal cavity. This is facilitated by using the laparoscope to illuminate the abdominal wall if it is thin, or choosing a spot where large vessels such as the inferior epigastric artery can be avoided. The safest area to place additional trocars is lateral to the epigastric vessels at a height most suitable to the procedure being undertaken. This placement not only minimizes the chance of vascular injury but also broadens the operative field, allowing more flexibility in the choice and use of additional instruments. Once more, the same technique of inserting trocars can be applied, this time under direct vision via the video camera, which has now been attached to the laparoscope.

Diagnostic laparoscopy consists simply of recording appearances within the abdomen and pelvis. These can be recorded either in the operation note or with digital images. The digital cameras currently in use can generate a number of images which can be stored or printed out and put into the patient's clinical record. These are of particular value in the recording of sterilization procedures and when wishing to discuss further more complex management which may be necessary following the diagnostic procedure.

Completing the procedure

Once the diagnostic laparoscopic procedure is complete, the laparoscope can be removed and gas released from the abdomen. Where a number of ports have been used, it is prudent to observe individual trocars being taken out to make sure that no untoward bleeding occurs and that there has been no inadvertent visceral injury. Finally, having released all the gas from the abdomen, the last trocar can be removed and the various incisions closed, usually with a single stitch for 5 mm laparoscopic procedures.

Problems and complications associated with laparoscopy

Although the basic procedure is simple in concept there are a number of traps and pitfalls that must be avoided, as follows.

• Failure to examine the patient prior to the procedure may result in missing uterine enlargement or masses in the pelvis which can be put in significant danger when the various instrumentation is being inserted into the abdomen.

• Failure to catheterize the bladder increases the risk of damage to that organ. As previously noted, if an excessive amount of urine is collected at this time (greater than 750 mL) and surgery is being undertaken for a simple large cystic midline mass, consideration should be given to obtaining an intraoperative ultrasound as the aetiology of the mass may have just been determined and the need for the laparoscopy eliminated.

• A tentative approach to the production of the pneumoperitoneum may result in gas being inserted in the fatty layer of the anterior abdominal wall. The Veres needle must be inserted through the abdominal wall at almost a vertical angle down towards the pelvis and not at a shallow angle, as this will generate problems. The double 'click' of the disposable Veres needle is reassuring. The use of Palmer's point will markedly reduce the risk of failure to develop a pneumoperitoneum.

Many complications of laparoscopy have been reported, including bowel damage and vascular injury. These can most often be avoided by always being mindful of proper technique, respect for your patient and the potentially lethal instruments in your use, and assiduous practice.

Laparoscopic surgery for endometriosis

In many ways, the surgical treatment of endometriosis, whether undertaken using 'open' or 'closed' approaches, is more difficult than treating most gynaecological malignancies. Surgical planes are often obliterated secondary to the sclerotic, invasive nature of endometriosis. Nevertheless, it is in this area that one might argue MAS has its most important application for, with it, postoperative adhesions are minimized and, given many patients with endometriosis are undergoing surgery in order to enhance their chances of conceiving, this advantage cannot be overstated. Thus, despite some technical difficulty for the operating surgeon, the benefits to the patient require the application of these techniques to the treatment of endometriosis. In cases of suspected severe endometriosis, the patient should not only undergo preoperative bowel preparation but should be scheduled for cystoscopy and proctosigmoidoscopy to fully evaluate the lower urinary tract and gastrointestinal tract.

Ablation or resection of superficial peritoneal endometriosis is straightforward and can be accomplished using any number of monopolar or bipolar instruments widely available. The editors' preference is to use the argon beam coagulator (ABC) in this setting. As the penetration of the current is limited to approximately 1 mm there is little risk of damaging underlying organs. There is additional gain as the simultaneous instillation of argon gas often facilitates the dissection and resection of the involved tissues by lifting them off the underlying organs.

Much more difficult is the management of the obliterated posterior cul-de-sac and retroperitoneal spread of the disease or scarring in the area of the uterosacral ligaments, resulting in ureteral stricture if not complete occlusion.

Sound, basic techniques should not be omitted in a rush to address significant pelvic pathology when encountered, lest disease in other locations be missed. This cannot be truer than in the treatment of endometriosis and the need to explore the entire abdomen. Often there is spread to the gastrointestinal tract outside the pelvis, particularly the appendix, and sometimes disease can be found as distant as the subdiaphragmatic peritoneum. Disease in these locations must be addressed as well as the disease in the pelvis. The disease involving the diaphragm peritoneum can be ablated using the ABC as described above, and the appendix and/or small bowel resected using Endo-GIAs (Ethicon Endosurgery Inc.). Key to approaching the obliterated cul-de-sac and any ureteral involvement is to open and develop the retroperitoneal spaces. Using the ABC set at 80 watts with a gas flow rate 2–3 litres per minute the peritoneum over the psoas muscle is incised from just above the

pelvic brim to the round ligament. By using the ABC or a Stryker battery-powered irrigator placed through the midline suprapubic port site, the pararectal and paravesical spaces can be developed by moving either of these instruments from side to side instead of parallel to the iliac vessels. This will allow for quick identification of the ureter and, if the ovary is to be removed, the gonadal vessels secured by either endoscopic staples or the energy source of preference. Using hydrodissection in this area is most advantageous as the rapidly instilled water quickly separates the ureter from the medial leaf of peritoneum as well as the uterosacral ligament where the most significant fibrosis is usually encountered. Low-flow irrigators will not provide the force necessary to separate the ureter from the uterosacral ligaments when involved secondarily by endometriosis. Once the ureter is mobilized laterally, the ABC can now be applied to the lateral aspect of the uterosacral ligaments with the transection taking place from the lateral to medial direction. This is important as the most significant disease in the posterior cul-de-sac is usually encountered in the midline and it is in this location that the rectum is most often involved. As the midline is reached, taking the irrigator just lateral to the rectum and medial to the hypogastric vessels and advancing it posteriorly, the water can be used to develop the retro-rectal space. This might seem unnecessary, but this move will elevate the rectum out of the sacral hollow and into the operative field. Now a rectal dilator can be passed through the anus and a Gyne Tube (Paragon Imex Co.) inserted into the vagina. With these two instruments in place, the ABC can be used to continue to incise the peritoneal reflection in the midline. If there is nodular disease here, the irrigator can be passed deep to the point of posterior attachment. The involved segment of rectum has now been circumferentially isolated and, even if continued ablation and/or sharp dissection results in entry into the rectum, the amount of tissue needed to be removed will be minimized, usually resulting in the removal of a small section of anterior rectal wall. This can now be closed using an Endostitch device (Covidien Inc.) with either a running or interrupted closure with 0 Vicryl.

Less frequently, the anterior peritoneal fold is involved by endometriosis that penetrates the bladder, requiring resection and a two-layer closure using the Endostitch with 0 Polysorb (Covidien Inc.) in a similar manner to that described when closing the vagina during total laparoscopic hysterectomy.

Occasionally, the ureter is involved to the extent that it requires resection and reanastamosis or ureteroneocystotomy, both of which can be accomplished using MAS.

Once these difficult areas of endometriosis have been addressed, the surgeon can proceed with planned ovarian cystectomy, salpingo-oophorectomy and or hysterectomy as per preoperative discussions with the patient and her family. The importance of thorough preoperative counselling cannot be overemphasized in this setting as the meshing of disease management and the patient's desire to preserve reproductive capacity are often at odds. If an error is to be made, one should leave the reproductive organs *in situ* as reoperation is a manageable problem whereas the finality of removing the reproductive organs is not.

Laparoscopic surgery in gynaecological oncology

For many years after the introduction of laparoscopy the technique was almost entirely utilized in the management of minor gynaecological and infertility problems. The role of MAS has expanded, particularly in gynaecological oncology, and predominantly in the area of hysterectomy (simple and radical) and lymphadenectomy.

Not only has the feasibility of safely undertaking the wide range of surgical procedures required in the practice of gynaecological oncology using MAS been demonstrated in centres around the world, but MAS has been documented to be the equivalent to laparotomy on a technical basis. Recently published randomized prospective studies undertaken by the GOG in the USA have demonstrated a reduction in the length of hospital stay and complications with MAS when compared with laparotomy in patients with endometrial cancers. Earlier prospective feasibility trials from that group as well as many other centres worldwide made it clear that MAS would meet the modern requirements of both gynaecology and gynaecological oncology in terms of ease of access, reduction of impact of surgery on patients, rapid recovery and, in many western countries most importantly, an early discharge from hospital, thus reducing overall costs of surgery. This pressure to speed up the process

of care had to be tempered by the need to be effective and be certain that new technologies were at least equal in efficacy to previous open surgical techniques. There is little doubt that major proponents of minimal access surgery have been able to demonstrate the ease with which major and at times extremely radical procedures can be performed using MAS techniques. However, it is also clear that such techniques require a considerable experience of standard surgery. They require a prolonged period of training and the equipment which is necessary has to be of the highest order. All the services associated with surgical care, including anaesthetics, nursing and operating theatre skills, have to be comparable, and it is vital that surgeons accept that the same prolonged period of training will be required for MAS as is accepted for open surgery.

Hysterectomy of all degrees of radicality as well as pelvic and aortic lymphadenectomy are now widely accepted as being standard procedures in MAS. By definition, the acceptance of MAS in these procedures has meant that it is mainly used in the management of early stage cervical and corpus cancers. As early stage ovarian cancer is infrequently encountered there is not the abundance of literature on the use of MAS in this setting. That being said, there has been demonstration of the adequacy and safety of using MAS in restaging patients with apparent early stage endometrial, fallopian tube and ovarian cancers. In doing so, MAS has been shown to be a viable technique to complete an omentectomy and thoroughly evaluate the peritoneal surfaces of the abdomen. A few centres have incorporated MAS into the management of advanced ovarian cancer as these techniques can be used successfully in resecting small and large bowel, splenectomy and the removal of diaphragmatic disease. This practice has not been widely adapted, nor have the MAS techniques for lymphadenectomy in the groin in the management of vulval cancer.

Complications

Port site metastases

Just as in the case of incisional recurrences following laparotomy, there has been a small but important series of individual case reports and comments concerning the risks of port site recurrences associated with MAS in gynaecological oncology. The mechanism of development is uncertain; however, it is likely that the major problem is contamination of the port with material containing cancer cells, the so-called implantation theory. This theory, however, seems to fall down when it is noted how rarely the vaginal vault is involved in recurrences, particularly in the case of cancer of the cervix. Various gas pressure theories have also been promulgated, but, to date, there is no certain aetiology. Not coincidentally, the vast majority of port site recurrences have been reported in patients with advanced stage ovarian cancer, and the clinical significance of this is hard to determine as the term port site recurrence in this setting is hardly accurate. Nevertheless, every measure should be taken to minimize the contact of potentially malignant cells to the subcutaneous tissues as described above. Some authors have suggested irrigating port sites with iodine solution. There have also been reports of port site recurrences following the treatment of both cervical and corpus cancers, although complete staging was not undertaken in most of these reports. To this point, it should be noted that in a recently published, prospective, randomized trial in patients with early stage endometrial cancer conducted by the GOG in the USA in which over 2500 patients were randomly assigned with a 2:1 bias in favour of laparoscopy there was not a single port site recurrence noted.

Port site hernia

Port site hernias continue to be a debilitating but rare problem for a small number of patients. The result of extensive study has shown the highest risk of hernia is associated with the use of larger ports. The result of these studies is that many experts now consider that closure of the large ports (larger than 7 mm) is of value and would be the recommendation of the editors to do so.

Port site haematoma

Port site haematomata can be extremely debilitating, slowing recovery and causing considerable pain and distress. Avoidance of large vessels such as the inferior epigastric is mandatory. However, when the lateral ports are inserted through a muscular abdomen, particularly through the rectus muscle, damage to contained vessels may be unavoidable. Damage to these vessels may result in a haematoma developing or may manifest itself as continuing pain after the procedure or even, in extreme cases, a significant drop in haemoglobin in the days following surgery.

Postoperative recovery

In general terms the most significant characteristic of the postsurgical period following MAS is the rapid and progressive recovery of the patient. Any patient who does not do so or who suddenly develops new pain or symptomatology must be carefully examined for complications. Early discharge of such a patient is a formula for progressive and sometimes long-term problems, including litigation. Patients should understand that part of their responsibility upon discharge from the hospital is to notify the surgeon of any untoward outcome immediately. Of particular importance is new onset of pain or fever or a new or unusual vaginal discharge.

Further reading

Litynski GS. Raoul Palmer, World War II, and transabdominal coelioscopy. Laparoscopy extends into gynecology. *JSLS* 1997;1:289–292.

Sandor J, Ballagi F, Nagy A, Rákóczi I. A needle puncture that helped to change the world of surgery. Homage to János Veres. *Surg Endosc* 2000;14:201–202.

Royal College of Obstetricians and Gynaecologists. *Preventing Entry-related Gynaecological Laparoscopic Injuries*. Green-top Guideline no. 49. London: RCOG, 2008.

6 Postoperative care and complications

The postoperative period is a time when the surgeon must not let down his guard. Patients recovering from complex surgical procedures need to be monitored closely, and those recovering from routine surgery may develop unexpected problems.

It is often the culmination of the preoperative assessment, counselling, consent and preparation followed by the eventual surgery that determines a successful outcome or not. Any deficiency in the preceding activities will become evident now. It is during this time that the surgeon's experience often counts and, for this reason, it is imperative that each surgeon keeps a record of his outcomes. It is the surgeon in whom the patient entrusted her own well-being; it is the surgeon who accepted that trust and the responsibilities beholding it; and it is the surgeon who must ensure a satisfactory outcome at all times.

Pain relief

Epidural anaesthesia has been shown to be most effective for postoperative pain relief. Not only does it provide relaxation of muscles during surgery and less blood loss through a reduction in venous and arterial pressure, continuation of the epidural anaesthesia reduces the risk of postoperative thromboembolic events and provides an excellent form of pain relief. In many institutions, the epidural can be

managed in the comfort of a standard ward rather than a high-dependency unit, where the possibility of peaceful recovery and relaxation is undermined by the constant activity of the nursing and medical staff and the increased risk of hospital-acquired infections.

An alternative analgesic option is patient-controlled analgesia, in which a controlled infusion of opiates can be administered based upon the patient's requirements. This can be combined with the use of local injection of the wound with local anaesthetic agents immediately before or after the surgery. Early recourse to non-opioid analgesics allows minimization of the associated side-effects such as drowsiness, nausea and vomiting, confusion and hallucinations.

Thromboprophylaxis

The role of thromboprophylaxis has been described in detail in Chapter 2. This section is simply to emphasize the need to continue prophylaxis until the patient is fully ambulatory or is ready for discharge. Following major surgery, the subcutaneous injection of low-molecular-weight heparin commenced immediately before or after surgery should be continued for at least 5 days or until the patient is mobile. The patient should be strongly advised to continue using the compression stockings postoperatively for at least 4–6 weeks until fully mobile.

It is always important not to overlook complaints of shortness of breath, and one should respond with the appropriate work-up to rule out pulmonary embolism including arterial blood gas and spiral CT.

Bonney's Gynaecological Surgery, 11th edition.
© Tito Lopes, Nick Spirtos, Raj Naik, John Monaghan.
Published 2011 by Blackwell Publishing Ltd.

Antibiotics

Other than prescribing intraoperative antibiotics, the editors do not recommend the routine use of postoperative antibiotics unless, as rarely occurs, there has clearly been considerable faecal soiling during the surgery or a confirmed infection has been identified preoperatively.

Catheterization

The editors' current practice relating to bladder catheterization is to use transurethral catheterization inserted immediately prior to major surgery and to remove the catheter on the second postoperative day when the patient can be expected to have recovered reasonably from the surgery and patient mobilization is to be encouraged. Radical abdominal hysterectomies, radical abdominal trachelectomies and urinary incontinence procedures are best managed by suprapubic catheters which are clamped on day 5, and the patient taught intermittent self-catheterization in the presence of high residual volumes.

Mobilization and physiotherapy

The need for early mobilization cannot be overemphasized and requires the nursing staff to 'bully' the patients out from their beds. Physiotherapists who concentrate more on motivating patients with breathing and lower limb exercises and early mobilization rather than vigorous documentation in notes are to be encouraged.

Outreach teams

Critical care outreach teams are to be congratulated for their expertise and manner in which they ensure adequate postoperative pain relief and identification of patients who are deteriorating through development of complications. Complete reliance on their activities, however, serves to de-skill the remaining nursing and junior medical teams and they should be seen as a useful educational resource rather than a replacement of an already established service.

Wound monitoring

There can be no excuse for the surgeon not monitoring the surgical wounds of his own patients during the postoperative period. Much can be learnt from this simple practice. Nursing staff, despite significant experience at managing wounds, often still require the need for support from their medical colleagues to ensure that difficulties do not arise and that optimal methods are being utilized.

Although the editors currently cover all abdominal and groin wounds with self-adhesive dressings immediately after the surgery is completed, these are generally removed on the second or third postoperative day when the wound is allowed to air and can be cleaned and dried with a shower-head and a dryer.

Stoma therapists

This service provides a valuable adjunct to the surgical team in terms of both patient education and proper placement and management of the stoma in the immediate postoperative period. This function is facilitated by a preoperative evaluation in patients in whom diversion of the urinary or gastrointestinal tract is being considered.

Complications

Infection

Postoperative infections are all too common in today's surgical practice. Pyrexia in the early postoperative period (less than 24 hours) is usually due to atelectasis rather than infection, and the trainee should resist the commencement of antibiotics unnecessarily. Thereafter, urinary, wound, chest, intra-abdominal, skin and line infections (including peripheral and central) as well as bowel infections including *Clostridium difficile* need to be diagnosed and treated early. Full blown sepsis/bacteraemia secondary to antibiotic-resistant organisms requires close cooperation from the antimicrobiological team, whose advice can often be invaluable. These events are all quite distinct from cellulitis, which may or may not require Gram-positive antibiotic coverage given parenterally or orally based on severity of the infection.

Wound breakdown

Occasionally, input from the tissue viability nurse provides useful advice regarding the need for vacuum-assisted closure (VAC) therapy and dressings which have been shown to provide speedier recovery of large wounds. Close liaison with the community nurses ensures that these patients are discharged in a timely manner and that their care is not interrupted or disadvantaged.

It is often the editors' practice, especially with perineal wounds, which have a tremendous blood supply, to leave the wound open to heal by secondary intention. The results with good nursing care, which can be witnessed and documented postoperatively, can be astounding.

In all cases, the surgeon should have a low threshold to return the postoperative patient to the operating theatre in order to evaluate and possibly debride necrotic tissue surrounding the surgical incision. This is particularly true in cases of suspected necrotizing fasciitis. The need for early and regular debridement is an often overlooked part of the management of the postoperative wound.

Wound dehiscence

Superficial dehiscence

This occurs more commonly in obese patients. They are easily managed through regular cleansing. Taking of culture swabs ensures the early detection of significant infections and the appropriate use of antibiotics.

Complete dehiscence

This is often masked during the early postoperative period as the skin staples or subcutaneous sutures are still *in situ*. Often, the only sign is the occurrence of profuse serous fluid emanating from the suture line for no apparent reason. It is only when the staples are finally removed that evidence of a complete dehiscence become obvious. Immediate application of large, wet, sterile packs over the open wound and preparation for urgent recourse to the operating theatre should be made. The sheath should be repaired with continuous or interrupted non-absorbable sutures, taking large bites of the sheath, and separate deep tension sutures can be added depending on the surgeon's preference. Antibiotics should be given intraoperatively and continued if there is any evidence of infection. Patients

particularly prone include the obese, malnourished, those on long-term steroids and those with chronic cough and severe constipation.

Urinary tract

Infection

Urinary infections occur more commonly following catheterization, ureteric stenting or bladder injury. The routine collection of a catheter specimen/midstream specimen of urine during the postoperative period should be mandatory to ensure that asymptomatic cases are identified and treated appropriately.

Fistulae

Vesicovaginal fistulae The women complain of being continuously wet. The fistula can be confirmed by the injection of methylene blue into the bladder through a urethral catheter and seeing whether a tampon inserted into the vagina turns blue. Confirmation can also be made by a cystogram or cystoscopy. Most cases will heal spontaneously if managed conservatively with long-term indwelling catheterization. Only occasionally is further surgical repair required.

Ureteric fistulae As with a vesicovaginal fistula, the patient may complain of being continuously wet. If the patient has enough fluid leaking out of the vagina, it can be collected and sent for a creatinine level. If it is significantly elevated above the patient's serum creatinine, the diagnosis can be suspected after a vesicovaginal fistula has been ruled out as above. An intravenous urogram (IVU) or CT urogram may also be useful in making a diagnosis, but a definitive diagnosis may be made only with a bilateral retrograde ureteropyelography (to exclude bilateral fistulae).

Referral to a urologist should be made for further management. Conservative management with insertion of a retrograde ureteric stent may be possible. Surgical options are described in Chapter 26.

Gastrointestinal

Ileus

Ileus is usually a result of excessive bowel handling during surgery. It is managed by minimizing oral intake and ensuring adequate hydration and electrolyte maintenance with intravenous fluids and supplementation. There is no value in routinely starving patients postoperatively after straightforward cases, even after bowel surgery, and this practice in general should be discouraged. Most, if not all, motility issues following surgery are related to improper emptying of the stomach and routine use of metoclopramide may facilitate emptying and reduce complaints of nausea. There is a significant body of literature on immediate feeding of patients in the recovery room using needle-catheter jejunostomy, making it clear that feeding immediately after surgery is almost always limited by gastric emptying.

Obstruction
Obstruction during the postoperative period usually occurs some weeks after surgery and is usually the result of surgically induced adhesions. Initial management should be conservative as most cases will recover spontaneously after a period of rest. Rarely will further surgery be required and often a band of tissue or adhesion of the small bowel to the pelvis or anterior abdominal wall is identified as the source of the obstruction. A simple excision of the band resolves the problem without the need for bowel surgery.

Leaks and fistulae
Gynaecological oncology procedures may often require the need for bowel surgery and, in some cases, the large bowel is anastomosed without a defunctioning stoma. The commonly accepted rate of anastomotic leaks or fistulae is less than 10%.

An attentive mind is therefore required during the postoperative period to ensure that any disturbance to expected recovery is not the result of an anastomotic leak, which often presents between the 7th and 10th postoperative day. A proactive approach, a thorough examination and early use of investigations including radiographs and CT scan for immediate detection are imperative to recover the situation whether the further management is to be conservative with drainage and antibiotics or surgical repair. Close relationships with colorectal colleagues ensure that an accepted approach is adopted.

Sepsis

Overwhelming postoperative sepsis is a rare event. All possible sites need to be inspected, examined and investigated to ensure adequate diagnosis and treatment. Blood culture investigation is mandatory and regular communication with the antimicrobiological department imperative. Broad-spectrum antibiotics are the mainstay of treatment. Detailed abdominal investigation to exclude anastomotic leaks, unidentified bowel injury and localized collections which may require drainage are also required.

Prolonged surgical times, hypotension, disseminated intravascular coagulopathy and excessive blood loss are all associated with the development of acute respiratory distress syndrome. As a result, every effort should be made to avoid these problems from occurring.

Co-morbidities

Often, it is the association of co-morbidities that determines the overall outcome. Many such patients succumb to cardiovascular or cerebrovascular events which to a large degree are unavoidable despite the best of surgical interventions. Maintenance of a consistent blood pressure and an adequate urine output with appropriate fluid resuscitation throughout the intraoperative and immediate postoperative period play a large role in ensuring that these complications are reduced to an absolute minimum. The rest is dependent upon adequate preoperative assessment and luck!

Part 2: Anatomical

For the general gynaecologist and gynaecologist in training

7 Operations on the vulva

Vulval biopsy

Biopsy of the vulva is a simple procedure not requiring general anaesthesia, special preparation or complicated instruments. It must be performed with precision in order to provide the pathologist with an adequate and representative sample of the vulval abnormality. It is the most important determinant of malignancy and, no matter how expert and experienced the operator, a biopsy confirming vulval cancer is mandatory prior to radical surgery. The biopsy is also used to confirm numerous dermatological conditions such as lichen sclerosis, lichen planus and vulval intraepithelial neoplasia (VIN). The use of colposcopy with dilute acetic acid or the application of toluidine blue can be of value in identifying areas to biopsy. The clitoris and labia minora should be avoided unless essential as they are sensitive and important in sexual function.

The biopsy is most easily obtained by using a dermatologist's (Keyes) punch, which will give a full-thickness biopsy of the vulval skin, allowing adequate comment to be made by the pathologist on the nature of the lesion. Sharpness of the cutting edge is most important and the disposable Keyes punch is ideal. For diagnostic biopsies a 3–4 mm diameter Keyes punch is more than adequate, although larger ones can be used to excise lesions completely.

Analgesia is required and is best produced by infiltrating below and around the lesion using a 27 or 30 gauge needle with 1 or 2% lidocaine with added epinephrine for haemostasis to extend the period of analgesia.

The Keyes punch is pushed into the skin, rotating it once or twice on its axis to assist its penetration of the skin and subcutaneous tissue, the depth of excision being controlled by the operator. The plug of tissue is then grasped and separated at the base, using scissors or a disposable scalpel (Fig. 7.1). The hole remaining is small and will only occasionally require touching with a silver nitrate stick to stop any bleeding. The need for a suture is extremely rare with the 3 mm Keyes but may be required for larger diameters.

Excision or incision biopsy using a scalpel may be performed using the same technique of analgesia followed by the cutting of an elliptical strip of tissue, taking care to remove the full thickness of the dermis. Excision biopsy is appropriate for small or localized lesions such as naevi, and incision biopsy for larger areas when a specimen should be removed from the growing edge.

The defect can then be closed using a fine absorbable suture on a cutting needle. Vicryl Rapide is ideal because of its quick absorption, but it can be removed after a few days if it causes any discomfort or irritation.

Treatment of Bartholin's cysts and abscesses

The most common large cyst of the vulva is the Bartholin's cyst, which arises as a result of an obstruction of the duct. In premenopausal women, if it is asymptomatic and small, no treatment is required. If

Bonney's Gynaecological Surgery, 11th edition.
© Tito Lopes, Nick Spirtos, Raj Naik, John Monaghan.
Published 2011 by Blackwell Publishing Ltd.

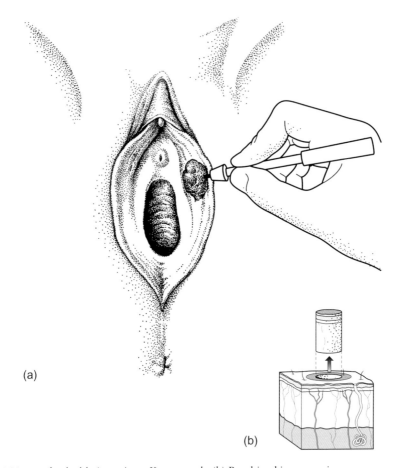

(a)

(b)

Figure 7.1 (a) Biopsy of vulval lesion using a Keyes punch. (b) Resulting biopsy specimen.

it is large, symptomatic or infected, it should be drained, and if there is any concern about malignancy it should be excised.

Incision and drainage

This is performed for the first episode of an acute abscess or for large or symptomatic cysts and will give immediate relief of symptoms. It can be performed under local anaesthetic.

A sterile field is prepared and the patient is preferably placed in a lithotomy position. Lidocaine is then injected into the skin at the same site using a dental syringe. Ideally, a local anaesthetic cream such as EMLA (eutectic mixture of lidocaine and prilocaine)

cream should be applied to the vestibular mucosa just distal to the hymeneal ring and left for about 30 minutes. A small 5 mm stab incision to a depth of 1–1.5 cm is made with a scalpel (no. 11 blade) where the cyst or abscess appears closest to the mucosal surface. A charcoal swab is used to break down any loculations and then sent for culture. A gauze wick or preferably a Word catheter is inserted into the cavity. This catheter is similar to a short paediatric catheter but without a lumen. The balloon of the catheter is inflated with 2–3 mL of normal saline and the free end is inserted into the vagina. The catheter is left in place for 4 weeks, if tolerated, to allow epithelialization of the tract, creating a new duct opening. The catheter is removed by deflating the balloon.

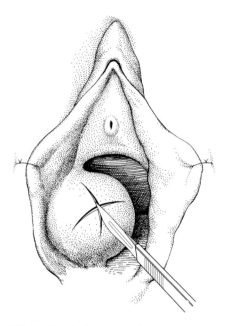

Figure 7.2 Cruciate incision over abscess.

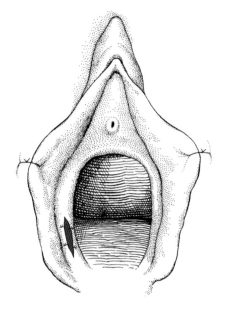

Figure 7.3 Wall of abscess sutured to skin.

Marsupialization

If the cyst or abscess recurs despite the use of a gauze wick or Word catheter then marsupialization should be performed. The procedure is very similar to that already described and can be performed under local or general anaesthetic. A 1–1.5 cm cruciate incision is carried through into the cyst, releasing its contents (Fig. 7.2). The four segments of skin and cyst wall formed by the incision are excised leaving a circular opening. The cyst wall is sutured using interrupted stitches to the skin edge allowing free drainage of its secretions to the exterior (Fig. 7.3). The new tract will slowly shrink over time and epithelialize, forming a new duct orifice.

Excision

A cyst that recurs despite repeated incision or marsupialization or one suspicious of malignancy should be excised. This should not be performed if there is active infection.

Preparation of the patient

As for vulvovaginal operations.

Instruments

Two Allis or Littlewood tissue forceps, toothed dissecting forceps, fine dissecting scissors.

The operation

• *Skin incision.* The incision should run along the long axis of the vestibular mucosa distal to the hymeneal ring over the cyst (Fig. 7.4). The skin will draw naturally apart, revealing the tense surface of the cyst.
• *Enucleation of the cyst.* The tissue plane around the cyst is now developed using a separating action of the scissors; occasional strands of fascia may need to be cut. If the gland has been involved in previous episodes of infection this dissection may not flow smoothly and more sharp dissection will be required (Fig. 7.5). Tiny blood vessels can be diathermied or cut and tied. The base of the cyst is a common place for bleeding because of the venous channels of the vestibular bulb and underlying glandular tissue. Dissection across this area may be best handled with a right-angled clamp and tying of the pedicles followed by complete removal of the duct and gland (Fig. 7.6).

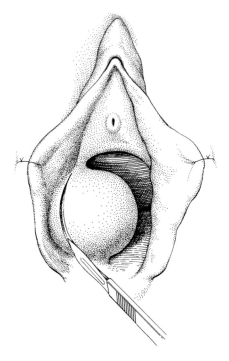

Figure 7.4 Incising over the Bartholin's cyst.

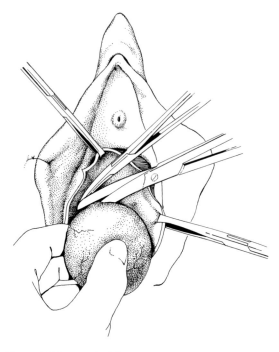

Figure 7.6 Removal of the cyst.

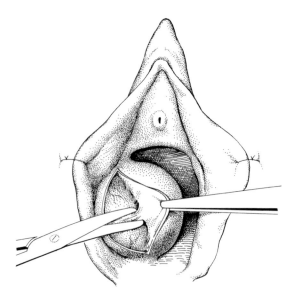

Figure 7.5 Enucleation of the cyst.

• *Obliteration of the cavity.* It is essential to completely close the cavity with fine absorbable sutures as venous oozing frequently occurs if a space is left, producing a haematoma which may be the nidus for infection and will significantly delay healing (Fig. 7.7).

• *Skin closure.* The cut edges of the wound are now apposed using interrupted sutures (Fig. 7.8). Continuous or subcuticular sutures are appealing but should be avoided so that any serous or sanguinous ooze can escape. A drain is not usually necessary but may be inserted and recorded if the procedure has been unusually bloody.

Simple vulvectomy

Indications

Simple removal of the vulval tissues is most commonly performed for the treatment of extensive VIN, or at the end of failed medical treatment for vulval dystro-

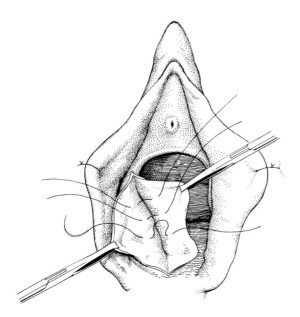

Figure 7.7 Obliteration of the cyst cavity.

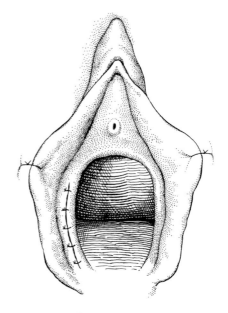

Figure 7.8 Closure of the skin.

phies. Other indications include massive hypertrophy of the clitoris or labia, intractable pruritus vulvae or Paget's disease. The removal may be total or partial depending on the extent of the disease; important sexual structures such as the clitoris may be preserved if not involved in the pathological process.

Patient preparation

No special preparation is necessary except to shave the vulva. It is useful to colposcope the vulva preoperatively in those patients in whom VIN is present to outline the full extent of the lesion or lesions, remembering that this problem is frequently multifocal. The vulva can be washed with toluidine blue or dilute (3% or 5%) acetic acid to identify the areas involved. The most important caveat being that, frequently, the acetic acid must be applied for a longer period of time before the characteristic changes appear.

Anaesthesia

A general anaesthetic is usually used although, for removal of small parts of the vulva, local infiltration techniques may be appropriate.

Instruments

The general gynaecological set is required (see Chapter 3).

The operation

The patient is placed in the lithotomy position and colposcopy performed where indicated to outline the lesion.

The incision for a total simple vulvectomy is shown in Fig. 7.9; it should be elliptical to include the clitoris, both labia and the fourchette. The inner limits are usually the vaginal mucocutaneous junction and a point a short distance above the urethral orifice. The exact limits will vary depending upon the extent of the lesion or lesions to be removed.

If the anterior part of the skin to be removed is grasped with Littlewood forceps and drawn down, the incisions can be deepened to the deep fascia. The entire vulva is then removed by peeling and cutting simultaneously in a posterior direction (Fig. 7.10).

Three major bleeding areas will be found: the first when the clitoral vessels are cut, and the second and third when the terminal branches of the internal pudendal arteries are cut on either side of the

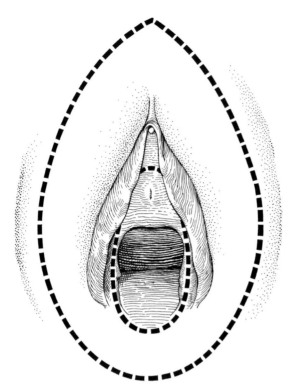

Figure 7.9 The incision for simple vulvectomy.

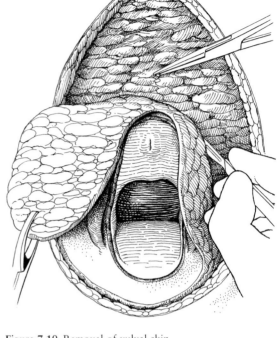

Figure 7.10 Removal of vulval skin.

fourchette. These vessels may be clipped and dealt with by inserting a crossed or square mattress suture which will pick up all the small vessels, especially around the base of the clitoris. Surprisingly few other vessels require individual treatment.

Resuturing requires a good eye in order to produce a symmetrical closure. The anterior part of the incision should be brought together using an interrupted vertical mattress suture in order to remove dead space below the skin. This area should be sutured down to a point a short distance above the urethral orifice so as not to hood the opening. Thereafter, the remainder of the vulva can be covered by apposing the two cut edges, taking care to sew evenly so that 'dog ears' are not produced (Fig. 7.11). Rarely, difficulty may be found in bringing the edges together; this can be obviated either by using short releasing incisions posteriorly alongside the anus, as in the radical vulvectomy operation, or by dissecting the vaginal mucosa off the rectovaginal fascia to create a vaginal advancement flap (see Fig. 8.2).

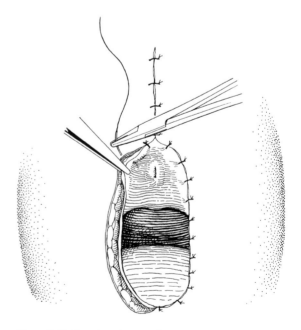

Figure 7.11 Suturing the cut edges.

At the end of the procedure, it is usual to insert a catheter into the bladder and maintain it for the first 3 days; this helps to keep the vulva dry in the immediate postoperative period.

Postoperative management

The patient must be rapidly mobilized and encouraged to bathe and use the bidet frequently. It is important to dry off the vulva after bathing and not to use creams or talc.

Usually, the wounds heal well and sutures can be removed after 7 days. Occasionally, haematomas may develop and should be treated conservatively unless they are large and painful, when drainage and tying of the vessels involved is necessary. Infection should be carefully watched for and guarded against by meticulous nursing and frequent vulval swabbing with a simple antiseptic substance.

For the patient who has suffered chronic pruritus vulvae the nights after operation come as a blessed relief.

Flaps and grafts

When the extent of disease is so wide that primary reapproximation of the vulva is not possible, rotational skin flap procedures or a skin graft can be applied. For skin grafts a wound vacuum device can be applied for 4–5 days following the excision, allowing for the development of an adequate base of granulation tissue, at which point a split-thickness skin graft is applied. The graft is harvested from the buttocks or anterior/lateral thigh using a CO_2-driven dermatome. A graft thickness of 0.3–0.4 mm is harvested and then stapled or sutured to the host site. The donor site is treated with thrombin spray and covered with a large Opsite or Tegaderm dressing. These dressings can be left *in situ* either until they fill with fluid, requiring replacement, or until they simply peel off over time.

Variations

These are legion, from partial procedures through hemivulvectomy to skinning vulvectomy whereby only the epithelium is removed. This last procedure has been performed using the CO_2 laser. The use of argon beam coagulation has also been reported in the treatment of multifocal VIN III.

Further reading

Wechter ME, Wu JM, Marzano D, Haefner H. Management of Bartholin duct cysts and abscesses: a systematic review. *Obstet Gynecol Surv* 2009;64:395–404.

8 Operations on the vagina

Vaginal cysts

Most cysts found in the vagina are embryological remnants, usually Wolffian. They are most commonly situated either in the anterior part of the lower vagina or in the lateral part of the upper vagina. They vary in size and are usually noticed because they interfere with intercourse or the insertion of tampons or surgical instruments. They rarely produce symptoms and even more rarely become infected. Cysts throughout the length of the posterior part of the vagina are commonly inclusion dermoids developing after childbirth, trauma or vaginal surgery.

It is important to determine the size and position of the cyst prior to surgery as some may extend for a considerable distance towards the pelvic sidewall, and what begins as a minor procedure may well turn into a major one. If the cyst is found to have a long communicating tract it is better to allow the cyst to drain into the vagina and then to identify the tract using radiology, including MRI, or by inserting dye at the beginning of a procedure where facilities for opening the abdomen are available.

Instruments
The gynaecological minor set of instruments described in Chapter 3 is adequate with the addition of a small number of malleable probes.

Bonney's Gynaecological Surgery, 11th edition.
© Tito Lopes, Nick Spirtos, Raj Naik, John Monaghan.
Published 2011 by Blackwell Publishing Ltd.

Patient preparation
If the full extent of the cyst is known to be small, no special preparation is required. If there is any likelihood of the abdomen being opened, the patient should be fully prepared and an appropriate consent form signed.

Anaesthesia
If the cyst is small and accessible the procedure may be performed under local analgesia; however, for the majority of cysts, it is much easier for the operator and kinder to the patient to use a general anaesthetic.

The operation
• *Position.* The patient is placed in the lithotomy position and the vulva prepared and draped.

If the cyst is on the anterior vaginal wall, a Sims speculum is inserted; for cysts in other positions, the area is exposed by the assistant holding a lateral vaginal retractor.
• *Skin incision.* The tissue overlying the cyst is grasped with Allis tissue forceps at the upper and lower ends of the cyst and an ellipse of skin is removed without cutting into the cyst. The cyst may then be enucleated by dissecting the surrounding tissues away using fine dissecting forceps. If the cyst cannot be enucleated it should be opened and the lining peeled away, leaving a clean cavity. Small vessels may bleed and require individual attention.
• *Precautions.* Great care should be taken during the dissection, which should be predominantly 'separate and cut' rather than 'sharp'.
• *Closure.* If possible, the cavity should be obliterated, closing the skin with interrupted stitches. If the

cavity is large or there has been much haemorrhage or previous infection, it is wise to simply suture around the edge of the cavity and allow it to granulate.

Postoperative care
No special care is required except for those patients in whom the cyst has been infected, when a course of antibiotics is prescribed, or when the cyst has been left to drain, in which case the patient should be warned that there may be continued vaginal loss.

Procedures for enlargement of the vaginal introitus

Having eliminated congenital causes for apareunia or dyspareunia, the gynaecologist must consider surgical means to facilitate the act of intercourse. This should include advice on the use of graduated dilatators. Some patients, however, find these techniques too painful or distasteful and the surgeon must consider operative methods. Common indications for the following procedures include scarring resulting from a previous episiotomy repair/surgery procedure or as a result of long-standing lichen sclerosus.

Fenton's operation

Instruments
Similar instruments to those used for the excision of a Bartholin's cyst will be required.

The operation
• *Skin incision.* A pair of Littlewood or straight Spencer Wells forceps are used to grasp the skin at the junction with the vagina. The skin may be incised or a narrow strip removed with the scissors (Fig. 8.1).
• *Development of the flap.* By slightly undercutting the skin on the vaginal aspect of the incision, a short flap can be developed. Care must be taken not to make this flap too long or to 'buttonhole' the skin (Fig. 8.2).
• *Perineal incision.* A vertical incision is now made towards the anus. All structures must be divided except for the external sphincter (Fig. 8.3).
• *Division of the hymen.* If the hymen is thick posteriorly then it must be divided by making two small cuts approximately 1 cm apart. Traction on the two forceps laterally flattens out the flap.

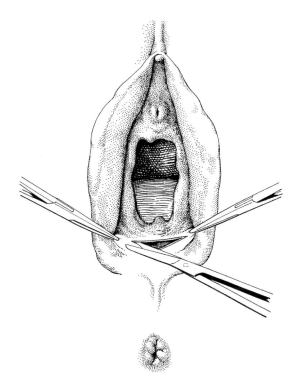

Figure 8.1 Incising the introital skin.

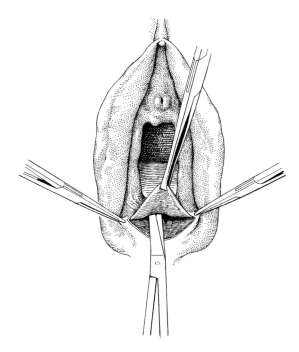

Figure 8.2 Developing a flap of vaginal skin.

67

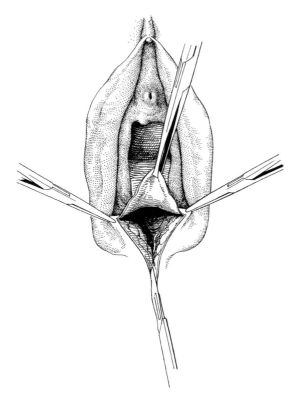

Figure 8.3 Making the posterior vertical incision.

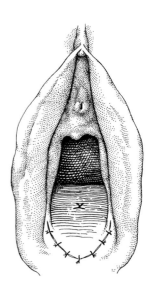

Figure 8.4 Obliterating the space under the flap.

• *Fixation of the flap and reconstitution of the introitus.* By passing a Vicryl suture into the base of the flap close to the midline and anchoring it to the fibromuscular tissue of the perineal incision, two purposes are served. The first is to anchor the flap and keep it in place if the skin sutures are too rapidly absorbed and the second is to obliterate the space under the flap and reduce the risk of haematoma formation (Fig. 8.4). The skin of the divided perineum is now sutured to the flap (Fig. 8.5) using interrupted stitches so that any ooze beneath the flap can escape. An absorbable Vicryl suture is used for these stitches. Absorption may be incomplete and the patient should be seen 7 days postoperatively for removal of any retained sutures.

Variation in technique

A simplification of the operation is to divide the perineum and lower vagina vertically and then to resuture transversely. On the rare occasion when there is

Figure 8.5 Suturing the skin edges together.

severe dyspareunia interfering with coitus due to pain and fissuring of the skin at the posterior fourchette/ perineum, the skin around this area can be excised as the releasing incision described above is performed. The posterior introitus and perineum is then refashioned, resulting in enlargement of the vaginal entrance and removal of the affected skin. If good attention has been given to patient selection, the results can be extremely rewarding to the patient who has often previously suffered many years of abstinence and ineffective treatments.

Dressing and postoperative care
Infections are common following surgery to the vagina or vulva. The patient should be advised of the benefits of regular cleansing using a detachable showerhead and allowing the area to dry with gentle dabbing with a towel. It is not the editors' practice to use prophylactic antibiotics as a routine, although these are often required should infection develop. The patient should be encouraged to begin to engage in intercourse as soon as the wounds have healed.

Congenital absence and partial development of the vagina

Congenital absence of the uterus or vagina is due to a failure of fusion and canalization of the caudad mullerian ducts. The ovaries, tubes and uterine ligaments are formed but the uterus is present as rudimentary horns and the vagina is absent. Lesser degrees of vaginal atresia also occur, varying from failure of canalization of the lower part to a complete failure of development, but with a normal uterus or uterus didelphys present. In these latter cases, cryptomenorrhoea will occur.

Uterovaginal atresia occurs in 1 in 5000 women. The most common presentation is that of a young girl (15 years of age) being brought to see the gynaecologist by her mother because she has failed to begin to menstruate. The girl has normally developed secondary sexual characteristics, including breast, pubic hair and vulval growth. As these girls are usually very nervous, examination in the outpatient department should be limited to the external structures. The mother should be fully informed of the need for a full vaginal and rectal examination of the child under

general anaesthetic. An MRI provides good assessment of the pelvic structures and an intravenous urogram (IVU) may be of value as there is an associated urinary anomaly in up to 30% of girls who have maldevelopment of the vagina and uterus.

Under anaesthesia the external genitalia are inspected, the vaginal dimple explored and, most valuable of all, a rectal examination is carried out. A laparoscopy can also be performed if previous radiology has been indeterminate.

Transverse septum of the vagina (imperforate hymen)

Patients with this problem will present with amenorrhoea but having had many of the signs of menstrual activity, including premenstrual symptoms and intramenstrual discomfort. It is not uncommon to find evidence of endometriosis present on laparoscopy, due possibly to retrograde menstruation. Rarely, the patient will present as an emergency due to obstructive symptoms of the urinary or bowel tract produced by the dilated vagina.

The septum usually lies just above the hymen with the hymenal remnants stretched over it. Occasionally, the septum lies higher in the vagina and is thicker.

The low septum frequently bulges outwards and is discoloured by the dark blood shining through; rectal examination confirms distension of the vagina and uterus.

Instruments
The gynaecological minor set is required.

Patient preparation
No special preparation is needed, although it is important to put the patient on broad-spectrum prophylactic antibiotics during and after the procedure.

Anaesthesia
A light general anaesthetic is required.

The operation
The procedure is simplicity itself: the bulging membrane is incised vertically and the retained blood allowed to drain. Once drainage has eased, another incision at right angles is made to form a cross; the edges of the skin flaps are now removed, and any bleeding dealt with by clipping and ligation.

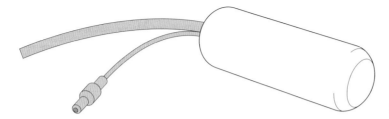

Figure 8.6 Vaginal stent.

Postoperatively, vulval hygiene is important but vaginal douches must be avoided.

Longitudinal vaginal septum

Patients who are free of dyspareunia may still benefit from excision of a longitudinal vaginal septum, which can cause obstruction at the time of delivery. After emptying the bladder, the septum is held with a clamp, and gentle traction is applied. Attention is required to avoid excess traction as this can draw the urethra, bladder or rectum into the area of excision. The septum is then incised at its inferior and superior attachments from the posterior and anterior vaginal walls, respectively, and the defects repaired using interrupted or continuous absorbable sutures.

Vaginal atresia

A superficial examination of the patient may suggest that the vagina is present but imperforate. The hymen can be seen at the upper part of a small vaginal dimple. However, on rectal examination and laparoscopy it is clear that the vagina is not developed and the uterus is present as widely displaced streaks of tissue leading to the ovaries. A diagnostic feature is the ability to trace the uterosacral ligaments uninterruptedly across the front of the rectum. Although the diagnosis is usually made when the girl is in her teens, treatment may be delayed until she wishes to embark on intercourse. The chances of producing a useful communication with the uterus are small and the prospects for procreation infinitesimal. However, a functioning vagina can be made using one of two techniques – Williams's and McIndoe's.

Owing to the rarity of the condition, most gynaecologists will have little if any experience of these procedures. They are best managed in specialist paediatric surgical centres and their descriptions have been retained in this chapter for the sake of the interested gynaecologist.

Instruments

The instruments in the gynaecological major set will be required, together with the plastic surgery instruments for cutting the graft (for McIndoe's procedure) and a vaginal stent such as the Heyer Schulte vaginal stent (Fig. 8.6).

Patient preparation

The patient is prepared as for any major vaginal procedure; shaving is essential to cut down the risk of infection, and the lower large bowel should be completely empty.

Anaesthesia

A general anaesthetic is required.

Williams's operation

Although this operation is of great value to the patient who has vaginal atresia, it is also of enormous benefit to the patient who has shortening or stenosis of the vagina following surgery or radiotherapy. It is a simple procedure producing a pouch of skin lying along the vulva rather than in the axis of the vagina. The postoperative period is short (10 days), and good results are obtained. Arthur Williams first described the operation in 1964 and again in 1976.

The patient is draped and catheterized (Fig. 8.7); the incision in the labia is made (Fig. 8.8), and deepened. The inner edges of the incision are now sutured together with interrupted Vicryl sutures (Fig. 8.9). An obturator is then placed in the pouch to check the size of the vaginoplasty; if it is satisfactory, the levators are sutured together using two interrupted stitches (Fig. 8.10). The operation is now completed by closing the skin with a series of interrupted stitches (Fig. 8.11).

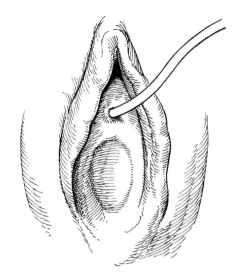

Figure 8.7 The vulva showing the vaginal dimple.

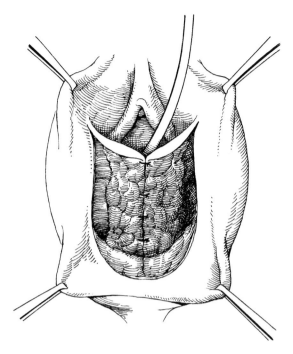

Figure 8.9 Suturing the inner edges of the labial incision.

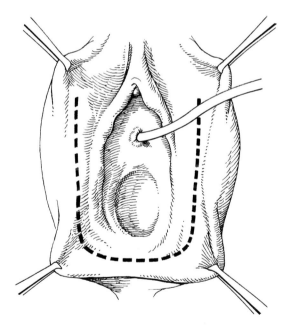

Figure 8.8 Incising the labia.

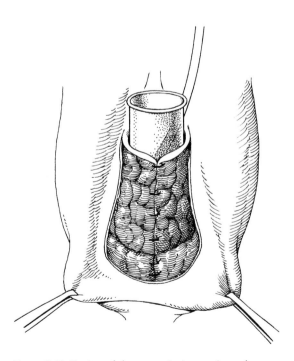

Figure 8.10 Testing of the neovagina's capacity and suturing levators.

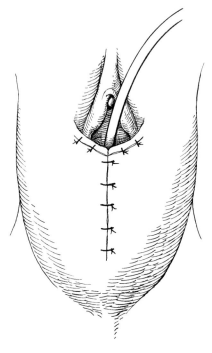

Figure 8.11 Closing the outer layer of skin.

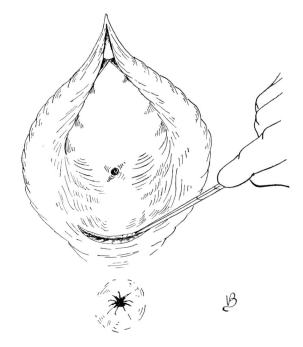

Figure 8.12 McIndoe's operation: incising the posterior part of the vaginal dimple.

McIndoe's operation

The first generally successful procedure to be described for the formation of an artificial vagina was that of McIndoe. The operation involves the formation of a space between the bladder and rectum which is filled with a mould, over which has been placed a skin graft from the patient's thigh.

The operation is usually performed in conjunction with a plastic surgeon, who prepares the graft and places it over the mould.

- *Developing the space for the neovagina.* The patient is placed in the lithotomy position. The skin is incised transversely at the posterior part of the vaginal dimple (Fig. 8.12). This incision is then deepened so that the soft areolar fascia between the rectum and bladder is identified. This level is often easier to find if a finger or blunt obturator, such as a large dilator, is inserted into the rectum. The plane dissects remarkably easily and the peritoneum is rapidly reached.

Using two index fingers, the cavity is developed (Fig. 8.13) so that the chosen mould can fit easily

within it. It is important to do this before cutting the graft. Meticulous haemostasis is necessary, although if the correct plane is found there is surprisingly little bleeding.

It should be noted that this surgery can be facilitated by using laparoscopy to help identify and develop the proper space between the rectum and the bladder

- *Cutting the graft.* A full-thickness skin graft rather than a split-thickness graft is taken from the inner thigh as this can be closed easily. The graft is now draped over a Heyer Schulte vaginal stent, which is inflatable and has a central drain in such a way that there is very little overlap; excessive skin should be trimmed away.
- *Inserting the stent.* The stent, covered by the graft, is now inserted into the cavity, where it should lie snugly but without any pressure contact points (Fig. 8.14).
- *Retention of the stent.* The stent must now be sutured in place. This is best done by mobilizing the labia via an incision made as shown in Fig. 8.15. The

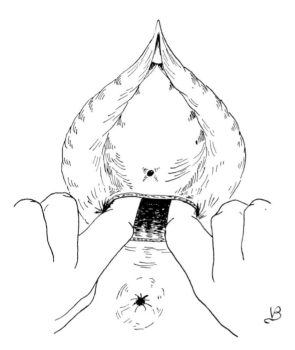

Figure 8.13 Stretching the cavity anterior to the rectum.

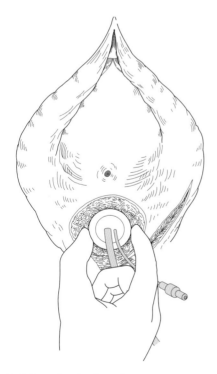

Figure 8.14 Inserting the draped stent.

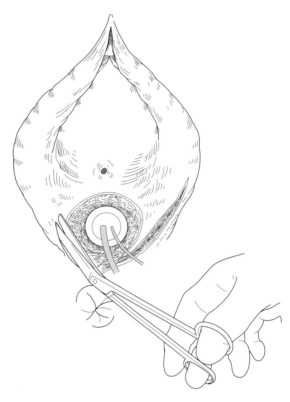

Figure 8.15 Incising the labia.

similarities between this incision and that of the Williams's procedure are obvious. The inner edges of this incision are now sutured together so as to form a shelf to retain the stent (Fig. 8.16). This is then reinforced by suturing the outer line of the incision (Fig. 8.17).

The stent is maintained in the new vagina for approximately 3 months; some patients demand that it be removed earlier but this should be resisted. It is important to keep the neovagina open and elastic; if the patient is not regularly practising intercourse she must dilate the vagina frequently using plastic or glass dilators. Any areas of granulation tissue can be touched with silver nitrate to promote rapid epithelialization.

Vaginectomy: partial and complete

Vaginectomy, or colpectomy, is an operation which is rarely performed but which has very clear indications and very significant benefits. The procedure is most

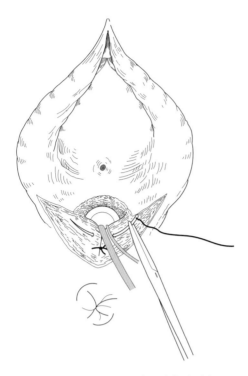

Figure 8.16 Suturing the inner edge of the incision.

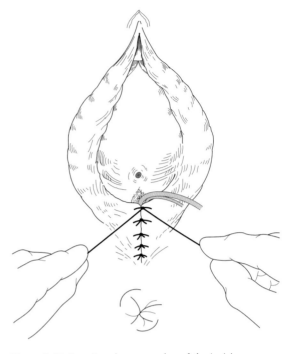

Figure 8.17 Suturing the outer edge of the incision.

commonly indicated when there is residual vaginal intraepithelial neoplasia (VAIN) in the upper vagina after hysterectomy. Unfortunately, a considerable number of women will continue to have hysterectomies performed for cervical premalignancy without the benefit of preoperative colposcopy to localize and delineate the disease. As a consequence, in a small number of women, there will be incomplete removal of the lesion, resulting in persistently abnormal smears in the postoperative period. If hysterectomy is indicated for cervical intraepithelial neoplasia (CIN), then ideally this should be performed vaginally in conjunction with colposcopy to reduce the likelihood of the CIN and associated VAIN being incompletely excised. If the lesion or lesions can be seen and fully outlined then an excisional procedure performed vaginally is the best management method (see below). If the lesion cannot be fully visualized or it extends into the 'dog ears' at the angles of the vaginal vault then a more extensive surgical procedure via an abdominal approach is the only realistic choice. Some authorities have recommended radiotherapy, but the editors feel that this is not indicated as there is the potential for

significant vaginal morbidity after treatment, often without clearance of the vault lesion, whereas with partial colpectomy there is a good prospect of a reasonable return to normal function.

Colpectomy is not an adequate procedure for invasive carcinoma of the vagina but is of great value in treating microinvasive lesions. In those patients with an upper vaginal lesion and who have a uterus, a hysterocolpectomy is performed – a much simpler procedure than colpectomy after hysterectomy.

The vaginal procedure

Instruments
The instruments in the general gynaecology set will be required.

The operation
• *Identification of the lesion.* The patient is placed in the lithotomy position, cleansed, draped and the bladder emptied. A bimanual and rectal examination is performed to exclude the possibility of a discrete invasive lesion lying above the suture line at the

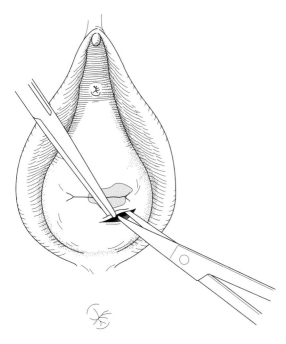

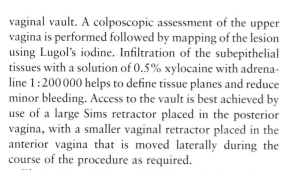

Figure 8.18 Releasing the vaginal edges.

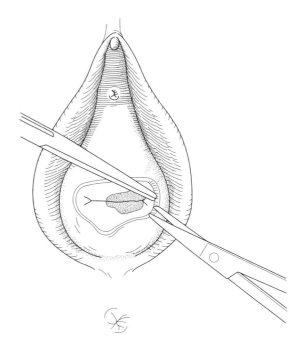

Figure 8.19 Excising the vaginal skin at the vault.

vaginal vault. A colposcopic assessment of the upper vagina is performed followed by mapping of the lesion using Lugol's iodine. Infiltration of the subepithelial tissues with a solution of 0.5% xylocaine with adrenaline 1 : 200 000 helps to define tissue planes and reduce minor bleeding. Access to the vault is best achieved by use of a large Sims retractor placed in the posterior vagina, with a smaller vaginal retractor placed in the anterior vagina that is moved laterally during the course of the procedure as required.

• *The incision.* A 2 cm epithelial incision is made just inferior to the posterior margins of the lesion. A toothed dissector is used to apply traction to the skin flap anteriorly, while the blunted scissors are used to develop the subepithelial plane further towards the vaginal vault and laterally (Fig. 8.18). The skin edges are incised further around the circumference of the mapped lesion as the development of the tissue planes continues. Attention is required not to 'buttonhole' the specimen, as this will increase the possibility of leaving diseased tissue remnants behind. Eventually, the incision is completed around the entire lesion, with the only attachment remaining being a thin strip at the vaginal vault with underlying scar tissue. Applying

firm traction to the vaginal skin, the attachments at the vaginal vault are now boldly cut from right to left including the 'dog ears' within the specimen, eventually releasing the entire specimen and without damage to the underlying structures (Fig. 8.19). In leaving the scarred tissue at the vaginal vault and 'dog ears' until last, the risk of injury to the underlying rectum, bladder and ureters is kept to an absolute minimum, while increasing the likelihood of achieving complete excision of the entire lesion with a single specimen.

• *Dealing with the denuded vault.* If the peritoneal cavity has been entered at the vaginal vault during the procedure then this can be either left open or closed using a continuous stitch. Individual vessels can be dealt with using a combination of sutures or diathermy. Once haemostasis is achieved, the denuded tissue at the vaginal vault is left unsutured to regranulate, and a bacteriostatic-soaked vaginal pack and indwelling transurethral urinary catheter inserted for 24 hours.

Postoperative care
No special attention is required, and the patient can be discharged home the following day.

The abdominal procedure

Instruments

The instruments outlined in the general tray will be required.

Preoperative preparation

This should be as for a radical hysterectomy, with the additional procedure of marking the inferior aspect of the lesion with a marker stitch, which will be useful later during the operation to confirm adequate excision. A firm vaginal pack is essential to facilitate dissection of the vagina from the bladder and the rectum, and an indwelling catheter with a small balloon should be inserted into the bladder.

Anaesthesia

It is a great advantage if this procedure can be carried out under epidural or spinal analgesia as a considerable reduction in small vessel oozing can be achieved.

The operation

Frequently, adhesions from previous surgery have to be cleared before it is possible to fully visualize the pelvic structures. As in the radical hysterectomy procedure, a self-retaining retractor should be used but without the lower blade, which should be replaced by a Morris retractor held by the second assistant. This allows the peritoneum and the bladder to be manipulated in order to give better vision and access. As a result of the previous surgical intervention, there can be considerable scarring, particularly at the angles of the vaginal vault overlying the ureters.

• *The incision.* The abdomen is opened via a longitudinal midline incision; low transverse incisions give more limited access and should not be used.

• *Identifying the ureters.* After clearing obstructions and adhesions from previous surgery, the ureters should be identified as they pass along the pelvic sidewall behind the peritoneum. The peritoneum at the brim of the pelvis is opened along a line between the remnant of the round ligament and the infundibulo-pelvic ligament. Using the fingers, the retroperitoneal space is opened and the ureter identified and separated from the overlying peritoneum (Fig. 8.20).

• *Dealing with the scar tissue at the angles of the vault.* The uterine artery should be identified as far

laterally as possible and then divided and drawn medially (Fig. 8.21). This will have the effect of identifying the entrance to the ureteric tunnel at its lateral end. This area is often surrounded by dense scarring from the previous surgery; however, if the ureteric tunnel can be accurately defined, the scar overlying it can be cut with confidence and without trauma to the ureter.

• *Identifying the medial end of the ureteric tunnel.* Now, the uppermost point of the vagina must be palpated and a transverse incision made in the peritoneum so that the bladder can be separated from the anterior surface of the vagina. It may be necessary to use sharp dissection in order to identify the correct plane. Once this has been identified, the bladder should be pushed down in the midline; this will have the effect of making the scar tissue and the fascia overlying the ureteric tunnel laterally more prominent.

• *Incising the roof of the ureteric tunnel.* Frequently, the ureter can be identified as it passes into the bladder. If this is possible, Bonney scissors should be gently introduced over the upper surface of the ureter and, using a separating movement without cutting, the scissors are gently insinuated laterally to appear at the lateral end of the ureteric tunnel. This dissection may be performed from medial to lateral or in the reverse direction. It is important not to kink or to nip the ureter in the edges of the scissors; the simple manoeuvre of lifting the scissors while in the tunnel will allow a good view of the entire length of the ureter. A medium, straight, tissue forceps is then placed over the scissors and the ureteric tunnel and the scar tissue incised (Fig. 8.22). The pedicle is then tied, as it carries some veins and small arteries to and from the bladder. At this point, there may still be a few strands of fascia passing across the ureter; these should be divided and the tissue plane between the ureter and the vagina identified. The cardinal ligament is now visible below and medial to the ureter. Sharp dissection may still be required if there has been extensive scarring from the previous surgery. The upper vagina is revealed very quickly and the ureters dislocated laterally. The firm pack in the vagina greatly facilitates this dissection.

• *Releasing the vagina posteriorly.* An incision is made in the peritoneum at the upper posterior part of the vagina (Fig. 8.23). This incision is then extended laterally over the remnants of the uterosacral ligaments. The rectum is now easily pushed away from

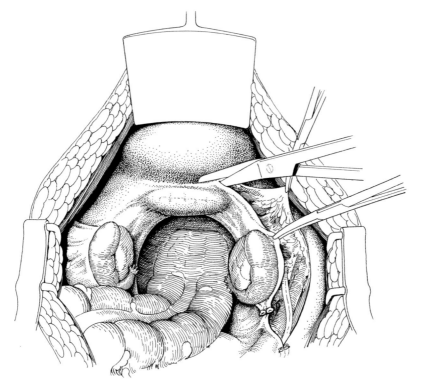

Figure 8.20 Identifying the ureter in the right retroperitoneal space.

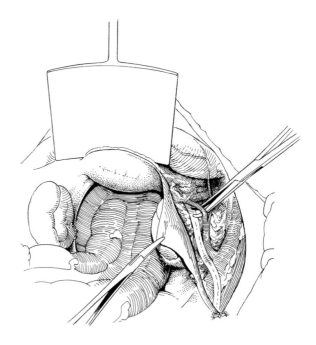

Figure 8.21 Dividing the uterine artery at the pelvic sidewall.

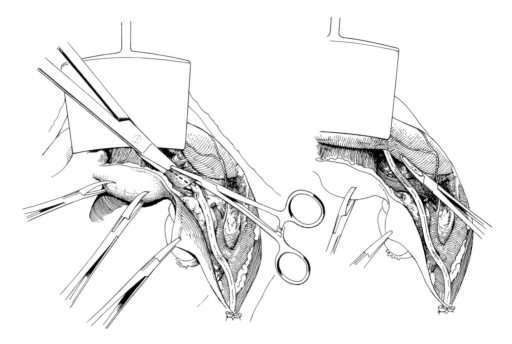

Figure 8.22 Dividing the roof of the ureteric tunnel.

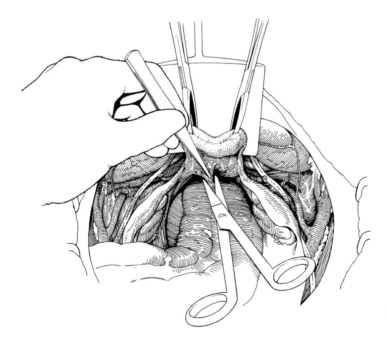

Figure 8.23 Incising the peritoneum between the uterosacral ligaments.

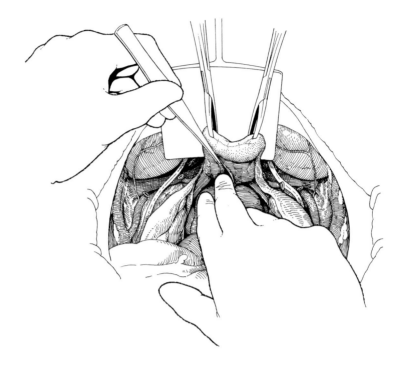

Figure 8.24 Developing the rectovaginal space.

the posterior surface of the vagina by passing the fingers down into the rectovaginal space (Fig. 8.24).
• *Removing the vagina.* At this point, having released the ureters laterally, the bladder anteriorly and the rectum posteriorly, the surgeon can decide just how much vagina to remove. The uterosacral and then the paracolpos is grasped and clamped in hysterectomy clamps and the chosen length of vagina removed (Fig. 8.25). If the requirement is to remove the upper part of the vagina to excise VAIN, no further dissection is necessary and the vagina can be opened at this point to confirm placement of the original marker stitch and adequate excision of tissue. If a total vaginectomy is necessary, the abdominal dissection should be extended down the vagina to the pelvic floor. Thereafter, the patient is put in the lithotomy position and the lower vagina dissected free from the urethra and bladder anteriorly and the rectum posteriorly. Great care should be exercised when dissecting below the urethra as the fascia is very dense and the dissection must be very accurate. Having joined up with the abdominal dissection, the entire vagina can be removed. A little bleeding is seen around the pelvic floor but is not of great trouble.

• *Draining the vagina.* The space left behind after vaginectomy will vary in size depending on the extent of the procedure. Following partial vaginectomy there is no need for special drainage procedures except to leave the vaginal remnant open. However, after total vaginectomy either a vaginal passive drain or a suction drain should be put in place. This may be augmented by a pelvic suction drain brought out abdominally if it has been necessary to perform an extensive dissection in the pelvis.

Complications
The main postoperative problems following this procedure will be similar to those following radical hysterectomy, particularly bladder dysfunction and difficulties in initiating micturition (see Chapter 21).

Postoperative care
Patients should be managed in the same manner as those undergoing radical hysterectomy, with particular emphasis being placed on bladder care and on the long-term continued surveillance of any remnants of vaginal tissue remaining.

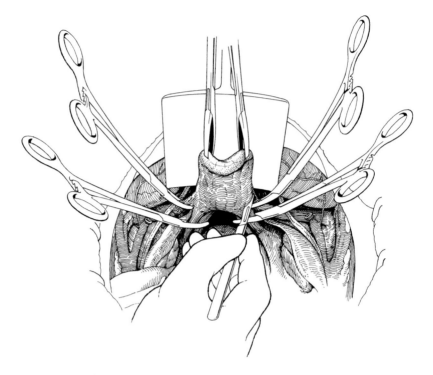

Figure 8.25 Removing the vaginal remnant.

Further reading

Edmonds DK. Congenital malformations of the genital tract and their management. *Best Pract Res Clin Obstet Gynaecol* 2003;17:19–40.

McIndoe AH, Banister JB. An operation for the cure of congenital absence of the vagina. *J Obstet Gynaecol Br Commonw* 1938;45:490–494.

Williams EA. Congenital absence of the vagina: a simple operation for its relief. *J Obstet Gynaecol Br Commonw* 1964;71:511–514.

9 Operations on the cervix

The cervix is the organ most subjected to surgical intervention and potential abuse in gynaecology. Dilatation of the cervix, as the preliminary step in numerous operations, is the most frequent surgical procedure in gynaecology. In countries with cervical screening programmes, colposcopy with its associated cervical biopsies and loop excisional procedures have developed into industrial proportions.

With the increasing trend among some gynaecologists to perform subtotal hysterectomies there is a proportional rise in the need to remove the cervical 'stump', an uncommon procedure, because of symptomatic reasons, the presence of cervical intraepithelial neoplasia (CIN) and even cervical cancer.

Dilatation of the cervix

This is the most frequently performed surgical procedure in gynaecology and, as such, should be carefully learned and practised, with close attention being paid to the potential pitfalls and complications. Although usually a fairly minor procedure, because of the sheer numbers performed and the risk for complications if executed badly, it is appropriate to describe the technique and potential complications in detail as they are rarely covered in other tomes.

Bonney's Gynaecological Surgery, 11th edition.
© Tito Lopes, Nick Spirtos, Raj Naik, John Monaghan.
Published 2011 by Blackwell Publishing Ltd.

Indications

Dilatation of the cervix is an important preliminary to many gynaecological procedures, including curettage, hysteroscopic procedures, surgical termination of pregnancy, evacuation of retained products of conception, endometrial ablation and intracavitary radiotherapeutic procedures. There are now very few circumstances when dilatation is used alone except for postsurgical or atrophic stenosis of the cervix and for the relief of postradiotherapy pyometra.

Instruments

A prepacked hysteroscopy, dilatation and curettage set should be available in gynaecological theatres (gynaecological minor set; see Chapter 3). It should include a Sims vaginal speculum, a uterine sound, a toothed vulsellum and a single-toothed tenaculum, graduated uterine dilators, a polyp and a sponge forceps, and uterine curettes.

Preparation of the patient

There is no necessity to shave the patient preoperatively. She should be asked to empty the bladder immediately before going to theatre, as a full bladder may distort the pelvic anatomy and make examination more difficult and inaccurate. If there is doubt about the emptiness of the bladder it should be catheterized prior to the procedure.

A general anaesthetic remains the norm even though dilatation is part of a minor procedure; increasingly, intracervical and paracervical blocks are being used successfully for outpatient hysteroscopies.

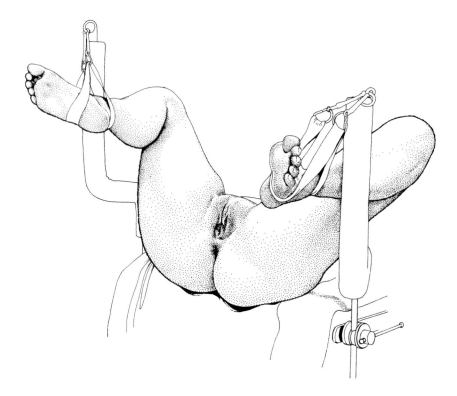

Figure 9.1 Lithotomy position.

The operation

Initial examination and assessment of the pelvis
The patient is placed in the lithotomy position with the buttocks projecting slightly over the end of the operating table (Fig. 9.1). The vulva and vagina are prepared, and the perineum draped. A bimanual examination is now performed. This is the most important part of the procedure as it allows the surgeon to fully examine the pelvis with the patient totally relaxed. Often, features which were not elicited in the consultation room are found and slightly worrying findings put into perspective. As with examination of the whole abdomen at laparotomy, the trainee surgeon should develop a habit of careful preoperative pelvic examination prior to even the most minor of procedures. The vulva is also inspected, the labia are gently drawn apart and the introitus viewed; the editors have seen early carcinomas of the vulva missed because the surgeon did not carry out this simple process meticulously. Two fingers of the right hand are now inserted into the vagina, and, with the left hand on the lower abdomen, the entire pelvic contents can be assessed.

Sounding of the uterus
The vaginal speculum is now inserted into the vagina, allowing access to the cervix. From the pelvic examination, the surgeon will have determined the size of the vagina and an appropriately sized speculum should be chosen. The anterior lip of the cervix is grasped with the vulsellum (Fig. 9.2) and, holding this in the left hand, the cervix is drawn down towards the introitus. This has the effect of straightening the endocervical canal and easing the passage of the instruments. It also allows the surgeon to assess the amount of uterine descent and, therefore, the potential for a future vaginal hysterectomy if required.

With a pregnant or recently pregnant uterus, a single vulsellum may easily cut out from the tissue of the cervix and multiple instruments may be required

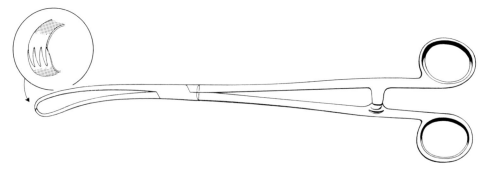

Figure 9.2 Cervical vulsellum.

to distribute the traction. The position of the uterus has already been noted at pelvic examination and is confirmed by the gentle passage of a uterine sound (Fig. 9.3). This allows measurement of the uterocervical length, which should be recorded.

Cervical dilatation

Dilatation of the cervix is now carried out using the graduated dilators in order, beginning with a size close to that of the sound, unless there is evidence of a patulous or partially dilated cervix. Remember that the larger dilators are potentially less likely to perforate the uterus than the smaller. The surgeon should be able to feel the dilator gently touch the fundus of the uterus as each one is inserted. The amount of pressure on the dilator calls for considerable judgement, which can be built up only by extensive practice. The pressure can be more easily controlled if the surgeon rests the heel of the left hand and lower forearm against the patient's right thigh and the heel of the right hand against the patient's left buttock (Fig. 9.4). The right and left hand are thus providing traction and countertraction, both of which are totally controlled. The dilator should be held in the right hand with the thumb posteriorly counterbalanced by the first three fingers along the length of the instrument. If this technique is adopted, considerable 'feel' can be achieved and any significant obstruction will cause the dilators to slide between the thumb and the fingers.

Another technique is to hold the dilator with the index finger extended so that the tip of the finger is in contact with the dilator at the point approximately equivalent to the uterocervical length, as measured by

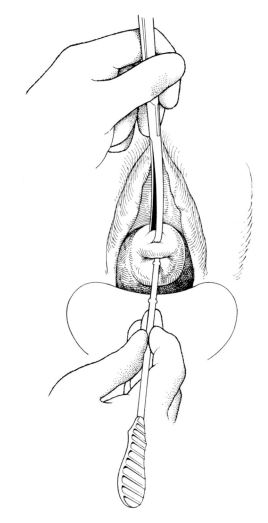

Figure 9.3 Passage of uterine sound.

83

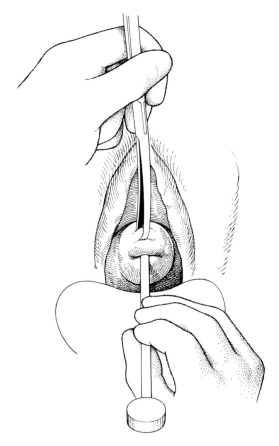

Figure 9.4 Dilatation of the cervix.

the sound. Using this technique, the finger prevents the dilator from perforating the uterus.

With either technique the surgeon should be building up in his or her mind a three-dimensional picture of the inside of the uterus, noting and mentally recording any obstructions or irregularities.

Extent of dilatation
The degree of dilatation will depend on the procedure to be performed. For most simple curettage procedures, the cervix will not require to be dilated to more than 7 mm, whereas for suction termination of pregnancy the optimum is 8–10 mm. Natural resistance of the cervix should be determined during dilatation to prevent fracture of the cervical integrity.

In nulliparous patients, the surgeon should consider inserting the smallest possible instruments through the cervical os to reduce the risk of trauma and long-term incompetence of the cervix.

For all patients, excessive force or roughness must be avoided.

Difficulties in performing the dilatation

Cervical stenosis
If the patient has a menstrual history, the os must be patent; patience and careful technique will almost always be successful. In cases with cervical stenosis, especially after a loop excision of the cervix, making a small incision in the dimple where the external os should be with a scalpel or diathermy or even repeating a small loop biopsy will often open the canal and allow easy sounding and dilatation. If no obvious dimple or os is identified, it is probably safest to abandon the procedure unless it is critical and the potential risks are acceptable.

Cervical rigidity or spasm
This problem manifests itself as an inability to proceed with the dilatation beyond a small dilator. The cure is to leave the maximum-sized dilator in the canal for a short while to allow the spasm to relax. If this is unsuccessful, the surgeon should warm the dilators in hot sterile water or lubricate them with a sterile lubricant. If the problem persists, it may be due to old scarring from previous surgery or childbirth, and the surgeon may then have to accept limited dilatation and modify his technique by using smaller instruments. If the problem is anticipated prior to the operation, 200 mg misoprostol can be inserted into the posterior fornix 8 hours prior to surgery.

Dilatation of a false passage or diverticulum
If this is not noticed, the end result may be perforation of the cervix or uterus. The procedure should be abandoned and if necessary repeated at a later date by a more experienced surgeon or after priming the cervix with vaginal misoprostol. This problem should be obviated if the surgeon meticulously follows the axis of the uterus as defined at bimanual examination.

Complications of dilatation

The majority of complications are inconsequential, such as minor lacerations to the cervix; relatively uncommon, such as perforation of the uterus; or extremely rare, such as haemorrhage. However, serious complications do occur and one of the editors recalls a patient with massive haemorrhage after dilatation of the cervix, for a presumed incomplete miscarriage. The young patient required a laparotomy, opening of the uterus and insertion of isthmal sutures to control the bleeding while preserving the uterus.

Injury to the cervix

Laceration is most likely to happen if excessive force is used, the cervix is dilated too widely or if spasm of the cervix is not allowed to relax before proceeding. Dilating the non-pregnant cervix beyond 7 mm probably results in minor lacerations of the endocervical canal and internal os. The pregnant cervix is at risk of laceration of the ectocervical portion by the excessive traction on the vulsellum. It is also at risk of laceration from the process of dilatation when the surgeon attempts to dilate the cervix to excessive levels, i.e. greater than 12 mm when undertaking a termination of pregnancy.

A sudden 'give' as dilatation is being carried out is very suggestive of a tear. Usually, these tears are small and out of sight in the endocervical canal; very rarely, they extend through the full thickness of the cervix into the vaginal fornices, or from the internal os into the body of the uterus, tearing through into the broad ligament. If the surgeon suspects that a significant tear may have occurred, he or she must cease dilatation immediately. If the laceration is visible, suturing will restore the anatomy and obviate bleeding developing later, but will probably not restore the functional integrity of the cervix if the internal os is damaged. Late complications of major laceration are bleeding, infection and cervical incompetence.

Perforation of the uterus

Perforation of the uterus occurs in up to 2% of cervical dilatations associated with curettage and hysteroscopy. It invariably occurs into the peritoneal cavity and does not usually cause any long-term problems. However, it can enter the broad ligament, the bladder or, more rarely, an adherent viscus, and very rarely can cause peritonitis or severe bleeding.

It is frequently related to dilatation of the pregnant or recently pregnant uterus, and of the uterus affected by carcinoma. However, it generally arises as a result of inexperience or carelessness, though, in rare instances, it cannot be avoided.

Careful assessment of the position and attitude of the uterus by bimanual palpation cannot be stressed enough in the prevention of this complication. Figure 9.5 shows the ease with which a perforation can be performed in the retroverted gravid uterus.

Perforation should be suspected if the sound extends beyond the clinical assessment of uterine size or if the dilator slips in much further than the previous dilator.

The uterine cavity should be checked with the hysteroscope if possible to identify any perforation or, if not appropriate, the procedure should be abandoned.

When the suspected perforation has occurred during a clean procedure, such as curettage for dysfunctional uterine bleeding, observation of the patient by half-hourly pulse and blood pressure is all that is necessary. If there is suspected infection, antibiotic cover should accompany the same observation and should be continued for at least 7 days. If malignancy is demonstrated, treatment at the earliest possible moment is essential because of the potential for dissemination.

Early bleeding

This may be of varying amounts; usually, it is slight if the tear is small and ceases as the cervix resumes its normal shape after dilatation has stopped. Rarely, significant haemorrhage may occur from a ruptured branch of the cervical arteries. This may be dealt with by direct suturing if a bleeding point is visible.

If the source of the bleeding is not identified, ribbon gauze or oxidized cellulose haemostats, such as Surgicel absorbable haemostat, can be inserted into the canal. Another option is to insert a transcervical Foley catheter to create an endocervical tamponade.

After conservative management, it is possible that the bleeding will continue, dilating the uterus or even extending into the broad ligament if the uterine lower segment has been damaged. It is therefore vital that the patient is carefully monitored in the postoperative period, with elevations of the pulse, lowering of the blood pressure and untoward pain being reported immediately. If a laceration has been suspected, the recovery room staff must be made aware of the possible consequences.

If the bleeding is considerable and coming from an invisible site in the upper cervix, the surgeon should contact the intervention radiologists, if available, to consider selective uterine artery embolization. If this

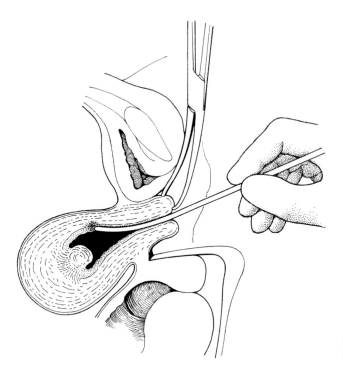

Figure 9.5 Damage of the anterior wall in a retroverted gravid uterus.

facility is not available, then deep lateral haemostatic sutures high in the ectocervix as described in the section on cone biopsy should be performed.

If unsuccessful, laparoscopy should be performed to exclude any intra-abdominal bleeding or injury, especially in the broad ligament. Very rarely, it may be necessary to open the abdomen and deal with the artery directly. However, the surgeon should remember the enormous collateral circulation, especially of the pregnant uterus, and realize that both internal iliac arteries may need to be tied off or a hysterectomy carried out if the haemorrhage fails to settle. Haematomas of the broad ligament will distort the anatomy, and the close relationship of the ureter must be remembered; failure to pay adequate attention may well turn a disaster into a tragedy.

Late bleeding
Very rarely, profuse secondary haemorrhage will occur, usually the consequence of an unnoticed laceration or haematoma becoming infected and rupturing a significant cervical or lower uterine blood vessel. Imaging with selective embolization should be considered. Broad-spectrum antibiotics should be given immediately following the taking of specimens for bacteriology. If the bleeding persists, the abdomen should be opened. Occasionally, ligation of the internal iliac arteries will suffice, but the surgeon should not expect this procedure to always produce the desired effect. Hysterectomy may be the final solution.

Perforation into the broad ligament
This complication is usually secondary to laceration of the cervix at or close to the internal os. Progressive dilatation then causes the laceration to deepen as the dilators are thrust deeper into the tear, culminating in lateral rupture of the uterus into the broad ligament. If the tear has not involved large vessels or has not occurred in the presence of infection or carcinoma, the problem often resolves with conservative treatment. However, all too often, the uterine arteries or their major branches are damaged, resulting in significant haemorrhage into the broad ligament. Pain is the commonest initial symptom accompanied by the usual signs of acute blood loss; examination

reveals a growing doughy mass in the broad ligament. If the haemorrhage is torrential, the patient will become rapidly shocked with signs of retroperitoneal haemorrhage, including gross intestinal dilatation due to disruption of the splanchnic nerves. Rapid emergency management, including fluid and blood replacement and uterine embolization or laparotomy, is essential.

Peritonitis

Most perforations produce no major or long-term sequelae. However, when associated with infection, perforation may progress to peritonitis. This is due to direct transfer of pathogens either to the peritoneal cavity or to the opening of the infected area allowing access. Symptoms may not develop for 12–24 hours, appearing as abdominal pain and discomfort with muscle rigidity and pyrexia. The classic signs of gas under the diaphragm may not be present and laparoscopy is of enormous value in order to accurately determine the diagnosis.

Peritonism

The most common cause of peritonism is irritation by escaped blood, the patient complaining of extreme and persistent lower abdominal pain in the postoperative period. If the patient has been lying in a slight Trendelenburg position, shoulder tip pain may also be a feature and is almost diagnostic. If the bleeding persists, features of a pelvic haematocele supervene with tenesmus, frequency and a bearing-down sensation accompanied by backache. Treatment may initially be conservative with antibiotics if there is any evidence of infection. However, if the patient shows evidence of progression, more active management, including laparoscopy and laparotomy, must not be delayed. The laparotomy must include a full inspection of the bowel, particularly the small bowel, which may have been lying close to the uterus as well as the genital organs.

Bowel damage

Reports of bowel damage following perforation still occur and should serve to warn the operator of the consequences of a careless approach to the seemingly simple process of cervical dilatation. If the operator suspects that the bowel has been damaged, an immediate laparotomy should be performed, the entire bowel inspected and any trauma dealt with.

Pelvic cellulitis and parametritis

It is not uncommon following minor procedures on the cervix to see evidence of inflammation and minor infection of the tissues alongside the cervix and uterus (parametritis). This is manifested as pain in the lower abdomen and back with associated dyspareunia and pain on pelvic examination and movement of the cervix. Occasionally, a thickening of the parametrium may result. The treatment is conservative with antibiotics and analgesics. If a mass is palpable, an ultrasound scan and drainage of any collection should be performed.

Removal of endocervical polyps and extruded fibroid polyps

Endocervical polyps

Most endocervical polyps are symptomless and are found at routine gynaecological examination, such as the performance of cervical cytology, and occasionally are associated with an abnormal cytology result. Less commonly, they produce symptoms such as intermenstrual and postcoital bleeding.

When the polyps are small (<2 cm), they can usually be easily avulsed in the clinic by grasping them with a small polyp forceps and rotating the forceps until the polyp falls off (Fig. 9.6). The specimen should be sent for pathological examination. When polyps are large or have broad sessile bases, the procedure may require to be carried out under general anaesthesia. The polyp should be grasped and the base diathermied. The placing of a suture prior to removal of the polyp should be considered as it is not uncommon for the base to retract into the endocervical canal making haemostasis difficult.

Fibroid polyps

From time to time the uterus extrudes submucosal fibroids through the cervical canal and they remain pulled up against the ectocervix; if large, they obliterate the cervix from view. The patient presents with pain, bleeding and discharge and, as the fibroid is often infected and ulcerated, it is often mistaken for an exophytic cervical cancer. In this situation, the gynaecologist should feel for a cervical rim above the mass and the presence of a pedicle extending from the mass into the endocervical canal.

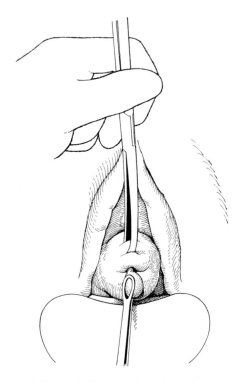

Figure 9.6 Removal of small endocervical polyp.

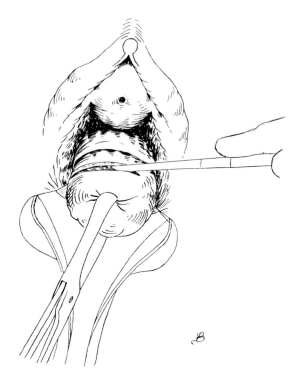

Figure 9.7 Removal of a large myomatous polyp: incising the capsule.

If the mass is large and distends the cervix, it is best to try and identify the base and then to gently diathermy or incise around the base, clamping bleeding points as necessary. It is extremely rare to have to enucleate the fibroid, as described by Bonney, to render access easier and then deal with the pedicle (Figs 9.7–9.10).

Ablative procedures

The majority of ablative procedures performed today are for cervical ectropians or CIN. Directed punch biopsies should be performed before any ablative techniques because of the small risk of CIN, even in the presence of a normal smear.

Cryosurgery

Cryosurgery has to a large extent superseded electrocautery as the optimal treatment for symptomatic cervical ectropians and is occasionally used for low-grade CIN, although the editors do not generally recommend this.

The principle

Cryosurgery depends on the cooling effects of a rapidly expanding gas. This is achieved by venting the gas through a narrow jet into a space behind a probe tip and then exhausting the gas via a large-diameter port (similar to the Venturi effect). The subsequent cooling is transferred to the cervix through the metal cryoprobe. The resultant cooling and indeed freezing of the cervical epithelium extends inwards for a depth of between 4 and 7 mm and is adequate for killing cells to that depth.

Instruments

There are many cryosurgical sets available, all with similar characteristics. A variety of probe heads are available which are interchangeable and can be sterilized, and an appropriate one should be chosen prior to engaging in treatment. A large Cusco or Sims speculum is necessary so that the entire cervix can be

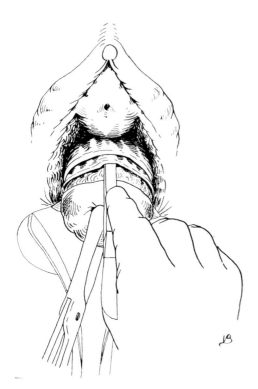

Figure 9.8 Reflecting the capsule.

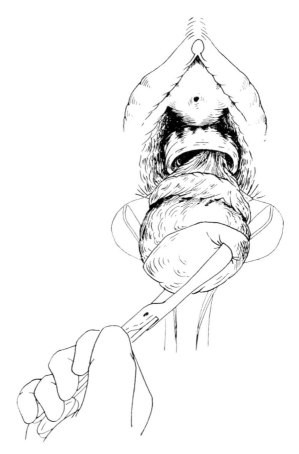

Figure 9.9 Enucleation of the tumour.

exposed with an adequate clearance around the cervix; in this way, the vagina is not involved in the treatment.

Anaesthesia
Cryosurgery has a very high patient acceptability, with patients usually only describing a discomfort similar to a period cramp. Therefore, neither anaesthesia nor analgesia are usually necessary. Almost all procedures are performed on an outpatient basis.

The operation

Exposing the cervix
The patient is placed in the lithotomy position and partially draped for her own modesty. No preparation of the vulva or vagina is necessary. The largest comfortable Cusco speculum should be used so that the entire cervix can be visualized, and the vagina held away from the edges of the cervix.

Defining the lesion
If the patient has low-grade CIN confirmed on histological assessment, colposcopy must be performed in order to outline the lesion. Treatment should not be performed unless the entire limits of the lesion are visible and accessible.

Cryosurgery
A cryoprobe head is chosen which will cover the entire lesion. If this is not possible, the lesion should be divided into segments and treated piecemeal. The cryoprobe head is gently pressed against the cervix and freezing begins. Within a few seconds the probe will be felt to 'stick' to the cervix as the ice crystals form on the back of the probe. The probe should be kept clear of the vagina to avoid unnecessary damage.

89

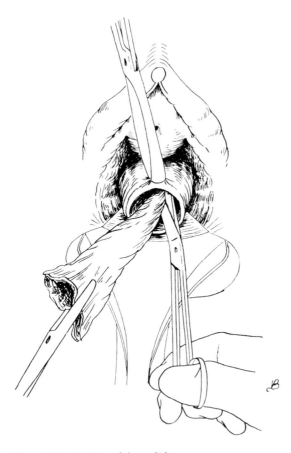

Figure 9.10 Excision of the pedicle.

Timing of the freeze
For a benign lesion a single freeze of 60 seconds will suffice, whereas for treating CIN a freeze–thaw–refreeze technique of 120 seconds on–120 seconds off–120 seconds on has proved to be most effective. The timing should begin from the moment the operator can see a clear rim of frozen tissue around the cryoprobe head.

Post-treatment care
No special precautions are necessary; the patient should be given a sheet of instructions informing her that:
• she should expect to have a profuse watery vaginal discharge which will last for 2–3 weeks
• she should avoid sexual intercourse and the use of tampons for 3 weeks

• any untoward pain or bleeding must be reported to her doctor.

Factors which influence success of cryosurgery
The most important factors to determine successful treatment of precancerous lesions are:
• size of the lesion
• irregularity of the cervical surface
• cryoprobe tip selection
• nitrous oxide bottle pressure.

Cold coagulation

The Semm cold coagulator was introduced into gynaecological practice in 1966. Initially, it was used for the local destruction of benign cervical lesions but many authors have confirmed its wide applicability to the treatment of CIN. The equipment works by raising the temperature of the surface epithelium of the cervix to approximately 110°C.

Instruments
The Semm cold coagulator is required together with a large Cusco or Sims speculum as for cryosurgery.

Anaesthesia
This procedure can usually be performed without anaesthetic, although the cervix can be infiltrated with local anaesthetic if the patient complains of discomfort.

As with cryosurgery, the thermoprobe is available in various sizes depending on the size of the lesion. The probe is applied to the lesion and may require more than one application for large lesions. The thermoprobe heats the tissues to between 110 and 120°C; thereby, literally boiling the tissues. Cell death is virtually instantaneous and the results of treatment are comparable to those following a radical electrodiathermy and laser ablation.

Complications are as for cryosurgery, laser ablation or electrodiathermy.

Cauterization of the cervix

Cauterization of the cervix may be superficial for the treatment of ectropions or radical for the treatment of CIN. The technique of radical cauterization using a needle and ball electrode is now rarely used in the management of CIN, having been superseded initially by carbon dioxide (CO_2) laser ablation in the 1980s and, since the 1990s, by the use of loop diathermy excision. Superficial cauterization using a ball electrode for the treatment of an ectropian has largely been superseded by the cryoprobe and cold coagulation as these can be performed as outpatient procedures without local anaesthesia. However, if the patient is having a general anaesthetic for another procedure, it is often simpler to treat a symptomatic ectropian with superficial cautery, which is more readily available in an operating theatre.

The operation

Do not use any antiseptic containing alcohol in the preparation of the patient as accidental burns to patients because of this error are indefensible. The cervix is exposed by inserting a Sims speculum into the vagina and then drawing down the cervix using a toothed vulsellum. The ball electrode is moved over the area of ectopic columnar epithelium, taking care not to touch the vagina and clearing the char from the electrode during the procedure. Modern Teflon-coated electrodes reduce the build up of char.

Laser ablation

The CO_2 laser became widely used during the early 1980s, mainly for the local treatment of intraepithelial lesions of the cervix, vulva and vagina. With the introduction of large loop excision of the transformation zone (LLETZ) in the early 1990s for the treatment of CIN, the laser has been almost universally replaced except possibly in a few centres.

Description of the instrument and the techniques for ablation can be found in the previous edition of this book.

Complications common to all local ablative treatment methods

Pain

Pain appreciation varies considerably from one patient to another and it does not appear to be possible to forecast which patients will or will not feel pain. In general, the higher the temperature of the treatment and the longer the application, the greater the pain. Thus, electrodiathermy, which utilizes extremely high temperatures, produces intolerable

pain and must be used under local or general anaesthesia, whereas cold coagulation and cryocautery rarely require analgesia, especially when supported by a 'chatty' nurse. A confident team of doctors and nurses produces the best results.

Pain occurring after treatment in the healing phase is usually due to infection of the cervix or the pelvic organs and should be investigated by pelvic examination, inspection of the cervix, culture of a high vaginal swab and midstream specimen of urine. Chronic pelvic inflammatory disease may flare up after treatment and must be actively managed with antibiotics and surgery if necessary.

Discharge

Almost all patients have a discharge, often profuse after cryocautery, which lasts for 2–4 weeks.

Bleeding

This problem is rarely seen after cryosurgery, but spotting can occur after cold coagulation or cautery.

Complications of healing

The squamo-columnar junction is frequently re-sited in the lower part of the endocervical canal; therefore, follow-up of CIN will often rely on cytology, since colposcopy is frequently unsatisfactory.

Narrowing or stenosis of the cervical os can occur but are rare in premenopausal women and rarely give problems during menstruation or pregnancy. The external os can often be opened by incising it with a scalpel or diathermy, or even performing a small loop biopsy. Occasionally, it may require dilatation under general anaesthesia, especially if there is evidence of a haematometra or the patient complains of dysmenorrhoea since the procedure.

Menstrual alteration

The menstrual period following local ablative treatment may be early, delayed or even missed and the flow may be greater or lighter than usual. Intermenstrual and postcoital bleeding associated with the healing process can occur but other gynaecological causes must first be eliminated.

No particular ablative technique is more prone to this complication than any other, and patients should be advised to consult their own doctor or to return to the clinic if they are concerned about significant alterations in menstrual pattern.

Subsequent obstetric performance
Patients who have had local ablative therapy are no more likely to develop obstetric complications than the normal population except if treated with radical diathermy.

Patient information
Patient concerns can be markedly reduced if they are kept fully informed about likely problems associated with the procedure. This should be complemented by the use of video colposcopy during diagnosis and information sheets explaining potential complications following treatment. The information sheet must warn the patient of any discharge, pain or abnormal bleeding which may occur and, where appropriate, advise against intercourse or the use of intravaginal tampons and creams for a short period after therapy.

Excisional techniques

The use of excisional techniques has been for many years the mainstay of the management of CIN. In the past, the predominant technique was the cold knife cone biopsy and to this was added the laser cone biopsy. Since the early 1990s, LLETZ has all but replaced the other excisional techniques.

Large loop excision of the transformation zone (LLETZ)

Small wire diathermy loops were used for many years to remove small lesions from the cervix, and it was not until 1989 that the use of larger loops (LLETZ) was first described by Prendiville. LLETZ has the advantage of ablative therapies with the added bonus that a large specimen can be obtained for pathological assessment. The technique in conjunction with colpo-scopic assessment has proved to be the most popular technique for treatment for CIN.

Patient preparation
The preparation of the patient is as for local ablative techniques. The vast majority of large loop excisional procedures are carried out in the outpatient depart-ment under local anaesthetic. The patient is colpo-scoped in the usual manner. In those circumstances where the patient is referred with a high-grade cytol-ogy, a loop diathermy can be used in a 'see and treat'

policy as, in these circumstances, it is possible to confirm the existence of a significant lesion on the cervix consistent with the high-grade cytological abnormality, and to effectively diagnose and treat it with the one procedure. LLETZ is also used to treat women with high-grade CIN confirmed by directed biopsies.

The equipment
The electrocautery systems used provide blended cut modes which provide flexibility through varying degrees of haemostasis. Although a wide variety of shapes and sizes of loops are available, in broad terms these consist of an insulated barrel inserted into a standard diathermy handpiece with buttons for cut and coagulation available to the operator. A stainless steel wire is made in either a thin flexible form or a thicker more rigid form. The rigid form is easier to use but does produce more thermal damage to the specimen. The fine flexible wire requires a delicate touch and an understanding of the memory facility of the wire so that a satisfactory loop specimen can be generated.

The operation
As with other conservative techniques the patient is advised of the procedure and consent taken. The patient is positioned on the colposcopy couch in a lithotomy position and a Cusco speculum with a smoke extraction facility attached is inserted. The cervix is exposed and colposcopy performed in the standard manner. The limits of the lesion are identi-fied with acetic acid and, if necessary, with Lugol's iodine. At this point, a local anaesthetic with a vaso-constrictor is injected directly into the cervix, giving adequate analgesia and reducing blood loss. The agent is delivered with a fine dental syringe at 3, 6, 9 and 12 o'clock. It is important to inject superficially so that blanching of the epithelium occurs, and this can be combined with deeper infiltrating when a loop cone is to be performed.

An appropriately sized loop is chosen to encompass the entire lesion so that the specimen can be removed in one block. In the editors' experience, it is rarely necessary to use more than one sweep; in a series over a 10 year period in which a total of 4944 loops were performed, 80% were made with a single sweep, 15% required two sweeps and the remaining 5% required more than two sweeps.

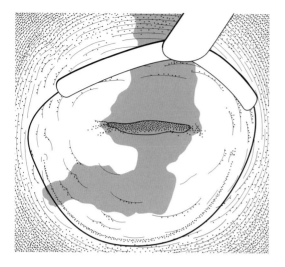

Figure 9.11 The loop is laid over the transformation zone to encompass the lesion.

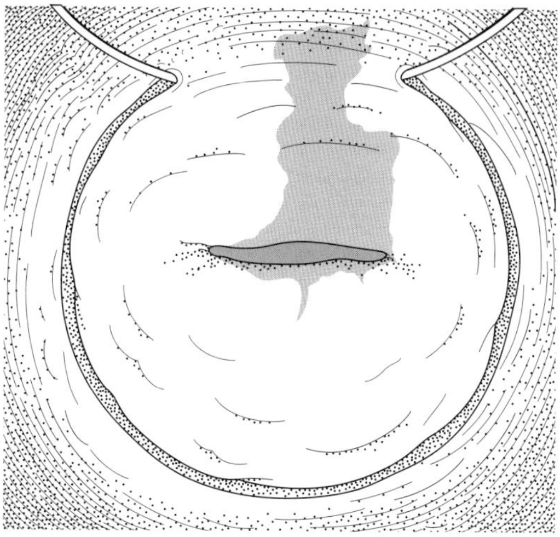

Figure 9.12 The wire is then 'followed' rather than pushed through the cervix.

The loop is laid over the transformation zone so as to encompass the lesion comfortably. If the fine wire loop is used, slight pressure is put on the loop so that it adopts a curved attitude to the cervix. The 'cut' button on the handpiece is pressed, and after a few seconds the wire begins to enter the cervix (Fig. 9.11). The surgeon should then follow the wire very gently as it cuts through the cervix, taking out a scoop of tissue to the required depth (Fig. 9.12). It is also possible to cut deeply into the cervix by inserting the wire in the long axis of the cervix so as to cut directly in, and then it is gently drawn backwards so that a much deeper scoop is performed.

At the end of the cut, the block of tissue, which usually sits in the cervix, can be removed. Minimal bleeding is experienced and the base and the edges of the loop can then be diathermied using a ball electrode. At the end of the procedure, the patient is allowed home with appropriate written instructions.

Complications

These tend to be minimal and are similar to local ablative techniques, most commonly that of bleeding, discharge and, occasionally, infection. Stenosis of the cervix can also be seen especially in the postmenopausal patient.

The trainee must be cautious of the rapidity at which the loop cuts and the need to obtain adequate exposure of the cervix. Lacerations of the lateral walls of the vagina, which result in pain and often heavy bleeding, are a complication seen during a trainee's learning curve. The sheer number of LLETZ procedures performed as a result of national screening programmes ultimately results in a variety of uncommon complications such as injuries to the bladder, rectum and uterine artery.

Numerous publications have shown an increased risk of preterm labour after excisional treatments for CIN, including LLETZ when performed greater than 10 mm in depth. Women planning future pregnancies should be counselled about the risk.

Laser cone biopsy

The CO_2 laser is an excellent instrument, not only as a vaporizing instrument but also when the spot size is reduced to 1 mm or less as a slow cutting device. This facility to reduce the spot size and thus increase the power density of the beam gives the surgeon a very accurate instrument with which to remove lesions from the cervix. In women in whom the ectocervix is flush with the vagina because of previous excisions or atrophic changes, it allows a narrow cylinder biopsy to be taken when a knife or loop cone would not be possible. Although the procedure is bloodless, the major drawback is the extreme slowness of the procedure; also, in inexperienced hands, there is a tendency to produce significant heat trauma to the specimen. With the introduction of LLETZ and its ability to perform loop cones, the CO_2 laser has all but become extinct. As with laser ablation, description of the technique can be found in the previous edition of this book.

Cold knife cone biopsy

Cold knife conization has not been used in Gateshead since the late 1980s. It was initially replaced by laser conization and then by loop conization following the department's publication in 1990 by Mor-Yosef showing that loop conization was feasible and adequate.

The technique described is as it was performed in Gateshead in the 1980s.

Instruments

The instruments required for this procedure are those described in the gynaecological minor set (Chapter 3). The knife itself may have a pointed blade, thus facilitating the formation of the conical excision.

Anaesthesia

This procedure is performed under general anaesthetic, although it is possible, though not in the editors' view desirable, to use a paracervical or wide local infiltration.

Patient preparation

The patient should be prepared as for any vaginal procedure. Shaving is not necessary. All cone biopsies should be carried out under colposcopic control to be certain of identifying the ectocervical limits of the colposcopic abnormality. Lugol's iodine may be used as an alternative. Usually, the cone biopsy is being performed because the endocervical limits of the lesion cannot be seen at colposcopy, or because there is a suspicion of invasive carcinoma.

The operation

Lateral haemostats

The patient is draped in the lithotomy position and an Auvard or Sims speculum inserted into the vagina. The cervix is visualized and colposcopy performed. Iodine may be applied as described previously. The

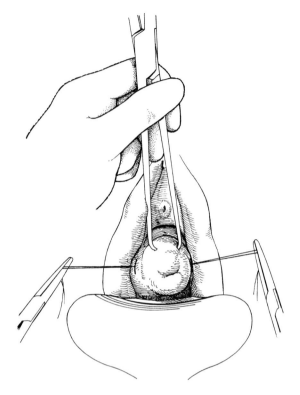

Figure 9.13 Placing the lateral haemostats.

cervix is then grasped above the anterior limit of the ectocervical lesion using a toothed vulsellum. By drawing the cervix to one side and then to the other, access is gained to place a deep lateral haemostatic stitch on either side of the cervix (Fig. 9.13). The stitch is inserted so as to ligate the descending branch of the uterine artery, which passes along the lateral side of the cervix deep to the epithelium. The stitches, usually of Vicryl, may be left long and attached to artery clips in order to manoeuvre the cervix later in the procedure.

An alternative for preventing bleeding is to infiltrate the cervix circumferentially with a vasoconstrictor either combined with a local anaesthetic as used for LLETZ or on its own.

Incising the cone

The cervix is now drawn down using the vulsellum and, taking a pointed blade scalpel, the cone is cut beginning at the posterior part and cutting around the

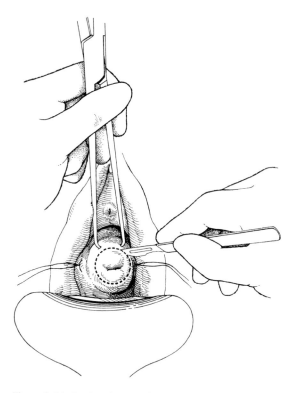

Figure 9.14 Cutting the cone biopsy.

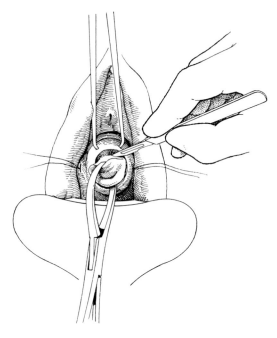

Figure 9.15 Grasping the cone biopsy.

anterior area (Fig. 9.14). As soon as the initial encircling incision has been made, it is a great advantage to grasp the specimen with a Littlewood tissue forceps so as to infold the ectocervical epithelium upon itself (Fig. 9.15). The deeper part of the cone can then be cut under direct vision. Holding the specimen in the tissue forceps also protects the ectocervical epithelium and produces an intact specimen for the pathologist. This is of particular importance when dealing with high-grade CIN as there appears to be reduced tissue adhesion between the dermis and the subdermal layers in this condition.

Repairing the cervix

For many years, the standard repair after cone biopsy was to insert Sturmdorf sutures, producing a very ugly cervix often with ectocervical epithelium infolded and hidden or epithelial cells drawn down stitch tracks, producing a potential danger of hidden precancerous change. Any bleeding of the cone base can be controlled by freezing the area with the cryoprobe or cauterizing with a 'ball' diathermy. Alternative methods include cautery with the argon beam coagulator or tying the lateral sutures over Surgicel (Johnson and Johnson Inc., New Brunswick, NJ, USA) or Gelfoam (Pfizer Inc., New York, NY, USA) soaked in thrombin.

In the rare cases when there is a persistent ooze the vagina is packed, and the bladder catheterized and the patient returned to the ward. Occasionally, it is necessary to augment this technique by using either isolated sutures to the edge of the cone or an encircling continuous suture around the edge. The great advantage of these simple methods is that the squamocolumnar junction is still accessible for future assessment for both cytology and colposcopy.

Dilatation and curettage

Many surgeons routinely perform this procedure with a cone biopsy. Unless there is a clinical reason, it should not be done and *never before a cone biopsy*.

This latter practice usually results in there being no epithelium left on the cone specimen and leaves the poor pathologist unable to make any realistic report.

95

There is also no advantage in attempting to dilate the cervix to reduce the risk of stenosis. Scarring and stenosis are more likely to occur after the enthusiastic insertion of Sturmdorf sutures.

Complications of cervical conization

Haemorrhage

Haemorrhage is the most important and common problem encountered. The bleeding may be primary or secondary, with the former usually occurring in the first 24 hours, and associated with reactive bleeding, the latter some 10 days postoperatively and often associated with infection. Vaginal packing is often all that is required, but the cervix should be inspected and any local bleeding points dealt with individually. Infection will occur from time to time, producing haemorrhage, discharge and occasionally progressing to pelvic infection. It should be actively treated by systemic antibiotics.

Cervical stenosis

Cervical stenosis may occur and should be treated by simple dilatation; rarely does it cause a problem in labour.

Pregnancy outcomes

As mentioned earlier, numerous publications have shown an increased risk of preterm labour after excisional treatments for CIN. Women planning future pregnancies should be counselled about the risk. However, it should be noted that women with CIN who are not treated are also at an increased risk of preterm labour, although not as high as those treated.

Trachelorrhaphy

A trachelorrhaphy is essentially a repair of a cervical laceration and has little if any role in modern gynaecological practice. It involves exposing the laceration, excising the edges and approximating them with interrupted absorbable sutures. A detailed description is available in previous editions.

It may rarely be necessary to repair cervical tears arising from childbirth, especially after an instrumental delivery, if there is heavy bleeding. It is important in these situations to grasp the cervix with sponge forceps and place a suture above the apex as this is often the source of the bleeding.

Cervical incompetence

Cervical incompetence or insufficiency is a difficult and confusing diagnosis in obstetrics. The diagnostic criteria are not well defined and the incidence is unknown. Classically, cervical incompetence was presumed in women with multiple painless second trimester miscarriages occurring earlier with each loss. Unfortunately, studies on the role of cervical cerclage have included lower risk women with previous preterm labours or cervical surgery such as conization. Cervical cerclage may prolong pregnancy in a woman who has had three or more unexplained second trimester losses or preterm labours but it is unclear whether this will improve neonatal outcome. These women have a 70% chance of delivering after 33 weeks even without a cerclage.

The use of ultrasound to measure cervical length and funnelling has provided a degree of quantification but has not improved appropriate selection of women for cerclage. A study on ultrasound measurement of cervical length in 47 000 women at 22–24 weeks gestation found that 1% had a cervical length of less than 15 mm. A number of these women were randomized to cervical cerclage with no observed benefit. The procedure may, however, benefit high-risk women who are also found to have a shortened cervix on scan.

There are only limited observational data supporting an emergency cerclage in a woman with a dilated cervix and no signs of uterine contractions.

In recent years, a cervical cerclage has been inserted at the time of radical trachelectomy for early cervical cancer as the majority of the cervix is removed at surgery. Numerous successful pregnancies have been achieved as a result of the procedure.

The procedure

There is no doubt that the name of Shirodkar will always be associated with this operation. However, in western practice, the simpler McDonald suture, which is described here, is used, predominantly because of its simplicity.

The operation is best planned when the patient is booked for delivery. It is usual to carry out the operation between 12 and 14 weeks gestation. It is important to perform an ultrasound scan in order to exclude fetal abnormality before embarking on the procedure. A variety of non-absorbable sutures such as Prolene, Ethibond or Mersilene tape with a large needle can be used. Monofilament sutures have the advantage of being easier to use, sliding through the cervical tissue with minimal trauma and less risk of infection than the tape. The disadvantage is that they tend to cut into the cervix more, making them more difficult to remove.

Instruments
The instruments required are found in the gynaecological minor set described in Chapter 3.

Patient preparation
It is of value for the patient to have a stat dose of prophylactic antibiotics and β sympathomimetics prior to surgery.

Anaesthesia
Either a light general anaesthetic or an epidural is ideal for carrying out this procedure.

The operation

Exposing and grasping of the cervix
The patient is placed in the lithotomy position and the cervix exposed by placing a Sims speculum in the vagina. The cervix is grasped using two or more sponge holders, one on the anterior and one on the posterior lip of the cervix. The cervix is gently drawn down, exposing the length of the cervix. By drawing the sponge holders first to one side and then the other, the lateral parts of the cervix can be easily reached with the needle.

Insertion of the suture
The McDonald suture is essentially a purse-string suture. The suture is placed circumferentially around the upper body of the vaginal part of the cervix in four separate 'bites', starting either posteriorly or anteriorly based on the surgeon's preference. To aid removal of the suture, it is advised to leave the threads about 4–5 cm long and create a knot before cutting the suture. This allows the thread to be hooked with a finger or instrument and the knot at the cervix cut. Placing the knot anteriorly makes it easier to remove

in late pregnancy. Practice will determine the correct tension, which should be tight enough to just close the os but not so tight as to produce a pallor of the cervix.

Removal of the suture
An anaesthetic is not required. Removal must be performed before labour becomes established and is easily accomplished by exposing the cervix, grasping the long end of the suture as described above and cutting the suture at any of the points where it is visible on the exterior of the cervix, and then by simply pulling the knot.

The patient must be informed of the importance of early attendance at the hospital if there is a suggestion of labour beginning. Management is particularly difficult when the patient goes into premature labour and the decision to cut the suture or to leave it and possibly conserve the pregnancy has to be made.

Potential complications
- Premature rupture of membranes.
- Chorioamnionitis.
- Cervical rupture if the suture is not removed before the onset of labour.
- Bleeding.

Excision of cervical stump

The term subtotal hysterectomy describes the procedure of removal of the uterine corpus while leaving the uterine cervix *in situ*. The procedure was initially advocated during the era before antibiotics and blood transfusion as it was associated with less morbidity and complications. It regained popularity when a Finnish study suggested that the procedure maintained coital satisfaction and orgasm compared with total abdominal hysterectomy, but this has been refuted by subsequent studies. Proponents of the procedure have redefined the procedure as supracervical hysterectomy, thereby obviating the term 'subtotal'.

Not too uncommonly, a subtotal hysterectomy may have been performed when a total hysterectomy would have been preferable, i.e. when an occult endometrial cancer is identified on histological examination of the subtotal hysterectomy specimen. In this instance, removal of the residual cervical stump is advocated. Other indications for cervical stumpectomy include abnormal cervical cytology, cervical cancer and persistent menstrual bleeding when the indication for the hysterectomy was menorrhagia!

The procedure of removal of the cervical stump is relatively straightforward when this is attempted by the vaginal route. Even when the subtotal hysterectomy was performed inadvertently as the novice surgeon encounters unexpected problems, access via the vagina to remove the stump can avoid many of the previously encountered difficulties.

Patient preparation is as with vaginal hysterectomy. An epidural or spinal anaesthetic is more than sufficient. The patient is placed in a lithotomy position and, after adequate cleansing of the perineum and vagina, the bladder is emptied. Insertion of a large Sims speculum and an additional anterior vaginal retractor gives good access to the cervical stump. Two Littlewood forceps are placed on the anterior and posterior cervical lips, and approximately 20 mL of 1:200 000 epinephrine in saline is injected into the subepithelial tissue. Traction is applied to the cervix as a circumferential incision is performed encircling the cervix. A toothed dissector is then used to grasp the anterior vaginal edge as the Monaghan scissors are used to enter and develop the cervicovesical plane and dissect the bladder off the anterior surface of the cervix. The cervix is then pulled anteriorly as the posterior vaginal edge is grasped with the toothed dissectors and the scissors

sharply dissect the tissues posterior to the cervical stump, allowing entry into the pouch of Douglas. The transverse cervical ligaments and any residual uterosacral ligaments are then clamped with a pair of hysterectomy clamps, cut and ligated. Additional lateral clamps are applied as necessary to allow release of the cervical stump from all but the remaining cranial adhesions and tissues. Attention must be given at this point to ensure that undue traction to the cervical stump is not applied so that the cervical stump can be sharply dissected off the superior aspects of the bladder and surrounding scar tissue without injury. A locking continuous suture is then inserted around the vaginal cuff, haemostasis is confirmed and the bladder is catheterized with an indwelling urethral catheter if this is considered necessary.

Further reading

Mor-Yosef S, Lopes A, Pearson S, Monaghan JM. Loop diathermy cone biopsy. *Obstet Gynecol* 1990;75: 884–886.

Prendiville W, Cullimore J, Norman S. Large loop excision of the transformation zone (LLETZ). A new method of management for women with cervical intraepithelial neoplasia. *Br J Obstet Gynaecol* 1989;96:1054–1056.

Singer A, Monaghan JM. *Lower Genital Tract Precancer: Colposcopy, Pathology and Treatment*, 2nd edn. Oxford: Blackwell Science, 2000.

10 Operations on the uterine cavity

Assessment of the uterine cavity remains a significant part of the work of the gynaecologist. Alterations in menstrual pattern in women over the age of 40 often require assessment and evaluation. Postmenopausal bleeding should be considered to be due to endometrial cancer until proven otherwise.

All such patients should be assessed with a comprehensive personal, menstrual and hormonal history. The patient's cervical cytology record must be reviewed.

A full pelvic examination should be performed including visualization of the cervix and palpation of the pelvic organs and all findings should be recorded. For many patients, particularly the young, bleeding problems are often associated with the use of hormonal contraception. Persistent postcoital bleeding requires colposcopy in the older woman and exclusion of a *Chlamydia* infection or ectropian in the younger.

Rapid access clinics

It is now commonplace for hospitals to run rapid access clinics for special problems which are amenable to ambulant or outpatient care. Rapid access clinics for menstrual disorders and postmenopausal bleeding are ideal as transvaginal ultrasound, endometrial sampling and even outpatient hysteroscopy lend themselves to this approach.

Bonney's Gynaecological Surgery, 11th edition.
© Tito Lopes, Nick Spirtos, Raj Naik, John Monaghan.
Published 2011 by Blackwell Publishing Ltd.

In England, patients with postmenopausal bleeding are required to be seen within 2 weeks as part of the National Institute of Health and Clinical Excellence referral guidelines for suspected cancer. Standard proforma faxes have been developed which cover all documentation required for rapid processing. Many clinics are run almost entirely by nursing and ultrasound staff who have been trained in history-taking, endometrial sampling techniques and abdominal and vaginal ultrasound.

As can be imagined such a complex system of care requires considerable organization and commitment of skilled individuals. There has to be a critical mass of patients with a special facility on one site. Equipment has to be of a high order with rapidly available and appropriate skills on tap. Cover for holidays and other absences dictates that the whole process is expensive to run but does provide an immediate high-quality service.

In many hospitals, the rapid access clinic concept is fragmented because of variable availability of skills and equipment. Many centres can provide elements of care, such as outpatient endometrial sampling with Pipelle or other systems linked to an ultrasound assessment of endometrial cavity structure and endometrial thickness measurement. However, drawing all these skills and facilities together may be difficult.

Following history-taking, visualization of the cervix and pelvic examination, a transvaginal ultrasound assessment of the endometrial thickness is performed. If the endometrial thickness is greater than 4–5 mm an endometrial sample should be taken. If it is greater than 10 mm, and if there is suggestion of endometrial polyps or the patient is on tamoxifen, a hysteroscopy and biopsy should be performed, preferably as an outpatient procedure to obtain a suitable histopathological assessment.

Sampling of the endometrium

There are numerous devices for sampling the endometrium in an outpatient setting with the Pipelle endometrial sampler being one of the most commonly used techniques.

The device consists of an outer tube measuring 3 mm in diameter, within which is a closely fitting rod; when the rod is withdrawn, it creates a vacuum that sucks in a section of endometrium sufficient to give a histological report on. The diameter of the whole instrument is such that for many patients it is easily introduced into the uterine cavity and a satisfactory sample obtained. Unfortunately, there can be difficulties in introducing the sampler particularly in the nulliparous and postmenopausal patients and the specimen generated is inadequate for pathological reporting.

The Tao brush, another instrument for sampling the endometrium, is associated with a lower incidence of inadequate samples and is better tolerated.

When outpatient sampling fails or the specimen is unsatisfactory then the gold standard assessment technique is hysteroscopy and curettage.

Outpatient hysteroscopy

In some centres outpatient hysteroscopy using either a low-viscosity liquid or a gas (CO_2) expansion technique has been developed. The technique involves the use of either fine rigid 30° hysteroscopes with a sheath diameter as small as 3.7 mm (Bettocchi Office Hysteroscope with a 2 mm lens) or flexible hysteroscopes with diameters of 3.1–4.9 mm. Although flexible hysteroscopes are less painful, the rigid scope provides superior optical qualities and has a higher success rate. In premenopausal women the procedure should be performed before day 10 of the menstrual cycle to avoid endometrial thickening. It can be performed without the use of local anaesthesia in the majority of women, but there should be a low threshold for the use of an intracervical injection of local

anaesthetic as pain is the main complaint regarding the procedure.

A comfortable couch, as used for colposcopy, should be used, preferably with controls for automatic positioning of the patient into a semi-reclined position.

A transvaginal 'no touch' approach described by Bettocchi involves using the irrigation fluid to fill the vagina, the cervix can then be located, inspected and the endocervical canal entered without the need to use a vaginal speculum, or grasp the cervix with a tenaculum. The continuous flow of fluid (normal saline) aids the opening of the canal and entry into the endometrial cavity. A constant pressure of 30–40 mmHg provides adequate distension of the endometrial cavity. The technique has been shown to result in less discomfort than when a vaginal speculum and cervical tenaculum are used. Diagnostic biopsies, excision of polyps and other operative procedures can be performed with the use of fine scissors, biopsy forceps or bipolar diathermy instruments, such as the Versapoint Bipolar Electrosurgical System, inserted through a 5 Fr. working channel available in some hysteroscopes. Manipulation or cautery of the myometrium should be avoided as this stimulates the muscle, causing discomfort.

Day-case or ambulant hysteroscopy

Although many patients have hysteroscopy performed as an outpatient procedure, hysteroscopy performed under general anaesthetic remains the norm in many hospitals, particularly where significant operative manoeuvres are involved.

The instruments

Hysteroscopes can vary in size from narrow diagnostic scopes to operative hysteroscopes and resectoscopes. The hysteroscope is linked to a continuous flow pressure system permitting continuous irrigation of the endometrial cavity. The procedure should be performed in a fully equipped day-case operating theatre with full recovery facilities available.

When an intervention is required, such as sampling of the endometrium, the gynaecological minor set is necessary (see Table 3.2). Excision of lesions identified can be performed either with a simple curettage or with endoscopic electrodiathermy resection equipment (resectoscopes).

The cavity of the uterus requires distension for the various procedures. CO_2 gas has already been described for the outpatient hysteroscopies. For diagnostic and minor therapeutic hysteroscopies, including the use of bipolar cautery, saline is cheap and safe.

However, whenever monopolar electrical energy is used within the uterus a non-conducting medium is essential, also a high flow rate of clean new fluid in and contaminated fluid out is essential. The two most commonly used are 1.5%vol. glycine and 5% sorbitol. Both these agents can cause hyponatraemia if excessive absorption occurs. Haemolysis is also possible. A meticulous account of fluid in and out of the systems is essential during any operative procedure.

The operation

In premenopausal women the procedure should be performed in the first half of the patient's menstrual cycle. The patient should be asked to empty her bladder immediately prior to going to theatre.

The patient is brought into the theatre and placed in the lithotomy position. The vulva and vagina are swabbed down with a non-alcoholic skin preparation. The legs and lower abdomen are draped.

The patient is examined using a bimanual technique to ascertain the shape, size, consistency and position of the cervix, uterus and adnexa.

A Sims speculum is inserted into the posterior vagina. The cervix is grasped on its anterior lip using a multi-toothed Vulsellum forceps. The cervix and uterus is then gently drawn down and forwards to place the uterus on slight tension. This effectively straightens the endocervical canal and provides countertraction when dilatation of the cervix is necessary. The cervical canal and uterus is gently sounded to determine the length of the cavity, the attitude of the uterus having already been determined. This length will be recorded in the notes. Some experts do not recommend sounding; however, the editors feel that the information gained is not disadvantaged by any potential risks of trauma.

For most parous patients, it will be unnecessary to dilate the cervix prior to inserting the hysteroscope. If the scope does not pass easily, gentle dilatation of the endocervical canal can be performed up to 6 mm. It is important not to overdilate the cervix as the uterine cavity will not be expanded owing to escape of the expansion medium.

The scope should be inserted gently along the anticipated line of the endocervical canal and the uterine cavity determined by the prior examination and sounding. The continuous flow of fluid should begin as the scope is inserted, aiding the opening of the canal. Visualization of this process is best achieved if the video camera is attached to the scope. Pressure to achieve expansion of the uterine cavity is produced either passively by elevating the bag of fluid at least 1 metre above the level of the uterus or by applying a pressure bag to the fluid, maintaining a pressure of 150 mmHg.

Once the hysteroscope is within the cavity of the uterus, after a short time any debris will clear giving a superb view of the entire field.

The findings should be described systematically, beginning with the endocervical canal, continuing into the cavity and ending with the tubal ostia. Positive and negative findings should be recorded. A full description with a drawing or ideally a photograph of the interior of the cavity is essential for adequate documentation.

Once the hysteroscopy is completed it is common for a sampling of the endometrium to be performed. This is best achieved using a curette.

Curettage

A small sharp curette is all that is required for the procedure. The small curette can be inserted without the need for further dilatation after the hysteroscopy. A systematic approach to sampling is required remembering that the uterine cavity consists of essentially an anterior and a posterior surface plus two cornu and a fundus. If the curette is gently but firmly scraped first length-wise down the posterior surface followed by the same down the anterior surface and finally scraping right to left and then left to right across the fundus, the whole surface will be effectively sampled. The action of curettage is a gentle one with the curette lightly held in the first three fingers and the thumb of the right hand (Fig. 10.1). As the surgeon's experience grows, a considerable amount of 'feel' will develop distinguishing irregularities, soft areas, septae and synaechiae seen on hysteroscopy. The specimens produced should be drawn out of the cervix and delivered onto a swab which has been placed just under the posterior lip of

101

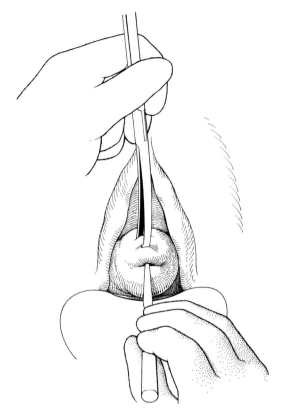

Figure 10.1 Curettage of the uterine cavity.

the cervix, in the posterior fornix. The swab is then taken, excess blood or mucus is removed and the curettings are immediately fixed in preservative.

At the end of the procedure the vagina is swabbed clean and a formal count of all swabs and instruments made and recorded.

Endometrial polyps

These are often identified at hysteroscopy and can be removed simply by inserting a small polyp forceps into the uterine cavity, grasping the polyp and avulsing it/them. If the polyp is large or sessile the use of a resectoscope may be necessary.

Fractional curettage

This technique has been largely superseded by the use of hysteroscopy, although it may have a value in

separately curetting the endocervical canal when localized cancer is suspected. Material generated from each separate area of curettage is placed in clearly marked pots for histopathological assessment.

Removal of retained products of conception

The most important aspect of this procedure is to remember the softness of the cervix and the body of the uterus and the use of utmost gentleness in all movements. The cervix should be grasped with one or two Vulsellum forceps but excessive traction should not be applied to avoid tearing the cervix. The curettage should be performed with a large blunt curette. Suction curettage can be used but is rarely required.

If there is any evidence of infection, bacterial swabs should be taken. All material should be sent for pathological examination, otherwise a molar pregnancy may be missed.

All pregnancy-related curettage should be performed using prophylactic antibiotic cover.

Complications and dangers

Trauma to the cervix and uterine wall are the commonest dangers and can be avoided with meticulous gentle technique.

Infection is a significant risk with pregnancy-related procedures

Endometrial ablation

Until recently, hysterectomy has been the standard treatment for women with menorrhagia unresponsive to medical treatment. However, since the 1980s, minimally invasive procedures to destroy the endometrium have been developed as an alternative. All of the ablative techniques rely on destroying the endometrium's regenerative capacity, which requires a depth of destruction of at least 4 mm. Pretreatment with hormones that decrease the endometrial thickness is invariably used to improve efficacy.

First generation

The first-generation techniques for endometrial ablation were essentially the Nd:YAG laser, the resectoscopic loop and the electrosurgical rollerball. All of these techniques are performed under hysteroscopic guidance. Although the techniques are effective, there are some drawbacks. They require a skilled hysteroscopic surgeon, and, despite having a lower morbidity than conventional hysterectomy, the incidence of uterine perforation ranges from 0.6% to 2.5%, and fluid deficits of greater than 2 litres range from 1% to 5%.

With the introduction of more conservative techniques for the management of menorrhagia such as the Mirena IUS and second-generation endometrial ablation techniques, the role of operative hysteroscopy with either the resectoscope or laser has diminished markedly. As a result, their main use is in the management of submucosal fibroids.

Second generation

Less invasive techniques have been developed for dealing with dysfunctional uterine bleeding. The advantages over resection are that there is no risk of fluid overload, the procedures are quick and simple, with a short learning curve, and are suitable as an outpatient procedure under local anaesthetic. The procedures are performed 'blind' without hysteroscopic visualization.

Current methods include:
- cryotherapy
- fluid balloon ablation
- hydrothermoablation
- microwave endometrial ablation (MEA)
- electrode: mesh
- laser interstitial hyperthermia.

The individual techniques vary in the size of endometrial cavity that can be successfully treated, and the majority except for MEA and hydrothermoablation require a regular cavity without pathology, such as fibroids.

Data on short-term effectiveness would suggest that second-generation ablation methods are comparable and are as effective as first-generation techniques.

Perforation of the uterus is rare but of concern as it may be undetected because the cavity is not visualized during the procedure. When activated, the perforated instrument may damage the bowel, leading to serious consequences.

Contraindications to second-generation techniques
- Previous uterine surgery or trauma resulting in a uterine wall thickness of <10 mm at any point.
- Previous classical caesarean section or transmural myomectomy.
- Previous ablative technique.
- Uterine fibroids distorting access to the entire uterine cavity.
- Current active pelvic inflammatory disease.
- Desire for future pregnancy.
- Known or suspected endometrial cancer.

Preoperative work-up
- Completed family and will use effective contraception other than an intrauterine device.
- A transvaginal scan.
- An endometrial biopsy in the last 6 months to exclude an endometrial cancer.
- Up to date with cervical smears.
- Preoperative preparation of the endometrium with a GnRH analogue 4 weeks before the procedure *or* oral progesterone for 10 days, 3 weeks before the procedure.

Hysteroscopic myomectomy

Submucous fibroids are the most common anatomical cause of excessive menstrual blood loss in women of reproductive age. Advances in operative hysteroscopy have enabled removal of these lesions with a significant reduction in morbidity compared with open abdominal myomectomy. Available instruments include the resectoscope, which, although usually monopolar, can be bipolar or 'cold', and the Nd:YAG laser. Disadvantages of the laser are the time taken to vaporize the fibroid, the lack of a specimen for histology and the cost of the equipment. Because of the costs and training required for the Nd:YAG laser, this is rarely used today except in specialist departments.

The ease of treatment, the technique used, and the success rate depends on the type of fibroid managed.

Classification of submucosal fibroids

- Type 0: fibroid polyp.
- Type 1: <50% contained within the myometrium.
- Type 2: >50% contained within the myometrium.

Fibroids developing completely within the uterine cavity (type 0) can be easily removed in a single procedure with the size of the fibroid representing the main limiting factor.

Resectoscopic slicing is the standard technique for treating such fibroids, as it is less expensive than laser treatment and quick to perform. Small type 0 and type 1 fibroids (with minimal intramural involvement) can be managed with the Versapoint as an outpatient procedure.

Resection of fibroids with intramural extension should be performed only by experts as it is technically difficult and has a higher risk of complications. Several techniques have been developed to completely remove such fibroids, all of them aiming at the transformation of an intramural fibroid into a totally intracavitary lesion, thus avoiding a deep cut into the myometrium.

Complications

Intravasation and electrolyte imbalance

The most dangerous complication during hysteroscopic myomectomy is intravasation of the fluid used to distend the uterine cavity. Severe fluid overload can cause pulmonary oedema, hyponatraemia, heart failure, cerebral oedema and even death. The procedure should be terminated if fluid intravasation is greater than 750 mL. It is therefore vitally important to have a meticulous technique for fluid inflow and outflow measurement.

The use of normal saline combined with bipolar energy reduces the risk of hyponatraemia, but excessive intravasation of greater than 1500 mL remains a risk and might cause cardiac overload.

Intrauterine adhesions

This is the major long-term complication and occurs in 1–13% of patients; one should avoid trauma to healthy endometrium and myometrium surrounding the fibroid.

Other complications include uterine perforation and uterine rupture during pregnancy.

Further reading

Bettocchi S, Ceci O, Nappi L, *et al.* Operative office hysteroscopy without anesthesia: analysis of 4863 cases performed with mechanical instruments. *J Am Assoc Gynecol Laparosc* 2004;11:59–61.

Di Spiezio Sardo A, Mazzon I, Bramante S, *et al.* Hysteroscopic myomectomy: a comprehensive review of surgical techniques. *Hum Reprod Update* 2008;14: 101–119.

11 Operations on the uterus

The number of hysterectomies performed in developed countries has fallen markedly as a result of more conservative measures for the management of dysfunctional uterine bleeding. In the 9-year period 1995–2004, there was a 46% reduction in the number of hysterectomy operations performed in NHS hospitals in England.

Once a decision to perform a hysterectomy has been made, the surgeon must decide and recommend to the patient the most appropriate route. The choices available currently include abdominal, vaginal, laparoscopically assisted vaginal, total laparoscopic and subtotal hysterectomy. The factors determining the choice depend on the pathology, the surgeon's ability and preference, and individual factors related to the patient such as obesity and co-morbidities.

Total abdominal hysterectomy

It is interesting that Berkeley and Bonney used the more correct title of abdominal total hysterectomy for the operation but, as with recent editions, the current editors have used the present form so that the accepted abbreviation of TAH is consistent. This operation remains the accepted basic procedure for removing the uterus in the management of benign disease; it is also used in oncological care for the management of cancer of the corpus uteri and ovary.

Bonney's Gynaecological Surgery, 11th edition.
© Tito Lopes, Nick Spirtos, Raj Naik, John Monaghan.
Published 2011 by Blackwell Publishing Ltd.

The technique described here is inevitably a melange of many influences upon the current editors, not least the previous editions of this book.

Instruments

The gynaecological general set described in Chapter 3 is used.

Patient preparation

The balance between late admission and reducing preoperative tension is a fine one. A good night's sleep before operation is advantageous, and this may best be achieved in the patient's own bed.

With patients commonly reviewed in pre-admission clinics, admission on the day of surgery is increasingly the norm.

It is essential that the patient fully understands the extent of the surgery intended, particularly in relationship to the removal or preservation of the ovaries. From time to time, fashions concerning preservation or removal of the cervix will appear.

Blood should be taken for a full blood count, grouping of the blood type and the sample saved in case a transfusion is required, although this is rare for most hysterectomies. The anaesthetist will review and counsel the patient about the anaesthetic and the options available for operative and postoperative pain relief such as epidurals and patient-controlled analgesia.

It remains traditional to shave the abdomen for an abdominal procedure; in the editors' view, this is necessary only for the visible part of the pubic hair.

It is important to perform any shaving as close to surgery as practicable; ideally, the hair should be clipped rather than shaved immediately prior to surgery as this has been shown to reduce the risk of infection. It is also unnecessary and potentially dangerous to overclean the abdominal wall with antiseptics as recolonization with more malign bacteria may occur prior to surgery.

Some patients may require sedation prior to surgery, whereas others will not.

The operation

Following general anaesthesia, the vulva and vagina are cleaned and the bladder catheterized and emptied. If the hysterectomy is being performed as the only procedure and the patient is fit, an indwelling catheter may not be necessary.

The use of intravaginal dyes or packs is superfluous. Suturing and occlusion of the cervix when dealing with corpus cancer is also unnecessary.

The incision
The choice of incision and the important preamble of exploring the abdomen and pelvis and packing the bowel is dealt with in Chapter 4.

Clamping and dividing the round and infundibulopelvic ligaments
The uterus is elevated by the surgeon placing his or her left hand into the pouch of Douglas and lifting the body of the uterus so as to put the uterosacral ligaments on the stretch. A medium-sized straight forceps is placed on either side of the cornu so as to include the origins of the tubes and the round ligaments approximately 1 cm from the uterine wall. When the handles of the two clamps are placed together and held in the left hand, the whole uterus can be manoeuvred. When the uterus is elevated, the round ligaments become prominent bands passing anterolaterally behind the peritoneum towards the inguinal ligament. The round ligaments are picked up at roughly their midpoints with a medium-sized clamp and then incised on their medial side (Fig. 11.1). This clamp is handed to the assistant, thus opening the anterior part of the broad ligament. The round ligament is the 'gateway' to the pelvic sidewall and, once divided, the soft areolar tissue within the leaves of the broad ligament are revealed.

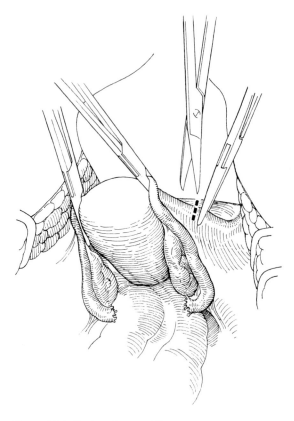

Figure 11.1 Cutting the round ligaments.

The editors recommend that, at this point, the simple manoeuvre of opening up the retroperitoneal space down the point at which the ureter is visible is an important practice which, once learned, can be applied to virtually all pelvic procedures. This technique allows the ureter to be visualized in the upper pelvic part of its course where it lies close to the infundibulopelvic ligament, a site of all-too-frequent clamping of the ureter. If there is any difficulty identifying the ureter, it is invariably found overlying the bifurcation of the common iliac artery and from here can be traced down the pelvis.

Once the course of the ureter has been identified, the index finger of the left hand can be used to elevate the infundibulopelvic ligament, allowing a clamp to be placed either on the medial or on the lateral side of the ovary, depending on whether these structures are to be preserved or removed (Fig. 11.2). If the ovaries are to be removed, they can be moved medially on the

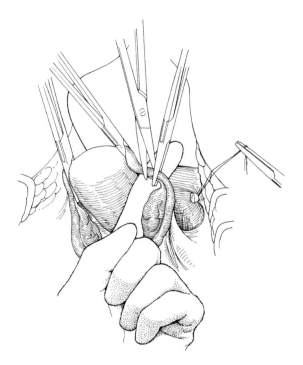

Figure 11.2 Cutting the ovarian ligament.

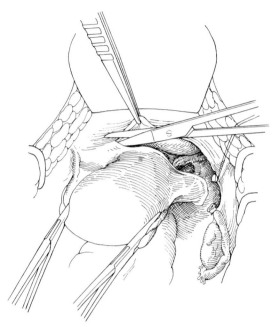

Figure 11.3 Incising the uterovesical fold.

index finger and a clamp applied directly to the vessels within the infundibulopelvic ligament. If the ovaries are to be preserved, the clamp is simply placed on the medial side of the ovary and the tube and ovarian ligament are cut.

Ligation of the round and ovarian/infundibulopelvic ligaments

It is useful to ligate these ligaments at an early stage in the procedure in order to leave the operative field as clear as possible. The pedicles may be stitch ligatured or simply tied, as is the editors' practice. The round ligament tie can be 'left long' and attached to a small Spencer Wells clip, thus maintaining tension on the peritoneum laterally and assisting in 'opening up' the lateral broad ligament space and providing improved access to the parametrial tissues. Note that a clip should never be left on a pedicle containing a blood vessel, such as the infundibulopelvic ligament.

Reflecting the bladder

It is logical to incise the peritoneum overlying the bladder along the line of the uterovesical fold at the same time as the round ligaments are divided. With the scissors in the surgeon's right hand and the assistant elevating the peritoneum over the bladder with a toothed forceps, it is very simple to run the scissors under the tented peritoneum, separating the bladder, and then to incise the peritoneum in a curved line across the front of the uterus to meet up with the round ligament on the opposite side (Fig. 11.3). If the level of the incision is too high, the peritoneum will not separate from the front of the uterus; if it is too low, bleeding will occur from the small vessels on the surface of the bladder.

Once this incision is complete, the bladder can be gently separated from the anterior surface of the uterus and then the cervix. The technique to achieve this manoeuvre will vary; the editors' preferred choice is to use the relatively blunt closed tips of the Monaghan scissors to gently push and occasionally incise the tissues attaching the bladder to the uterus. If the surgeon begins close to the midline and gently separates, staying close to the uterus and the cervix, a clean plane will be identified. A thin gauze swab over the finger may be used to push the angles of the

107

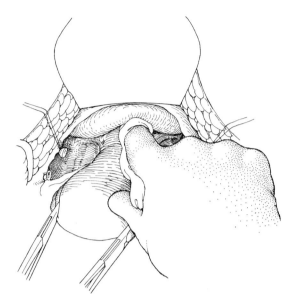

Figure 11.4 Separating the bladder.

bladder away from the cervix if preferred (Fig. 11.4). This entire process is assisted by the surgeon maintaining tension on the uterus by gently drawing it upwards using the clamps originally placed close to the cornu.

The lower limit of the cervix can be readily identified by observing the indentation and the longitudinal fibres of the vagina as the cervix ends and the anterior fornix begins. It is important to be sure that the lateral parts of the bladder are adequately reflected as the ureters are very close to the upper vagina at this point. If the patient has had a previous lower segment caesarean section, the dissection may be more difficult and will require significantly more sharp dissection in order to release the scar tissue; this sharp dissection is in fact less traumatic and fundamentally safer than blunt pushing of the tissues. Close attention should be paid to the tissue plane on the surface of the lower uterus and cervix, as this is the optimal and safest position for any sharp dissection.

If the uterus is a little immobile, it often helps if the surgeon puts his or her left hand into the pouch of Douglas, bringing the thumb around the uterus to the anterior part at the level of the junction between the corpus and the cervix; pressing the fingers of the left hand into the posterior fornix will cause the cervix to protrude forwards and the position of the anterior fornix becomes more obvious. The effect of this step is to make the application of clamps to the parametrium and the paracervical tissue easier as well as causing the bladder to drop 'below' the level of the cervix.

Clamping the uterine vessels and the vaginal angles
The uterine arteries arise from the anterior division of the internal iliac arteries deep in the lateral pelvis at the level of the obturator fossa. They then pass medially, overlying the ureter as it approaches the lateral part of the cervix. The artery divides close to the uterus at the level of the internal os into a descending and an ascending branch. The ascending branch, which is larger, runs close to the lateral sides of the uterus and can be seen as it passes in a tortuous fashion from below upwards, feeding small branches into the substance of the uterine corpus. This vessel is clamped by placing a pressure forceps with the tip abutting onto the myometrium at right angles to the long axis at the level of the isthmus (Fig. 11.5). The pedicle is divided as close to the forceps as possible. The same procedure is performed on the opposite side. A further forceps, ideally one with longitudinal ridges, such as the hysterectomy clamp, is now placed parallel to the cervix, squeezing the paracervical tissue off the side of the cervix. It is advantageous to incise on the medial side of the forceps before placing the one on the opposite side as this step reduces tension on the tissues, allows the forceps to be placed very close to the cervix and reduces the risk of the tissue sliding out of the forceps. This is particularly important if the cervix is bulky and access is limited. The forceps may be curved or straight (the editors prefer a slight curve as the forceps can be used to 'fit' the shape of the cervix to a very high degree). The forceps should be placed so as to reach the vaginal angles but should not include the tissue of the vaginal epithelium (Fig. 11.6). The tissue on the medial side of these forceps is now incised either with powerful scissors such as the Bonney or with a knife for greater accuracy.

An alternative is to open the vagina anteriorly first, extending the incision towards the angles and then inserting the anterior blade of the forceps in the vagina. Closing the forceps clamps the vaginal angle and uterosacral ligament together in the same clamp and avoids the need for a third clamp for the uterosacral ligaments as described below.

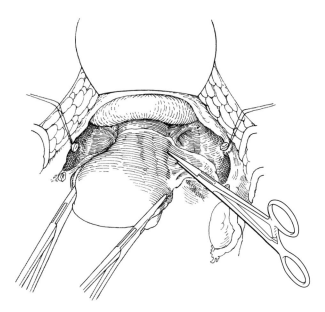

Figure 11.5 Clamping the uterine artery.

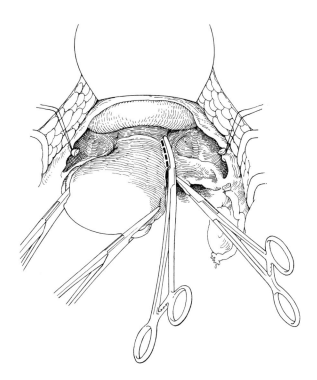

Figure 11.6 Clamping the parametrium.

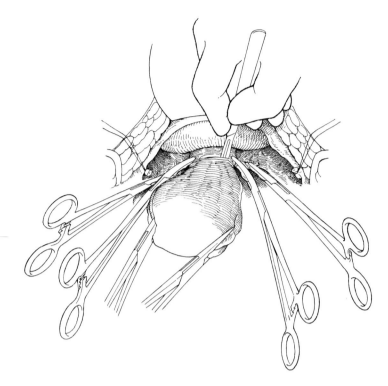

Figure 11.7 Incising the vagina (showing all clamps in place).

Clamping the uterosacral ligaments
It is not the editors' constant practice to clamp and divide the uterosacral ligaments. However, if the uterus is not mobile and is clearly bound down by contracture of these ligaments owing to scarring from previous endometriosis or infection then mobility can be advantageously achieved by clamping and cutting the ligaments using a curved hysterectomy or similar forceps.

Opening the vagina and removing the uterus
The surgeon should now draw up the uterus with the left hand and clearly identify the vagina using the techniques described above, making sure that the bladder is safely reflected. A knife is now plunged into the anterior fornix (Fig. 11.7), and then run to the right and to the left using the tips of the lowest forceps as the lateral landmark. The clamping of the uterosacral ligaments can take place at this point. This is done by passing the curved hysterectomy clamps backwards so that each blade comes to lie on either side of the vagina in the lateral part of the

posterior fornix. This has the effect of clamping the uterosacral ligaments close to their attachments to the posterior part of the cervix. The tissue in these last two clamps is incised and the uterus removed from the pelvis. The entire circumference of the vagina is now visible.

Ligating the lateral uterine and cervical pedicles
The two or three pedicles on either side are now stitch ligatured using a 1 Vicryl suture. It is important to obliterate any 'dead space' between pedicles as these may be or may become the site of troublesome bleeding in the intra- or postoperative period. Accurate placing of the sutures allows an overlapping technique to be used, obliterating any spaces.

Dealing with the vaginal edge
It is frequently recommended that the vaginal edge be grasped with a tissue forceps for identification and manoeuvring purposes. The editors recommend abandoning this technique and simply picking up the posterior edge of the vagina with the stitch that is to

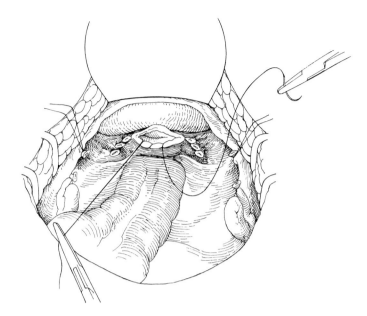

Figure 11.8 Suturing the vaginal edge.

be used to suture the vaginal edge. The long free end of the stitch can be grasped with a clip which is placed over the edge of the wound (Fig. 11.8) and used to place light tension on the vaginal edge, allowing the needle to be accurately placed as the edge is sutured circumferentially. Whether the vagina is left open or closed, this technique is simple and allows maximum access with minimal equipment in the wound. The excellent visibility can be further improved by adopting the following suture technique.

The posterior vaginal suture should be placed at approximately 5 mm intervals and the suture locked in a form of 'blanket' stitch. Once the angles of the vagina have been reached, carefully identified and sutured, the stitch should change to a 'rolling' pattern causing the edge to evert, thus making the inner edge of the vagina totally visible and accessible.

This part of the procedure can be performed without any active participation of the assistant. It has been the editors' practice to leave the vault of the vagina 'open', although there does not appear to be a great deal of evidence of the value of either 'open' or 'closed'. The advantages are that any unexpected bleeding will usually present early with vaginal bleeding and a pelvic collection can often be drained by gentle insertion of the index finger through the apex of the vaginal vault. The potential risk of bowel evis-

ceration has not been seen by the editors after routine hysterectomy, although it has been reported after robotic laparoscopic hysterectomy.

Closing of the abdominal peritoneum
The pelvis is finally checked. It has now become clear that there is no need to close the pelvic peritoneum and indeed there may be significant disadvantages. If the pelvic peritoneum is observed as the tension on the abdominal wall retractor is relaxed, it will be seen that the peritoneal edges lie close together transversely across the pelvis. All that is required is that the abdominal pack be removed and the sigmoid colon lain down into the pelvic cavity. It is superfluous to draw down the omentum as so many surgeons ritualistically do.

Drains should be only very rarely required following a hysterectomy if there is any concern regarding bleeding.

Closing the abdominal cavity.
This is described in Chapter 4.

Prophylactic antibiotics
Intraoperative antibiotics are the norm. It is important to be cognizant of any allergies and, to make sure that the manufacturer's time cover is observed, it may

111

be necessary to repeat the antibiotics if the surgery is unduly prolonged.

Variations in technique

There are many modifications to this technique. All surgeons should first learn a standard procedure from their chiefs and then, by dint of careful analysis and modification, develop their own 'style'. This analysis should take the form of constantly questioning the value of every move, determining whether the step can be eliminated or improved and made more efficient. This should always be with the aim of reducing tissue handling and improving patient recovery times.

Hysterectomy for a double uterus

The technique of hysterectomy for a double uterus does not differ materially from that for the single organ except in certain particulars. When two complete organs are present (uterus duplex), a pronounced fold of peritoneum exists (median raphe) which joins the bladder to the rectum in the middle line, separates the two corpora, and divides the uterorectal pouch into two lateral compartments. This fold should be divided by the same incision through the peritoneum that demarcates the anterior peritoneal flap, and the operator must make sure that the bladder is pushed well forward and the rectum well backward before proceeding with hysterectomy (Fig. 11.9).

With a double corpus and a single cervix (uterus bicornis unicollis) the fold may not be present.

In uterus duplex, the two cervices, although complete in themselves, are joined together by a block of tissue, which is continued downwards as a median vaginal septum. There is only one uterine artery to each half of a double uterus.

It is important to remember that uterine abnormalities are associated with urinary tract abnormalities and there may be duplex ureters or absence of ureters on at least one side. A preoperative intravenous urogram should be considered prior to surgery.

Subtotal hysterectomy

The editors have to declare that they do not see any indication or value in such a procedure. The recent

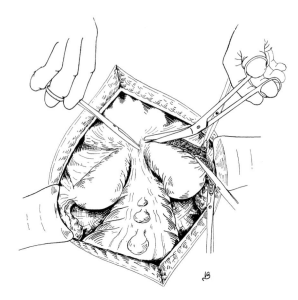

Figure 11.9 Hysterectomy for a double uterus: dividing the vesicorectal fold or median raphe.

fashion for this procedure is driven by a misguided belief that the procedure reduces the risk of post-hysterectomy prolapse and facilitates the orgasm, the evidence for which is lacking.

Vaginal hysterectomy

Although the main indication for vaginal hysterectomy is in the treatment of genital prolapse, it is a frequently used alternative to abdominal hysterectomy for other conditions. The objections to the procedure in the absence of prolapse have been on the grounds of limited access, but, with good technique, this objection can be overridden.

More practical relative contraindications are:
• a uterine size larger than the equivalent of a 12 week pregnancy
• endometriosis or pelvic inflammatory disease
• a narrow subpubic arch
• a long narrow vagina
• when it is essential that the ovaries are removed, such as in the management of corpus cancer (although vaginal hysterectomy may be the management of choice in grossly obese women).

Although a large uterus can be removed vaginally, either by splitting the uterus in two or by fragmentation of the uterus (morcellation), it is more simply managed abdominally. It is important that vaginal hysterectomy should be achieved simply and easily without considerable trauma or the need for excessive force. Endometriosis, or pelvic inflammatory disease, are sometimes encountered during the course of a vaginal approach and can usually be overcome, but, if diagnosed preoperatively, they generally indicate a preference for an abdominal approach. The last two relative contraindications (endometriosis and pelvic inflammatory disease) restrict access and render the vaginal route potentially difficult and more hazardous.

The indications for a vaginal hysterectomy other than for prolapse are usually benign, such as dysfunctional uterine bleeding or a small fibroid uterus. Premalignant conditions of the cervix, may, in the relatively rare circumstances when hysterectomy is indicated, be preferentially dealt with using the vaginal route. This is particularly important when there is a wide abnormal transformation zone, especially when it extends onto the vaginal fornices; in those circumstances when abdominal access may be difficult, increasing the risk of leaving behind premalignant tissue exists. Malignant conditions of the cervix when surgical treatment is chosen can be dealt with by the more radical vaginal procedures. However, the commonest indication for the use of vaginal hysterectomy is in patients with gross abdominal obesity in whom the production of an abdominal wound may render postoperative recovery more complex.

The advantages of vaginal hysterectomy over abdominal are that there is:
• no abdominal wound
• no transgression of the abdominal peritoneum
• no significant disturbance of the intestines
• usually less postoperative discomfort, easier mobilization and very commonly earlier discharge from hospital
• no risk of an abdominal wound infection.

The principles of the procedure

These are similar to those of abdominal hysterectomy. There are three main pedicles on each side of the uterus to be secured:

1 the cardinal and uterosacral ligaments
2 the uterine vessels
3 the tubo-ovarian, including the round ligaments.

The pelvic peritoneum is opened anterior to the uterus and posteriorly in the pouch of Douglas. Although in the past it has been reconstituted after removal of the uterus and strenuous attempts have been made to ensure that the pedicles are extraperitoneal, this is generally not now performed.

As with abdominal hysterectomy, care with the handling of the bladder and an observation of the position of the ureters must be made.

Instruments

Vaginal operations are more simply performed with two assistants, but this is not always possible and one assistant and the occasional help of a scrub nurse can be sufficient.

Although in the past narrow-bladed vaginal retractors have been used, it is the editors' preference to utilize a broad Sims speculum that can be further assisted by the use of right-angled vaginal retractors (Landon retractors). These retractors can be managed easily and it is important to instruct the assistants not to push too deeply with these retractors as this simply pushes the operative site further away from the surgeon.

The personal choice of suture materials varies enormously, with most clinicians preferring either Vicryl or Dexon. Some clinicians utilize simple pedicle needles; others clamp the tissues and then use stitch ligatures. It is the editors' preference to use cutting needles at all times in surgery, which some other experts would regard as anathema. Whatever system is used it is the accurate placing of sutures which is more important than the particular material or stitch system.

Preoperative preparation

This should follow the normal procedure for gynaecological operations. The patient is brought into hospital shortly before surgery, having had appropriate preoperative assessment performed. It is now standard to use antibiotics intraoperatively. The antibiotic cover should cover the full period of the surgical procedure. It is normally given intravenously at induction by the anaesthetist. It is not necessary to

113

perform extensive cleansing of the vagina and cervix prior to the patient coming to theatre.

Anaesthesia

The use of epidural or caudal anaesthesia either alone or in addition to a light general anaesthetic is helpful in reducing minor bleeding and is often used to relieve early postoperative pain. Simpler techniques such as the use of postoperative rectal analgesic suppositories will obviate the need for maintaining epidural catheters.

Vaginal hysterectomy, however, is an operation which lends itself perfectly to being performed under regional anaesthesia, which, once more, is an advantage for the grossly obese patient or the patient who has significant lung impairment.

Position

It is important that the normal lithotomy position is used with the patient's hips and knees hyperflexed, although some surgeons prefer having the patient's legs elevated and stretched out virtually straight. It is also very important to ensure that the patient's buttocks are right at the end of the table, but not hanging over, as, once more, this can make the performance of the surgery significantly more difficult.

The operation

As all patients should have emptied their bladder prior to being taken down to theatre, it is not necessary to perform catheterization at the beginning of the procedure. It is important to check the size and mobility of the uterus by performing a bimanual examination as this is an ideal opportunity to make sure there is no unexpected pathology.

Most surgeons use some form of subepithelial tissue infiltration. It is the editors' choice to use approximately 20 mL of bupivacaine with norepinephrine 1 : 200 000. This helps to define tissue planes and reduce minor bleeding. In order to facilitate this process, the cervix is grasped either by two Vulsellum forceps or by two Littlewoods forceps. The cervix is drawn down to put the vaginal tissues on tension and the infiltration is placed circumferentially approximately 2–3 cm above the cervical os into the soft tissues anterior to the bladder, around the cervix

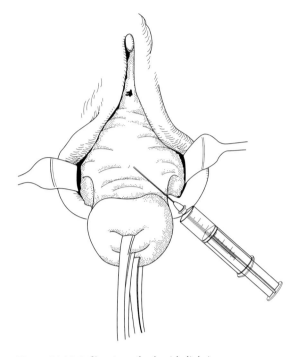

Figure 11.10 Infiltration of subepithelial tissues.

and into the soft tissues of the posterior fornix (Fig. 11.10).

The incision
The incision is carried circumferentially around the cervix over the area which had been infiltrated (Fig. 11.11). This incision may require development anteriorly into a teardrop shape if an anterior prolapse is present and correction of the prolapse is required. As the incision is made the infiltrate very clearly allows definition of the subepithelial layers and the epithelium is easily lifted up by a toothed forceps in the surgeon's left hand and, with angled scissors, the subcutaneous tissues can then be incised vertically down onto the anterior part of the cervix. It is important not to angle the scissors upwards as identification of the anterior surface of the cervix will make sure that no trauma occurs to the bladder base.

Division of the cervicovesical ligament
One of the assistants draws down the cervix using the attached tissue forceps. The surgeon lifts the anterior vaginal wall in his or her left hand with the toothed

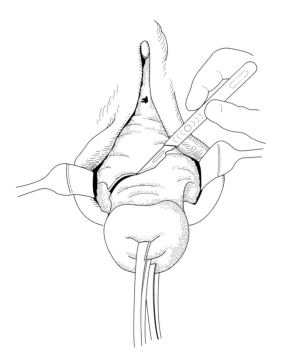

Figure 11.11 Incision around the cervix.

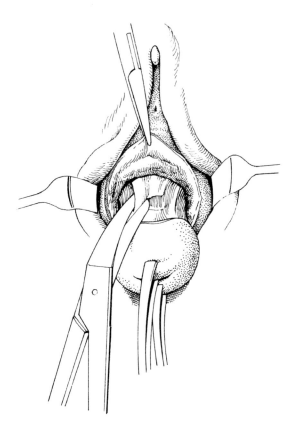

Figure 11.12 Division of the cervicovesical ligament.

dissectors and this allows definition of vertically running tissue (the cervicovesical ligament). This ligament is divided with Monaghan scissors (Fig. 11.12) and the bladder can now easily be deflected off the anterior part of the cervix using either the scissors themselves or blunt gauze dissection. It is the editors' preference to use the scissors which gently elevate the bladder, pushing it smoothly off the anterior part of the cervix. Usually, the uterovesical pouch of the peritoneum can be seen, but it may be necessary for the surgeon to insert his or her index finger to identify this sulcus, which can then be incised. The angles of the bladder can be gently elevated as this allows the ureters to be pushed upwards and outwards into safety.

Opening the pouch of Douglas
The cervix is now elevated and the forceps handed to one of the assistants and, once more using the tissue forceps in the left hand, the epithelium of the posterior fornix can be drawn down, putting the tissues behind the cervix on tension and, by boldly cutting up towards the back of the cervix, the pouch of Douglas is opened (Fig. 11.13).

Division of the cardinal and uterosacral ligaments
With the cervix drawn downwards and over to one side, the surgeon can now place his or her index finger of the left hand into the opening of the pouch of Douglas. Lying in front of this finger as it is drawn down will be the uterosacral and, anterior to that, the cardinal ligaments. These can be put on stretch tension by the left hand and a strong clamp placed over this pedicle (Fig. 11.14). This first clamp will include the uterosacral ligament and a significant part of the cardinal ligament. The tissues can be divided on the medial side of the clamp. It is important not to be overambitious and include too much tissue in this clamp as the risk of slippage is considerable and may generate a large number of postoperative problems. The clamp may be tied at this point using a stitch ligature technique (Fig. 11.15). The same procedure is performed on the opposite side and at this point, if the anterior peritoneum has not already been

115

BONNEY'S GYNAECOLOGICAL SURGERY

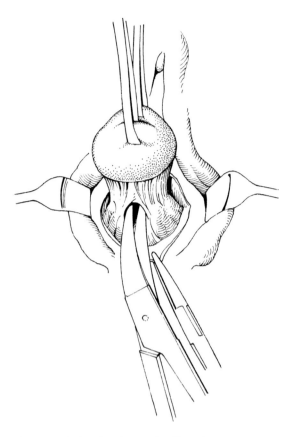

Figure 11.13 Opening the pouch of Douglas.

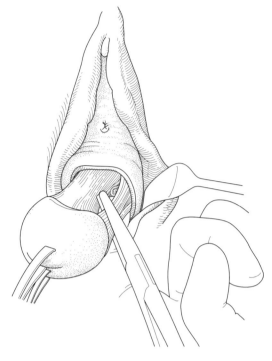

Figure 11.14 Clamping of the ligaments.

opened, it is possible to easily perform this procedure (Fig. 11.16).

Occasionally, a further clamp may be required to include the remaining part of the cardinal ligament and, at this point, the uterus is being gently drawn down to the introitus.

Division of the uterine vessels

The uterine vessels are now lying just above the last clamped pedicle. If the uterus is small, the descending branch of the uterine artery may already have been included in the last clamp. It is important to make sure that the next clamp to lie alongside the uterus will include the uterine vessels as they pass at right angles to the uterus and then branch and run up alongside the uterine body (Fig. 11.17). It is sometimes helpful to put the finger of the left hand behind

this pedicle to make sure that it is well identified and the softer area of the broad ligament noted above the clamp.

As mentioned earlier, if the uterus is normal in size it is usually possible to take the uterosacral and cardinal ligaments in one clamp and the uterine vessels in the next clamp. Although it is not the editors' practice, once the uterine vessels have been divided, they can be sutured together with the uterosacral and cardinal pedicles.

Division of the tubo-ovarian pedicles

All that remains supporting the uterus in the abdomen is the peritoneum of the broad ligament and the tubo-ovarian pedicles, which will include the round ligaments as well as the infundibulopelvic ligaments. At this point, the anterior part of the uterus may be delivered from the vagina, leaving the pedicles visible; this is known as Doderlein's manoeuvre. A firm clamp with longitudinally running grooves can be applied at this point (Fig. 11.18). Once the uterine side of the clamp has been divided, the opposite side clamp

116

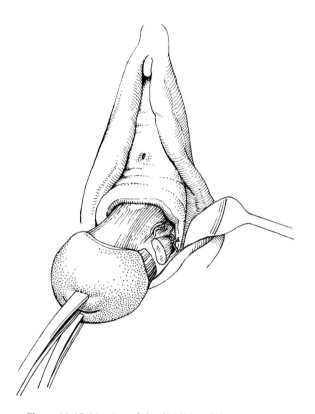

Figure 11.15 Ligation of the divided pedicle.

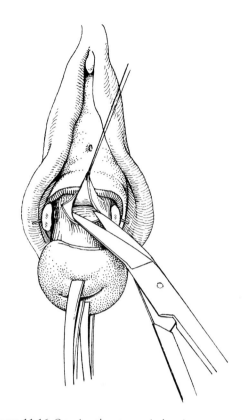

Figure 11.16 Opening the uterovesical peritoneum.

can be easily applied under direct vision. In other circumstances with a narrow vagina, it may be possible to remove the body of the uterus only once the pedicles have been completely divided. Once the pedicles have been divided, the uterus can be completely removed from the vagina, leaving behind only the long clamps which are holding the outer part of the ovarian and round ligaments. These are usually tied. Some surgeons would use a transfixion stitch at this point, but the danger of traumatizing small veins is significant and the editors prefer simply to tie with Vicryl.

Closure of the vagina

In the past, significant efforts have been made to draw together the various pedicles into a bunch at the top of the vagina with a view to reducing the risk of prolapse. There is no evidence of the value of this technique and, similarly, the meticulous closure of the

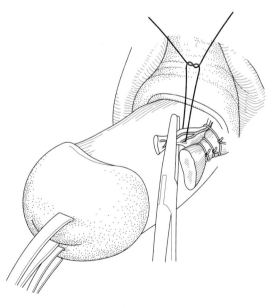

Figure 11.17 Ligation of the uterine vessels.

117

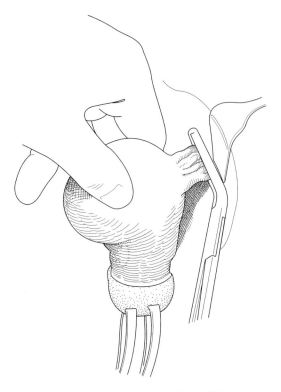

Figure 11.18 Clamping the tubo-ovarian pedicles.

peritoneal edges is also now no longer practised. All that is required at this point is to close the vaginal vault, which is normally carried out in an anteroposterior manner using a series of mattress sutures. A circumferential running suture leaving the vault open, as for the abdominal hysterectomy, can also be used. It is not normal to drain the retroperitoneal space and it has been the editors' practice to end the procedure by using an indwelling catheter for the first 12 hours postoperatively and a light vaginal pack soaked in acriflavine.

Complications

Complications are uncommon if the technique is meticulous. The commonest complication is that of a small haematoma above the vaginal vault, which at best may cause a mild pyrexia for a few days but at worst may cause a significant pelvic infection with marked morbidity.

Laparoscopic-assisted vaginal hysterectomy (LAVH)

The technique described is that developed in Gateshead in the early 1990s. The aim was to create a simple procedure that would not take much longer than a total abdominal hysterectomy and would guarantee the removal of the ovaries, which is not always possible at vaginal hysterectomy. The operation was used initially for benign pathology but became increasingly incorporated into the surgical management of gynaecological malignancies, especially in endometrial cancer where the women are often unfit and obese.

In the first 300 cases, the median operating time from commencing insufflation to completing the surgery was 60 minutes, with an interquartile range of 50–75 minutes and a range of 33–190 minutes.

Approach

The operation is performed with the woman in the lithotomy position. An 'in and out' catheterization is performed and, in patients with benign pathology, an intrauterine manipulator is inserted. A pneumoperitoneum with the intra-abdominal pressure at 15 mmHg is created following the insertion of a Veres needle. A 12-mm disposable trocar is inserted through an umbilical incision, followed by installation of the camera. After observation of the liver surface, pelvic organs and abdominal wall for spread of tumour and the presence of adhesions, two further 12-mm trocars are inserted 2 cm below and 8 cm lateral to the umbilicus. The course of the inferior epigastric artery is visualized prior to insertion of the trocar. An additional 5-mm trocar is inserted in the midline above the pubic symphysis if pelvic node dissection is intended.

Laparoscopic procedure

Peritoneal washings are carried out if required by instilling 20 mL of normal saline into the peritoneal cavity and aspirating the fluid using a 20-mL syringe.

The LAVH is performed by using an endoscopic stapling device; in most cases, two staples are used on each side, with the ovary and fallopian tube being drawn medially using the grasper. The first stapling device is applied to the broad ligament just lateral to the ovary to include the round ligament.

The uterovesical peritoneum is incised transversely at a point just above the upper border of the bladder using scissors. The bladder is reflected from the cervix by a combination of sharp and blunt dissection. The second set of staples is applied on each side from the apex of the initial staple line along the uterine body. This staple will frequently not include the uterine artery.

Vaginal procedure

The uterine excision is completed vaginally using the technique as described for vaginal hysterectomy. The cervix is grasped with two pairs of Vulsellum forceps and cervicovaginal tissue infiltrated with 20 mL of lidocaine with 1 : 200 000 norepinephrine. A circumferential incision is made around the cervix. The bladder is reflected away with a combination of sharp and blunt dissection until the peritoneal cavity is identified; the uterovesical peritoneum having been opened laparoscopically. The cervix is now pulled forward and the pouch of Douglas is entered. The cardinal ligament and the uterosacral ligament are clamped, divided and ligated. A straight clamp is applied to the remaining uterine pedicle to reach the edge of the staple with the aid of digital palpation. After the removal of the uterus, fallopian tubes and the ovaries, the vaginal vault is closed with interlocking stitches or left open with a running suture as with the abdominal hysterectomy. A urethral catheter and vaginal pack soaked in proflavine can be used if there is any concern regarding oozing.

Laparoscopic check

A final check is performed laparoscopically to confirm good haemostasis

Total laparoscopic hysterectomy

As the surgeon's laparoscopic skill set expands, so will the need to learn and undertake total laparoscopic hysterectomy. The application of this technique will allow the surgeon to radically expand the use of minimally invasive surgery in gynaecology. Patients with severe endometriosis, large leiomyomata uteri or pelvic inflammatory disease can now be managed using minimally invasive techniques.

The key components of the total laparoscopic hysterectomy that differentiate it from LAVH are:
• securing the uterine blood supply at both the proximal uterine artery as it branches from the internal iliac and the ascending branch of the uterine artery after it crosses over the ureter
• mobilizing the ureters
• transection of the uterosacral and cardinal ligaments
• circumferential incision of the vaginal cuff
• closure of the vaginal cuff.

Critical to successfully and safely completing this surgical procedure is an understanding of retroperitoneal anatomy. To begin, the peritoneum is incised over the psoas muscle using shears or the electrosurgical device of choice. Care should be taken to carry out this incision from the round ligament to just above the pelvic brim. The pararectal and paravesical spaces can easily be developed by using a probe or an argon beam coagulator. The key is to develop these spaces by moving the instrument right to left at right angles to the vessels, instead of parallel to the vessels. This move allows the surgeon to identify perforators from the iliac vessels to the midline structures. It also allows for easy identification of the ureters.

Once the ureter is identified, it is mobilized posterior to the ovarian vessels, which can then be transected. The medial leaf of the peritoneum is then grasped and the ureter dissected off laterally, down to the point it passes by the uterosacral ligament. In doing this, the ureter can quickly be traced to the point where it crosses under the uterine artery. At this point, the uterine artery and/or hypogastric artery can be clipped and proximal control of the pelvic vasculature secured. Once this has occurred, the likelihood of significant blood loss has been dramatically reduced.

Using argon beam coagulation or other energy sources, the bladder peritoneum can now be incised and the Gyne Tube (Paragon Imex Co., Menlo Park, CA, USA; see Fig. 21.12) placed into the vagina. This device serves multiple purposes, including distending the vagina; providing a ridge effect over which the bladder can be easily mobilized (the editors prefer using hydrodissection and argon beam coagulation at this point); and maintaining the pneumoperitoneum after anterior colpotomy. The vagina is then entered using argon beam coagulation and the anterior lip of the cervix grasped with a single-tooth tenaculum placed through the left lower quadrant 5 mm port site.

Countertraction on the cervix can be used to provide excellent exposure of the cervicovaginal junction, which can now be circumferentially incised along with the proximal cardinal and uterosacral ligament, using argon beam coagulation. At this point, the ascending branches of the uterine vessels will be stretched out with the ureters displaced laterally and posteriorly. The blood supply can now be secured with Endo-GIA staplers and a variety of energy sources, including the Gyrus PK device (Gyrus Inc., Southborough, MA, USA). The specimen is grasped and delivered vaginally with a single-tooth tenaculum passed through the diaphragm of the Gyne Tube device. The vagina is closed using an EndoStitch device with 0-Polysorb (Covidien Inc., Boulder, CO, USA). This closure is done by passing the suture through the posterior wall of the vagina and running the suture from back to front and back again, providing two layers of closure. Since adopting this method, we have had no cuff dehiscence, which has been reported to be occasionally associated with leaving the vagina open.

When undertaking hysterectomy for large leiomyomata, particularly when the uterus is 20-week size or greater, the most critical step is to learn how to identify, secure and transect the uterine artery at its point of origin as described above. Once the blood supply is secured and the vaginal cuff incised, the uterus can be morcellated with impunity, doing so vaginally or laparoscopically with a motorized morcellator such as that produced by Gynecare Inc. Care should be exercised so that all fragments of the morcellated fibroids are removed, as, if retained, they can cause infection, intestinal obstruction or, in rare cases, result in parasitic leiomyomatosis. The McCartney tube or Gyne Tube devices are ideal to place the cored fibroid fragments into, thereby minimizing the number of times the morcellator must be passed into and out of the abdomen.

A simpler method to complete a total laparoscopic hysterectomy with or without removal of the adnexa can also be utilized. This method does not allow one to secure the blood supply to the reproductive organs near its origin, and is not as safe when undertaking the resection of severe endometriosis as the ureters will not have been effectively mobilized lateral to the uterosacral ligaments.

The difference with this procedure is the fact that the retroperitoneum is not opened; instead, the ureter is visualized on the medial leaf of the peritoneum as it crosses over the pelvic brim and, after opening the avascular space of Graves, the ovarian vessels are then secured using either staplers or the bipolar energy source of choice. The round ligaments are then transected and the bladder flap developed as noted above. At this point, after inserting the Gyne Tube, the anterior colpotomy is created and, using either a Gyrus PK device or the Harmonic Scalpel (Ethicon Endosurgery Inc., Cincinnati, OH, USA), the vagina is circumferentially incised; when they are reached, the ascending branches of the uterine vessels are sealed or cauterized and transected, leaving the specimen to be delivered and vaginal cuff closed as previously described.

A word of caution – if the ureters are not dissected out as described previously, it is a mistake to apply Endo-GIA staplers parallel to the uterus or cervix in an attempt to secure the blood supply as the width of the stapler will inevitably lead to ureteral injury. If the blood supply is going to be secured in this manner then a smaller diameter bipolar instrument with minimal lateral thermal spread should be used. The Harmonic Scalpel and Gyrus PK device are two instruments that are appropriate for this.

Further reading

There are many textbooks and papers published describing the surgical techniques for hysterectomy by the various approaches. If there was one name which the editors would recommend to every trainee and gynaecological surgeon it would be that of Joel-Cohen. His writings always stimulate, and one can feel the enthusiasm exuding from the page.

Textbooks

Joel-Cohen SJ. *Abdominal and Vaginal Hysterectomy. New Techniques Based on Time and Motion Studies*. London: William Heinemann, 1972.

Journals

Bolger BS, Lopes T, Monaghan J. Laparoscopically assisted vaginal hysterectomy: a report of the first 300 completed procedures. *Gynaecol Endosc* 1997;6:77–81.

Nieboer TE, Johnson N, Lethaby A, et al. Surgical approach to hysterectomy for benign gynaecological disease. *Cochrane Database Syst Rev* 2009;(3):CD003677.

12 Uterine fibroids

Victor Bonney developed, in the course of his surgical career, a particular skill in dealing with fibroids in almost every site within the pelvis. In the original edition of this book, there were separate chapters for cervical fibroids, broad ligament fibroids, myomectomy and uterine fibroids complicating pregnancy. In this edition, the editors felt it more appropriate to describe the basic principles of surgery for uterine fibroids rather than providing extensive details on the surgery for every anatomical variation of uterine fibroids. The surgeon wishing greater detail on these procedures can review the previous editions of this book.

Uterine fibroids are the most common tumours in women, and are found in approximately 20–25% of women of reproductive age. They can occur as a single tumour but often are multiple.

Anatomical classification

• *Uterine body*
  – *subserosal myoma:* located just beneath the uterine serosa and generally growth occurs outward into the pelvic cavity; they may become pedunculated
  – *intramural myoma:* located within the muscular layer of the uterus, account for about 95% of fibroids

  – *submucosal myoma:* located just beneath the endometrial lining and generally growth occurs into the uterine cavity; they may become pedunculated.
• *Cervical:* located within the cervix, account for only 3% of fibroids.
• *Broad ligament:* located between the two layers of the broad ligament.

Symptoms

The majority of fibroids are small and asymptomatic. Symptoms include heavy and painful periods, pelvic pain, urinary frequency and constipation. They have also been noted to occur more frequently in women with subfertility, and retrospective studies have suggested the benefit of surgically removing fibroids to increase fertility.

Imaging

Ultrasound is useful in the detection and evaluation of uterine fibroids. MRI scans can be used for defining the anatomy of the uterus and may be helpful in planning myomectomy, or selective surgical removal of a fibroid.

Management

Surgery remains the mainstay of treatment for uterine fibroids; there is an increasing use of radiological

Bonney's Gynaecological Surgery, 11th edition.
© Tito Lopes, Nick Spirtos, Raj Naik, John Monaghan.
Published 2011 by Blackwell Publishing Ltd.

embolization, but this should not be used in women who wish to conceive.

Surgical management

Hysterectomy remains the most common surgical procedure for symptomatic uterine fibroids when retaining fertility is not an issue. For women wishing to conceive, myomectomy is the treatment of choice, with the laparoscopic approach being used for pedunculated and subserosal fibroids and the hysteroscopic approach for submucosal fibroids.

Hysterectomy for uterine fibroids

Approach

A uterus less than 12 weeks in size can often be removed vaginally, and, in experienced hands, this can be extended to a 14–16 weeks size uterus. Above 12 weeks the laparoscopic or open approach is more appropriate, but for a large uterus an open procedure is necessary.

Patient preparation

It is not the editors' practice to pretreat women with gonadotrophin-releasing hormone (GnRH) agonists prior to open hysterectomy. However, short-term use can result in a dramatic reduction in the total volume (up to 44% after 2 months of treatment), which can make the laparoscopic approach to hysterectomy feasible.

Abdominal hysterectomy

Incision
The surgeon should have a low threshold for using a midline incision for large fibroids. Surgery should be kept safe and straightforward, and adequate exposure to the pelvic sidewall is often crucial in these cases, justifying a vertical incision.

Orientation
The uterus can be markedly distorted by fibroids, and it is important that the surgeon identifies structures to allow orientation. The round ligaments, fallopian tubes and ovaries should be located; this may seem

logical, but it is surprising how difficult it may prove at times.

Healthy side first
With a difficult hysterectomy, the pelvic sidewall most easily accessed should be dealt with first. This is especially true with broad ligament fibroids affecting one side.

Vital structures
Despite the presence of fibroids, the hysterectomy can be straightforward, as described in Chapter 11. However, especially with cervical and broad ligament fibroids, this is unlikely and there is a high risk of injury to the ureters and uterine arteries and even the bladder. It is essential that every effort is made to identify these structures during the procedure.
- *Round ligaments.* These should be identified and divided, giving access to the pelvic sidewall.
- *Reflection of bladder.* If readily accessible, the uterovesical peritoneum should be divided at this stage to allow reflection of the bladder.
- *Ureters.* These should be visualized and if necessary mobilized away from any fibroids. If they cannot be identified at this stage, care must be taken until they have been located. With broad ligament fibroids, the ureter may be medial to the fibroid rather than lateral.
- *Ovarian vessels.* The ovarian vessels should now be clamped and divided; this will reduce the blood loss if a myomectomy is required and it should allow the ureter to be identified at its most consistent point, where it crosses over the bifurcation of the common iliac artery.
- *Uterine arteries.* The next step is to divide the uterine artery alongside the uterus, but this is often not possible because of the distortion. In this situation, it may be easier to ligate the uterine artery at its origin from the internal iliac artery or even ligate the internal iliac artery. Ideally, ligating the uterine arterial supply by any of these means should be performed before enucleating any fibroids as it will significantly reduce the blood loss.

Debulking
With a large uterus, debulking of the uterine mass should be performed by enucleating fibroids, bisecting the uterus, or performing an initial subtotal hysterectomy. Ideally, the uterine and ovarian vessels will

have been ligated prior to this step, but this is often not the case with the uterine vessels. The purpose of debulking the uterus is primarily to obtain access laterally to the pelvic sidewall and the vital structures there.

• *Enucleation.* When enucleating fibroids one should remove the largest, most accessible fibroid, which will result in greatest exposure laterally. These are often central when a vertical incision can be made over the bulge followed by identifying the plane between the fibroid and myometrium. The myomectomy screw (a large corkscrew instrument) is useful in holding and manoeuvring the fibroid. If adequate access is not obtained then the next largest fibroid should be removed.

The surgeon should be prepared for blood loss at this stage if the uterine arteries have not been ligated. For this reason, once the decision has been made to enucleate the fibroids, it should be deliberate and rapid. Access to and ligation of the uterine arteries should be performed once they are accessible.

At this stage with reasonable access and control of bleeding, the ureters should be identified, if this has not been possible previously, before removing any broad ligament fibroids and completing the hysterectomy.

• *Uterine bisection.* This technique is used more often with the vaginal approach to hysterectomy, but it is useful to access large intramural fibroids in the lower uterine segment or cervix.

• *Subtotal hysterectomy.* With large fibroids involving the uterine body, it is simple to remove the uterine body with the fibroids, making it much simpler to remove the cervix.

Myomectomy

The name of Victor Bonney will always be associated with the development of myomectomy so as to preserve uterine function. He demonstrated that fibroids could be removed, the uterus preserved and successful pregnancies achieved.

The sole purpose of myomectomy is to retain and improve fertility; it should never be used as a surgical exercise, nor to preserve the uterus in the mistaken belief that such an act will maintain the femininity or sexuality of the woman.

Submucosal fibroids are ideally excised hysteroscopically. Subserosal and pedunculated fibroids are readily removed laparoscopically, but intramural fibroids will invariably require an open approach.

Open myomectomy

Patient preparation
As with hysterectomy the patient can be pretreated with GnRH agonists prior to surgery to reduce the size of the fibroids.

Incision
The surgeon must assess the most appropriate incision for the size of the uterus and location and size of the fibroids.

Haemostasis
Various techniques have been developed to reduce blood loss during the procedure, which can be excessive.

Mechanical
• *Bonney myomectomy clamp.* Bonney devised a paracervical clamp with which he could temporarily cut off the blood supply to the uterus (Fig. 12.1). It is applied across the uterus at the junction between the body and the cervix, softly occluding the uterine arteries as they pass up the lateral side of the uterus.
• *Uterine and ovarian tourniquet.* Recently, the use of temporary tourniquets across the ovarian vessels and a further ligature around the ascending branches of the uterine vessels has been described.
• *Temporary atraumatic vascular clamp.* A simple technique used by the editors is to open the pelvic sidewall and apply an atraumatic vascular bulldog clamp on both internal iliac arteries and the vessels medial to the ovaries. At the end of the procedure, these can be removed with no harm to the blood supply to the uterus.

Vasopressin and other agents
The injection of dilute vasopressin (20 units in 50 mL of normal saline) into the stalk of a pedunculated fibroid or the bed of a subserosal fibroid will further decrease the blood loss during the myomectomy procedure. This solution can also be injected close to the origin of the ascending uterine artery bilaterally, taking care not to inject it intravascularly. If the procedure exceeds 30 minutes, the injection may be repeated.

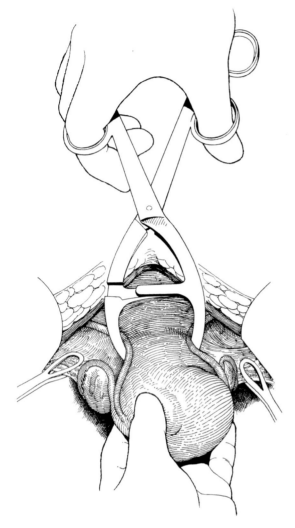

Figure 12.1 Bonney myomectomy clamp applied to the lower uterus.

A recent Cochrane review suggested that use of misoprostol, bupivacaine plus epinephrine, tranexamic acid, and chemical dissection with sodium-2-mercaptoethane sulphonate (mesna) may reduce blood loss during myomectomy.

Incision of uterus
The lower an incision is made in the uterus, the stronger will be the subsequent scar. A single midline incision should be used whenever possible, but invariably the optimal incision for a solitary fibroid is over the greatest bulge produced by it.

Removing the fibroid
The 'false capsule', the junction between the fibroid and normal myometrium, should be identified and, with a combination of blunt and sharp dissection, the fibroid can be 'shelled' out. When removing multiple fibroids, the surgeon should avoid multiple incisions of the uterus and avoid entering the endometrial cavity.

Obliterating the cavity
The cavity should be obliterated methodically using interrupted Vicryl sutures, in layers until the space is obliterated, and the serosal surface should be repaired with interrupted sutures.

Further reading

Victor Bonney never had children, his wife having had a hysterectomy soon after they were married for uterine fibroids. In his professional life he was an advocate for conservative surgery despite his reputation for radical surgery for cervical cancer. He was a doyen of myomectomy for uterine fibroids, performing over 700 cases in his professional life. The original edition of his textbook, which can be downloaded from the Internet, had several chapters on myomectomy.

Berkeley C, Bonney V. *A Text-book of Gynaecological Surgery*. London: Gassell & Co., 1912. See www.archive.org/details/textbookofgynaec00berkuoft
Bonney V. The fruits of conservation. *J Obstet Gynaecol Br Emp* 1937;44:1–12.
Chamberlain G. The master of myomectomy. *J R Soc Med* 2003;96:302–304.

Cochrane reviews

Griffiths AN, D'Angelo A, Amso NN. Surgical treatment of fibroids for subfertility. *Cochrane Database Syst Rev* 2006;(3):CD003857.
Kongnyuy EJ, Wiysonge CS. Interventions to reduce haemorrhage during myomectomy for fibroids. *Cochrane Database Syst Rev* 2009;(3):CD005355.

13 Operations on the fallopian tubes

Extrauterine gestation

Ectopic pregnancy remains a common cause of pregnancy-related death and is the most common direct cause of maternal mortality in early pregnancy in the UK. In the 2003–5 triennium, there were 32 100 ectopic pregnancies in the UK; these resulted in 10 deaths, seven of which were judged to be associated with substandard care.

The management of the collapsed patient exsanguinating from a ruptured ectopic pregnancy must be immediate, and relies on an experienced team of a gynaecologist, anaesthetist and haematologist with an early recourse to laparotomy. However, for the majority of cases, sensitive urinary and serum β-HCG tests and transvaginal ultrasound scanning have improved the possibility of early diagnosis. Up to 70% of all ectopic pregnancies will resolve spontaneously, and the majority of the remaining 30% can be managed medically.

The incidence of ectopic pregnancy is 11 : 1000 pregnancies, and this figure has remained static since 1994. Most (95%) ectopic pregnancies are located in the fallopian tube, with 55% being in the ampulla and 2–4% being cornual/interstitial. Other rarer sites are cervical, ovarian and abdominal implantation.

Aetiology

Ectopic pregnancy is a condition which has no single aetiological factor. Women at higher risk are those who:

- have a previous history of ectopic pregnancy
- have a previous history of pelvic infection
- have had previous surgery to the fallopian tubes, particularly sterilization procedures and reconstructive surgery
- have had assisted reproductive techniques
- have an intrauterine contraceptive device *in situ*
- become pregnant while taking progestogens, e.g. the progesterone-only pill or emergency contraception (Levonelle)
- have congenital malformations of the fallopian tubes or uterus.

Symptoms

Thirty per cent of ectopic pregnancies present before a period has been missed. Pain in the lower abdomen is usually the first symptom, and this can occur in either the iliac fossa or centrally. Vaginal bleeding, if it occurs, is often slight. There may be a missed period and signs of pregnancy. Diarrhoea and vomiting are atypical symptoms which should be remembered.

If the pregnancy has ruptured, bleeding can be profuse with features of shock.

Signs

There may be some lower abdominal tenderness and, if bleeding has occurred, there may be signs of peritonism. Vaginal examination may reveal cervical excitation or a tender fullness in one adnexum. However, many now recommend against vaginal examination when a transvaginal scan is available as it is said to add nothing to the clinical picture and may aggravate the bleeding.

Bonney's Gynaecological Surgery, 11th edition.
© Tito Lopes, Nick Spirtos, Raj Naik, John Monaghan.
Published 2011 by Blackwell Publishing Ltd.

Differential diagnosis

The proper diagnosis may be confused with a threatened miscarriage, appendicitis, salpingitis or complications of ovarian cysts.

Investigations

The most useful investigations are a transvaginal scan combined with quantitative assessment of HCG levels.

Surgical management

The indications for surgery are:
- *haemodynamically unstable patient*: immediate surgery indicated to stop the intraperitoneal bleeding
- *severe abdominal pain*: suspected tubal rupture
- *live tubal ectopic pregnancy*: high risk of rupture
- *large complex adnexal mass*: with significant free fluid and moderate to severe abdominal pain
- *patient not suitable for methotrexate (MTX)*: abnormal LFTs, U&Es, active lung/liver/kidney disease or the patient is unable to attend for follow-up
- *recurrent ectopic pregnancy of the same tube*: increased risk for further ectopic pregnancy, although not an absolute contraindication
- *patient's choice*: e.g. family complete
- *known severe tubal damage*: high risk of recurrence.

In the shocked patient, an immediate laparotomy should be performed to control the bleeding. Intravenous resuscitation is undertaken at the same time but should not delay surgery.

In the haemodynamically stable patient, a laparoscopic approach should be used in preference to an open approach. There is no significant difference in future ectopic or successful pregnancy with either approach, but the laparoscopic approach results in less operative blood loss and analgesic requirement and a shorter hospital stay, and convalescence and costs are less. A cornual or non-tubal pregnancy should be managed by laparotomy.

When the contralateral tube is healthy a salpingectomy should be used in preference to a salpingotomy. A salpingotomy should be considered as the primary treatment when managing tubal pregnancy in the presence of contralateral tubal disease and the desire for future pregnancies.

Where the tube has been preserved (salpingotomy/ 'milking' of the tube), there is a small risk (3–20%) of persistent trophoblastic activity and follow-up testing of the serum β-HCG level should be arranged weekly until it is <25 iu/L.

Emergency laparotomy

Opening the abdomen
The patient is anaesthetized quickly, the abdomen is cleansed and draped and a midline subumbilical incision is made. The peritoneum usually has a bluish tinge owing to the blood in the peritoneal cavity. As soon as the peritoneum is incised, blood and clots may pour out. Do not waste time mopping them away.

Stopping the bleeding
The surgeon should immediately reach into the abdomen and grasp the uterus with the left hand, bringing it up into the wound if possible. Squeezing the broad ligament adjacent to the uterus on the affected side compresses the ascending branch of the uterine artery, reducing the blood flow.

Identifying the source of bleeding
As the uterus is elevated, it is usually immediately apparent where the bleeding is emanating from. If the whole tube is involved, a total salpingectomy will be necessary. Rarely will a tubal abortion produce a massive bleed, but, if it has, when the contents of the tube have been milked out it may be possible to preserve the entire tube. If the bleeding is due to rupture close to the uterine part of the tube, it may be necessary to run a mattress suture into the substance of the uterine muscle in order to stem the flow.

Surgical procedure
The different surgical procedures are described later.

Peritoneal toilet
After the tubal operation has been performed, it is important to remove all blood from the peritoneal cavity, especially that which has tracked up into the paracolic gutters. Tilting the patient head-up will result in any blood in the upper abdomen draining into the pelvis for aspiration.

Closure of the abdomen
The abdomen is closed as described in Chapter 4, without drainage.

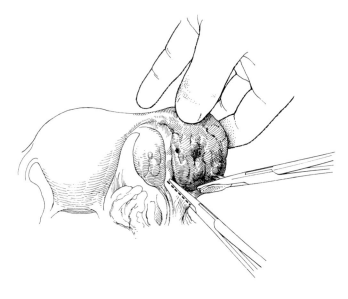

Figure 13.1 Total salpingectomy for a tubal pregnancy.

Salpingectomy

Having identified the source of the bleeding, the tube and its contents are elevated and separated from the ovary. Tissue forceps should now be applied serially along the mesosalpinx near the tube, as shown in Fig. 13.1. The tube is progressively removed using Monaghan scissors as each forceps is applied. Each forceps is stitch ligatured and complete haemostasis achieved.

Partial salpingectomy may be carried out if only a short section of the tube is involved. This procedure is useful where *in vitro* fertilization is unavailable as it allows the chance of later tubal surgery to achieve function in the future; the forceps are placed as shown in Fig. 13.2.

Laparoscopic salpingectomy can be performed using various techniques to divide the mesosalpinx such as mono- or bipolar diathermy, other energy sources, endoscopic staples or pre-tied ligatures. Endoscopic staples, although more expensive, allow rapid excision and control of a bleeding ectopic.

Conservation of the fallopian tube

Conservative surgery for ectopic pregnancy should adhere to microsurgical principles, avoiding trauma by gentle handling and constant irrigation, and maintaining meticulous haemostasis.

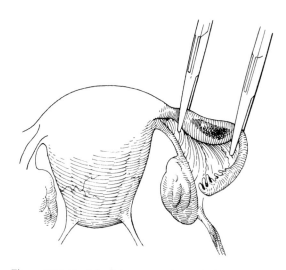

Figure 13.2 Partial salpingectomy for a tubal pregnancy.

Salpingotomy

When the fallopian tube has been fully mobilized, the surgeon steadies the tube in his or her left hand and a linear incision is made on the anti-mesenteric border over the length of the swelling (Fig. 13.3). The material contained within the tube is then extruded or gently scraped out with the scalpel handle. Bleeding points are carefully ligated as diathermy may damage the tube. Injecting the mesosalpinx with vasopressin

127

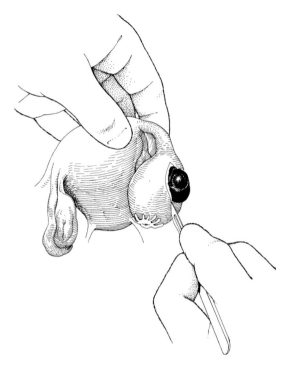

Figure 13.3 Removing an ampullary tubal pregnancy with conservation of the tube.

prior to the procedure reduces the blood loss. The tube is left to heal by secondary intention as primary closure has not been shown to be of benefit. Meticulous peritoneal toilet is then performed and the abdomen closed.

Laparoscopically, the anti-mesenteric incision can be made with scissors, needle diathermy or other energy sources.

Fimbrial expression (milking of the tube)
Milking of the tube is appropriate only if the trophoblastic tissue is already aborting through the fimbria. This is associated with an increased risk of persistent trophoblastic tissue and recurrent ectopic pregnancy.

Operative management of an intra-abdominal extrauterine pregnancy

In the very rare circumstances of this diagnosis being made, it is important to perform a laparotomy as soon as possible after the patient and the operating theatre have been fully prepared. Blood should be readily

available, the anaesthesia should be of the highest quality, and, if there is any prospect of extracting a viable child, full paediatric staffing is mandatory.

The operation
The abdomen must be opened with great care as the placenta may be attached to any intra-abdominal structure. Omental adhesions are also very common. A large incision to give good access is essential; the subumbilical midline incision is recommended. If the placenta is attached to the anterior abdominal wall, it is important to undersew large vessels and to try and choose a relatively avascular area to gain access to the abdominal cavity.

The fetus is delivered and the cord clamped and cut close to the placenta. It is important to resist the temptation to try to separate the placenta from surrounding structures as this can be disastrous. The placenta and the membranes will be absorbed once the fetus is delivered.

Operations on the fallopian tubes for female sterilization

In many parts of the world it has become commonplace for both men and women to choose some permanent form of contraception once they have achieved their optimal size of family.

Preoperative counselling is of utmost importance, and evidence of the discussions held with the patient, highlighting relevant points, should be clearly documented within the medical case notes. Also, it is imperative that consent forms detail the principles and pitfalls of the procedure. The editors also recommend obtaining an intraoperative photographic record of the appliances accurately placed on each fallopian tube for storage within the case notes and potential future use. Despite these recommendations, sterilization procedures remain a major cause of medical litigation.

In women, techniques to obstruct the fallopian tubes are the most popular. Methods available include:
• total salpingectomy
• ligation of the tube
• laparoscopic-controlled diathermy and cutting of the tube
• laparoscopic-controlled application of metal or Silastic clips and Silastic rings to the tubes

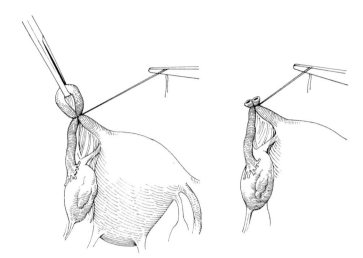

Figure 13.4 Ligation and resection of the fallopian tube.

• resection of a portion of the tube and tying or burial of the ends.

Resection of the fallopian tubes

This procedure is rarely performed except when there is evidence of unilateral tubal infection or ectopic pregnancy. It is not recommended as a sterilization technique.

Ligation of the fallopian tube

This simple procedure consists of grasping the tube close to its midpoint, elevating it and tying a ligature around the tube and the mesosalpinx (Fig. 13.4). A variation of the technique is to resect that part of the tube contained within the ligature, taking care not to cut too close to the ligature. This technique, which forms the basis of the Pomeroy operation, has the major disadvantage that it carries an unacceptably high failure risk, as the tubes have a tendency to recanalize after the ligature has been absorbed.

Laparoscopic methods

The technique of laparoscopy is described in Chapter 5. The ease with which the tubes can be visualized and manipulated has virtually eliminated the need to perform open tubal ligation procedures.

After introduction of the laparoscope and an additional trocar/introducer into the abdominal cavity, various appliances can be used to perform the tubal occlusion procedure.

Shortly after the first use of laparoscopy, there developed a great vogue for diathermy of the tubes and resection of the diathermied area. Although this technique has been successfully used to sterilize many thousands of women, it is potentially dangerous and has been superseded by the application of tubal occlusion devices to the tubes using applicators specially designed for this purpose.

The devices include the Falope-Ring, which is a small Silastic ring that is applied by drawing the fallopian tubes up into a hollow applicator and then releasing the ring from the end of the applicator so that the ring lies firmly around the loop of tube. These techniques carry the same disadvantages as the Pomeroy operation.

The Hulka and Filshie clips are small locking devices which are applied to the tubes using special applicators; if applied appropriately, they will seal the tubes completely. Despite common practice, it is not recommended that the clips be applied in pairs to each tube because of the potential risk of a symptomatic hydrosalpinx developing between the two clips.

The material of which all these devices are constructed is inert and the devices remain with the patient for the rest of her life; however, on occasion, following fibrosis of the surrounding tissues, they can dislodge from the fallopian tubes and can be seen lying within the pouch of Douglas.

It is said that the advantage of these mechanical obstructive devices is that they damage only a small portion of the tube so that it is relatively straightforward to reconstruct the tubes in the future, giving a realistic prospect of pregnancy. The editors would stress that it should not be the policy of any doctor to recommend sterilization techniques on the basis that they may be reversed; all patients embarking on a sterilization operation must do so in the knowledge that the procedure is permanent.

Operations for correction of infertility

Significant advances with *in vitro* fertilization (IVF) in recent years have largely left tubal reconstructive procedures to the history books. During their time, however, these techniques were masterly performed by their advocates, resulting in many pregnancies and the joy of motherhood for innumerable women.

Many of these advocates now strongly support the use of IVF, as few indications remain for tubal surgery. Those indications that do remain include adhesiolysis for minor adhesions involving the distal segment and fimbrial end of the tube, and reversal of sterilization in young women (less than 35 years) in whom the sterilization was performed using techniques that preserved the majority of the tube, i.e. Filshie or Hulka clips, as described above.

Adhesiolysis can often be performed laparoscopically depending on the severity of the condition. However, full use of microsurgical techniques is usually best achieved through an adequate transverse suprapubic incision. If IVF is planned and hydrosalpinges are present, current recommendations are that the patient should be offered salpingectomy, preferably by laparoscopy. Alternatively, proximal tubal occlusion should be considered.

As a result of IVF, tubal surgery is no longer a procedure for every gynaecologist and is limited to a number of specialists in tubal surgery with the appropriate equipment available to maintain an adequate service. A detailed description of the assessment and selection of patients, the surgery involved and the postoperative care can be obtained from the previous edition.

Further reading

Ectopic pregnancies

Lewis G (ed.). *The Confidential Enquiry into Maternal and Child Health (CEMACH). Saving Mothers' Lives: Reviewing Maternal Deaths to Make Motherhood Safer – 2003–2005.* The Seventh Report on Confidential Enquiries into Maternal Deaths in the United Kingdom. London: CEMACH, 2007.

Tubal surgery

National Institute for Health and Clinical Excellence. *Fertility: Assessment and Treatment for People with Fertility Problems.* NICE guideline no. 11. London: NICE, 2004.

Pandian Z, Akande VA, Harrild K, Bhattacharya S. Surgery for tubal infertility. *Cochrane Database Syst Rev* 2008;(3):CD006415.

Siassakos D, Syed A, Wardle P. Tubal disease and assisted reproduction. *Obstet Gynaecol (Lond)* 2008;10:80–87.

14 Operations on the ovaries

Ovarian cysts are said to be the fourth most common gynaecological cause for hospital admissions. They are classified as non-neoplastic functional cysts such as follicular or corpus luteum cysts, or neoplastic cysts. Their ratios vary with age but approximately:

- 25% are functional cysts
- 40% are benign cystadenomas
- 15% are dermoid cysts (benign)
- 10% are endometriotic cysts
- 10% are malignant cystadenocarcinomas.

The rapid development of ultrasound technology and its increasing use in routine medical practice has led to an increased diagnosis of ovarian cysts in women of all age groups. In premenopausal women, the majority of lesions are benign functional cysts which usually disappear with menstruation or can be managed conservatively by suppression of ovulation with the combined oral contraceptive pill. Persistent cysts or those suspicious of malignancy require surgical removal. In recent years, there has been an increasing use of the laparoscope for assessment and removal of adnexal cysts thought to be benign in nature.

Diagnosis of an ovarian mass

The normal ovary is usually palpable in the premenopausal woman but barely palpable in the postmenopausal one. Consequently, almost any enlargement should be looked upon with suspicion and warrants

Bonney's Gynaecological Surgery, 11th edition.
© Tito Lopes, Nick Spirtos, Raj Naik, John Monaghan.
Published 2011 by Blackwell Publishing Ltd.

further investigation. Transvaginal sonography is the investigation of choice not only in the detection of the ovarian cyst but also in the initial assessment of potential malignancy. Features such as multiple loculi, solid areas, papillae, thickened septae and bilateral lesions are indicative of potential malignancy, as is an increased blood flow on Doppler studies. In these cases, an abdominal ultrasound scan should also be performed to assess the upper abdomen (liver, omentum and para-aortic lymph nodes) for evidence of malignant spread.

The determination of serum levels of the tumour marker CA-125 is also useful in differentiating benign from malignant cysts, especially in the postmenopausal woman. The editors use the ultrasound findings combined with a serum CA-125 level and menopausal status to calculate the Risk of Malignancy Index (RMI) to try and differentiate benign from malignant lesions. Those with an elevated RMI of >200 are at increased risk of malignancy (70% will be malignant) and are managed by gynaecological oncologists, whereas those with an RMI <200 may be managed by the gynaecologist. Over 90% of primary ovarian malignancies can be identified using this simple method. A new marker, HE4, has been evaluated and may be incorporated with CA125 in the future as a more sensitive discriminator.

Surgery

The role of surgery for an ovarian cyst is its removal and histological diagnosis. In women under 40 years of age, benign cysts should be managed using ovary-preserving procedures, but above that age an oophorectomy may be more appropriate. If there is doubt about the nature of the cyst, frozen section of the cyst should be undertaken.

Laparoscopic surgery has become the gold standard in the treatment of benign ovarian masses in many centres, with laparotomy being reserved for the treatment of malignant tumours. In cases of unsuspected ovarian cancer managed laparoscopically, definitive surgery/staging procedures should be undertaken by a specialist gynaecological oncologist within 2–3 weeks and the trocar sites should be excised as part of the procedure because of the potential of port site implants. With careful preoperative assessment and appropriate selection of cases, the situation should arise infrequently.

The principles of laparoscopic surgery for ovarian cysts are similar to those at open surgery, but the approach and technique differ and have been described in Chapter 5.

Ovarian cystectomy

Victor Bonney gave this name to the procedure whereby the cyst is removed without compromising the function of the ovary. For ovarian cystectomy to be successfully carried out, the mass to be enucleated must have a capsule, which is a characteristic of most benign tumours.

The procedure should always be considered in young women in whom ovarian preservation is to be desired, particularly when the cysts are bilateral and total loss of the ovaries would produce a premature climacteric.

The operation (laparotomy)

Opening the abdominal cavity
This is described in Chapter 4. The decision to use either the transverse or the longitudinal incision will obviously depend on the size of the ovarian cyst and whether there is any possibility of the tumour being malignant. If there is any likelihood that the mass is malignant, a vertical incision must be carried out.

Exploration of the abdomen
The examination of the entire abdominal cavity is meticulously performed as described in Chapter 4, together with the collection of washings from the peritoneal cavity. If there is any free fluid in the abdomen, its presence should be recorded and sent for cytology. Washings are best carried out by instilling 50 mL of normal saline into the pelvis and along the paracolic gutters and then collecting the fluid using a large syringe. It is not unusual to find a small quantity (20-50 mL) of fluid in the peritoneal cavity in association with benign lesions.

Extraction of the enlarged ovary
If the cyst is large, it is easily delivered from the wound; if the cyst is relatively small, or the tubes and infundibulopelvic ligaments are resistant, the procedure can be performed within the abdomen, using a self-retaining retractor to give adequate access and carefully packing away the bowel to avoid contamination in the event of cyst rupture.

Incising the ovary over the cyst
It is often possible to identify the edge of the normal ovarian tissue running along the lower part of the ovary. If this is so, the knife should be lightly run along this line (Fig. 14.1); the plane of cleavage will

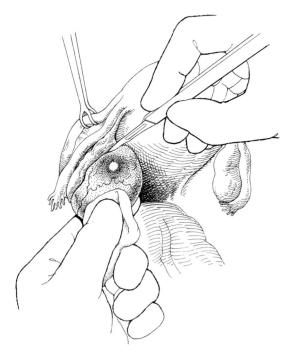

Figure 14.1 Incising the ovary over an ovarian cyst.

readily become apparent and should now be developed using blunt dissection either with the handle of the scalpel, or, as the editors prefer, with Monaghan scissors, using the blunt points to separate and develop the plane.

Carrying the incision further around the cyst
The cyst is gently peeled back from the normal ovarian tissue (Fig. 14.2) until all that is left is a thin strip of normal ovary which is cut with the scissors.

Repair of the remaining ovarian tissue
Usually, there is a thin rim of redundant capsule which should be resected back to the thicker normal ovarian stroma. The edges of the ovarian tissue are brought together using fine interrupted monofilament sutures.

Use of anti-adhesive agents
As discussed in Chapter 3.

Abdominal closure
The ovary is returned to the abdomen and the wound closed as described in Chapter 4.

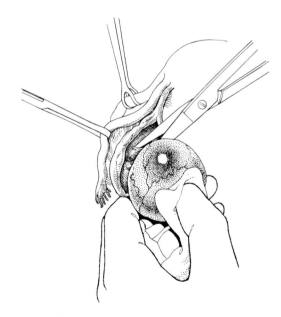

Figure 14.2 Removing the ovarian cyst intact.

The operation (laparoscopy)

Insertion of trocars
Unless contraindicated, a 12-mm trocar is inserted into the umbilicus either following insufflation using a Veres needle or by an open technique. The laparoscope is inserted and inspection of the pelvis and upper abdomen made. If laparoscopic surgery is feasible then two further 5-mm trocars are inserted either side of the lower abdomen for instrumentation; occasionally, a further suprapubic port may be necessary. Using a 5-mm laparoscope increases the flexibility as it can be inserted into any port.

Exploration of the abdomen
This is identical to the open approach, and washings should also be taken for cytology. If there is any suspicion of malignancy, a biopsy should be performed and the operation abandoned with referral to a gynaecological oncologist, or, if appropriate, converted to a laparotomy.

Incising the ovary over the cyst
Using laparoscopic scissors and forceps an attempt is made to find a plane of cleavage to remove the cyst intact. For large cysts and where there is difficulty finding a plane, the cyst may be punctured and the fluid aspirated. This should be performed in an Endobag inserted through the umbilical port to avoid leakage into the peritoneal cavity. The cyst lining is examined for any areas suspicious of malignancy and, if there is none, the cyst wall is excised. Haemostasis is obtained and there is often no need to repair the ovary.

Removal of the ovarian cyst
The ovarian cyst is placed in an Endobag and removed through the umbilical port, which may need to be extended or the cyst aspirated in the bag before removal.

Port closure
The port sites are closed in layers.

Removal of a retroperitoneal cyst

The majority of retroperitoneal (or broad ligament) cysts are ovarian cysts which have grown retroperitoneally. This is more likely to occur after hysterectomy

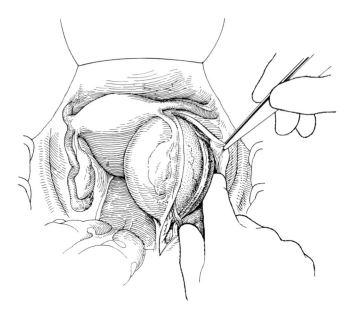

Figure 14.3 Opening the peritoneum and identifying the ureter.

with ovarian conservation when the ovaries frequently become retroperitoneal structures. Occasionally, one is dealing with a pseudocyst and no capsule will be identified. Left-sided lesions can be particularly problematic as the retained ovary and cyst can find itself buried under the sigmoid colon.

The exact position of the ureter will vary depending on the size and extent of retroperitoneal extension of the cyst, stressing the vital importance of identifying the ureter at an early stage in the procedure and following it for the full length of its course across the cyst. Clear identification and separation of the ureter will remove the most important danger in this procedure.

The operation

Identification of the cyst
Having opened the abdomen as described in Chapter 4, the cyst is palpated and its limits defined.

Opening the peritoneum and identifying the ureter
The safest area to open the peritoneum is between the fallopian tube and the round ligament. The peritoneum is lightly incised and the edges picked up (Fig. 14.3). The incision is now curved posteriorly so that, by separating between the cyst and the lateral pelvic

sidewall using the fingers, the ureter can be isolated as it courses in the peritoneum over the cyst. Usually, the plane of cleavage is easily found and the cyst is rapidly circumnavigated.

Enucleation
If the cyst is not ovarian in origin, it usually shells out without great difficulty, but if it has burrowed below the uterine artery this can be sacrificed together with small veins which lie in the same position. If oozing does occur, tissue must not be blindly clamped; the best technique is to gently insert a swab into the space and wait for 2 minutes, taking care to inform the scrub nurse that a swab has been inserted and is marked up. When the swab is removed the whole field is dry and the small bleeding points can be identified and ligated or diathermied. If the cyst is ovarian in origin one can perform either a cystectomy or oophorectomy.

Cutting away redundant peritoneum
After the cyst or ovary has been removed and haemostasis secured, no attempt is made to repair the pelvic peritoneum.

The abdomen is closed in the manner described in Chapter 4.

Further reading

Michel Canis from Clermont-Ferrand, France, has one of the largest experiences in laparoscopic surgery for adnexal masses, and has published widely on the subject.

Bailey J, Tailor A, Naik R, *et al.* Risk of malignancy index for referral of ovarian cancer cases to a tertiary center: does it identify the correct cases? *Int J Gynecol Cancer* 2006;16:30–34.

Canis M, Botchorishvili R, Manhes H, *et al.* Management of adnexal masses: role and risk of laparoscopy. *Semin Surg Oncol* 2000;19:28–35.

Canis M, Rabischong B, Houlle C, *et al.* Laparoscopic management of adnexal masses: a gold standard? *Curr Opin Obstet Gynecol* 2002;14:423–428.

Jacobs I, Oram D, Fairbanks J, *et al.* A risk of malignancy index incorporating CA 125, ultrasound and menopausal status for the accurate preoperative diagnosis of ovarian cancer. *Br J Obstet Gynaecol* 1990;97:922–929.

Moore R, McMeekin D, Brown A, *et al.* A novel multiple marker bioassay utilizing HE4 and CA125 for the prediction of ovarian cancer in patients with a pelvic mass. *Gynecol Oncol* 2009;112:40–46.

Royal College of Obstetricians and Gynaecologists. *Ovarian Cysts in Postmenopausal Women.* RCOG guideline no. 34. London: RCOG, 2003.

15 Caesarean section

Although caesarean section is now regarded as a 'safe' procedure for both mother and child, it should be remembered that it was not until 1793 that James Barlow working in a Lancashire town managed to carry out the procedure with subsequent survival of the mother. However, until anaesthesia had developed sufficiently the procedure was no more than a heroic method of trying to terminate an obstructed and doomed labour.

It is extremely important that all obstetricians carefully study the details of this procedure, particularly the features that can improve its safety, as caesarean section remains an important cause of maternal morbidity and mortality. Despite dramatic reductions, one of the most common complications associated with caesarean section mentioned in the 2007 *Report on Confidential Enquiries into Maternal Deaths in the UK*, covering the period 2003–2005, is thrombosis.

Despite the additional risks over vaginal delivery, the rates of caesarean section have increased dramatically in recent years, from 12% in 1990 to 24% in 2008 with no improvement in outcome for the baby. There are many reasons for this increase, which will not be addressed in this text. Maternal request for caesarean section, however, is currently not considered sufficient reason or indication in itself and, in such cases, the mother should be wisely informed of the merits of avoiding surgical delivery.

The Confidential Enquiry into Maternal and Child Health (CEMACH) reports continue to provide valuable and contemporary information on maternal mortality and have greatly contributed to the improvements in safety associated with surgical delivery. All trainee and specialist obstetricians should be guided by their recommendations and advice.

The National Institute for Health and Clinical Excellence (NICE) has, in recent years, provided a comprehensive document relating to caesarean section. This document and the associated algorithm is a culmination of many years of research and investigation into the indications, preparations and techniques associated with surgical delivery. The CORONIS trial, which is currently ongoing, is expected to provide useful answers relating to controversial areas of surgical technique including:
- blunt versus sharp dissection for abdominal entry
- exteriorization of the uterus for repair
- single-layer versus double-layer closure of the uterine incision
- catgut versus polyglactin for uterine incision repair
- closure versus non-closure of parietal and visceral peritoneum.

Lower segment caesarean section

This procedure is the standard method for the surgical removal of the fetus from the uterus. The lower segment of the uterus is that lower part of the anterior

Bonney's Gynaecological Surgery, 11th edition.
© Tito Lopes, Nick Spirtos, Raj Naik, John Monaghan.
Published 2011 by Blackwell Publishing Ltd.

uterine wall which is covered by the loose peritoneum of the uterovesical sulcus or pouch.

The lower uterine segment incision has become accepted as the standard approach because it has certain distinct advantages over the classical operation:
• The lower segment is less vascular than the upper part of the uterus.
• The risk of rupture of the uterine scar in subsequent pregnancies is greatly reduced.
• Postoperative complications such as ileus and peritonitis are much reduced.
• The risk of adhesions and postoperative obstructions is greatly reduced.
• As the incision is made in a relatively inactive part of the uterus, haemostasis is easily achieved and healing occurs readily.
• In those cases in which there is already infection present, the lower segment operation markedly reduces the risk of contamination for the remainder of the peritoneal cavity.

Instruments

The instruments included in the gynaecological general set described in Chapter 3 are required with the addition of a Doyen curved retractor and four large Green Armytage tissue forceps.

Patient preparation

Anaesthesia during delivery is potentially extremely dangerous; the risks of inhalation of gastric contents are significant. If this problem arises, the damage to lung tissue by the acid gastric fluid may result in Mendelson's syndrome, a potentially lethal pneumonitis. It is, therefore, vital if the patient is to have a general anaesthetic that steps are taken to reduce this risk. Two procedures may be effective: the first is to give antacids and H2 receptor antagonists before induction; the second is that all patients must have endotracheal intubation.

It is now commonplace to use epidural analgesia in labour with an epidural catheter *in situ* that can be 'topped up' as required. This technique has significant advantages as the patient is still conscious and retains her cough reflex, therefore reducing the risk of inhalation of vomit. The 'block' can also be rapidly and conveniently extended if an emergency caesarean section has to be performed.

Prophylactic antibiotics have also been shown to significantly reduce the risk of postoperative infective morbidity, and should be given immediately prior to the procedure commencing.

Anaesthesia

There is little doubt that the risks of general anaesthesia are far greater than those of local techniques, including epidural and spinal analgesia. The advantages of having a patient with her cough reflexes intact is considerable at a time of high risk of vomiting and inhalation problems.

The induction of a safe general anaesthetic in a pregnant woman at term, especially after a prolonged labour, can be a major test of skill for even the most experienced of anaesthetists. Intubation is often difficult and may be time-consuming, whereas the risks of performing the procedure without intubation are enormous and of the severest gravity. Delay in performing the operation may also seriously jeopardize the fetus owing to anoxia or complications arising from those indications that led to caesarean section. Finally, a significant contributory factor to the problems which may occur during caesarean section will be the relative inexperience of both the surgeon and the anaesthetist. It is thus of vital importance that the obstetrician is confident of his or her role in this procedure and allows the anaesthetist to perform his or her task without impedance or interference.

Syntocinon is traditionally given by the anaesthetist at the time of delivery of the fetal head. The syringe containing 5 units of Syntocinon must be drawn up and available before the procedure is commenced.

The operation

Preparation and catheterization
The anaesthesia for the mother and fetus should be light and for as short a period as possible. To this end, the vulva and vagina should be cleansed and the bladder catheterized prior to induction of a general anaesthetic. The surgeon then completes his gowning while the patient is anaesthetized; he is then ready to begin the operation as soon as the patient enters theatre.

Opening the abdomen
The choice of incision is between a subumbilical midline and a low transverse Pfannenstiel incision.

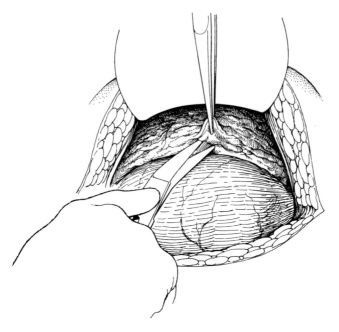

Figure 15.1 Reflecting the peritoneum over the lower uterine segment.

The decision should be based upon the speed of entry into the abdomen that is required.

For most caesarean sections and probably for all elective procedures, the Pfannenstiel incision has considerable advantages. The wound heals rapidly, it is relatively comfortable in the postoperative period, it is not unsightly, the risk of ventral hernia is low and rupture is rare.

The subumbilical midline incision should not be totally dismissed. It is simple and quick and is often the incision of choice when a placenta praevia is present or when the uterus has been the site of previous surgery, such as myomectomy or classical caesarean section.

The midline incision should not be extended too far into the hair-bearing area, as this does not improve access, may cause unnecessary bleeding and is often very uncomfortable when healing.

It is also important not to 'cross' incisions as the site of the crossing often heals badly owing to damaged blood supply and may be the site of an irritating and persistent infection.

The length of the incision is usually from the line of the pubic hair to 1 cm below the umbilicus in the midline and 10–12 cm long for the Pfannenstiel.

The abdomen is opened as described in Chapter 4 with special care being taken to avoid the bladder

when the midline incision is used as it may be drawn upwards by the growth of the uterus. The peritoneum should be incised in the upper part of the wound.

Packing around the uterus
In the past it was common practice to pack off the bowel around the edge of the uterus to prevent soiling of the abdominal cavity by liquor. With increasing use of epidural and spinal analgesia this has been abandoned as it causes discomfort. Any fluid can be aspirated or gently removed with swabs after delivery when the uterus has contracted and access to the pelvis and abdomen is easier. If packs are used they should be marked with large forceps attached to the tapes which lead out from the abdomen. The insertion of the packs is recorded on the swab count board.

Reflecting the peritoneum over the lower segment
The curved Doyen retractor is now inserted into the lower end of the wound so that easy access is obtained to the lower segment (Fig. 15.1).

It is important not to pick up the peritoneum overlying the uterine segment too close to the uterine attachment as the peritoneum does not separate easily and troublesome bleeding will occur. If the peritoneum is picked up using toothed dissectors at the correct level, it will immediately begin to separate from the underlying lower segment (Fig. 15.2). The fold is incised and carried laterally towards the round ligaments on either side. The index fingers of each hand are then inserted into the fascial plane, which is revealed, and the bladder is completely separated from the lower segment along this relatively avascular plane (Fig. 15.3). The ureterovesical angles are separated and dislocated laterally and downwards, rendering the incision into the lower segment safe.

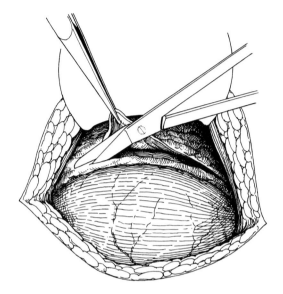

Figure 15.2 Incising the uterovesical fold.

Incising the lower segment
The lower segment is now incised by stroking gently with the knife over a length of approximately 2–3 cm. The amniotic sac frequently bubbles through like an inner tube on a thin bicycle tyre if the membranes are still intact, or the hairs on the head of the fetus become visible as the lower segment thins.

The surgeon inserts the index fingers of each hand into the incision, which is extended laterally so that the presenting part can be delivered from the wound (Fig. 15.4). It is preferable to use the fingers for this separation rather than to cut the lower segment with scissors as the fingers push the uterine vessels to one side rather than cut them.

Delivery of the presenting part
When the incision in the lower segment is complete the Doyen retractor is removed and the presenting part delivered. If the head presents, the surgeon will insert the hand below the head to disimpact it from

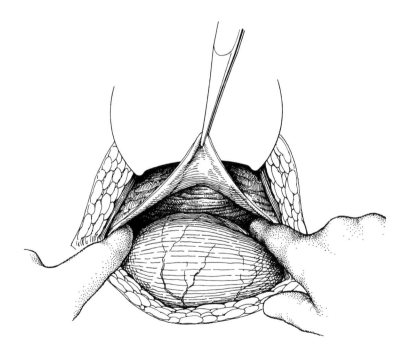

Figure 15.3 Separating the bladder from the lower segment.

139

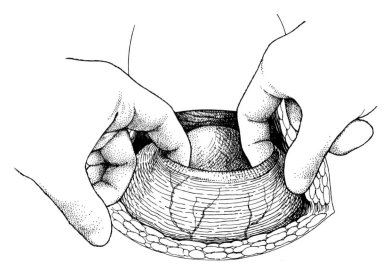

Figure 15.4 Extending the lower segment incision.

the pelvis. Release of atmospheric pressure will ease this process; the assistant applies fundal pressure when the head is brought into the incision and the fetal head delivered.

Once the head is delivered, the respiratory passages are cleared of mucus, blood and liquor. It is at this stage that the anaesthetist gives the patient the Syntocinon (5 units) intravenously. The use of forceps are rarely required for delivery and should not be used routinely.

If the presentation is breech, the arms may be delivered by the Lovset manoeuvre and the head then follows. Care should be taken to maintain flexion by jaw traction when necessary.

The cord is then clamped and cut and the newborn passed to the paediatrician in attendance.

Removal of the placenta

The placenta and the membranes are now removed. If the uterus is contracting normally following injection of the Syntocinon, then traction on the cord together with fundal pressure will usually deliver the placenta from the wound. The membranes should be grasped with a sponge holder and gently drawn out, taking care not to tear them and leave fragments within the uterine cavity. If the uterus is soft and placental separation has not quickly occurred, then manual removal may be necessary, but this should not become the preferred method of removal; if the surgeon exercises patience and deals with

blood loss from the wound by applying the Green Armytage forceps he or she will not encounter many problems.

Controlling the bleeding

The abdominal wound can now be held open by inserting a Balfour self-retaining retractor. Blood and clots mixed with liquor are now scooped out of the lower segment by the surgeon and the assistant, enabling the identification of the edges of the lower segment. The Green Armytage forceps are then attached to the lateral edges of the lower segment incision anteriorly and posteriorly so as to gently occlude the most common and significant sites of haemorrhage (Fig. 15.5).

Suturing of the uterine wound

In previous editions it was recommended that the uterine cavity be explored and blood removed; this procedure was also accompanied by dilatation of the cervical os in elective sections so as to improve drainage. These procedures should be avoided as they increase the risk of infection with no benefit to the patient.

The Green Armytage forceps are now gently elevated and the extreme corners of the wound clearly identified; the uterine lower segment is sutured in two layers using a continuous absorbable suture material. It is important to insert the first stitch a short distance lateral to the corner of the lower segment incision in order to be sure of achieving haemostasis at the angles. Although it is impossible to identify two separate layers, the surgeon should close the lower segment (Fig. 15.6a) and then oversew the line of sutures with a continuous stitch (Fig. 15.6b). A small amount of

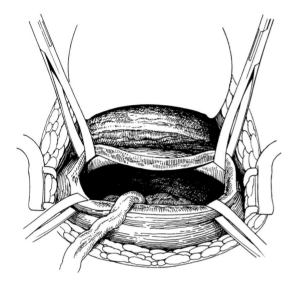

Figure 15.5 Attaching Green Armytage forceps to the lateral edges of the lower segment wound.

ooze will often respond to pressure for a few minutes, or the application of a hot pack to the suture line.

Suturing the lower segment peritoneum
There would appear to be no value in suturing the lower segment peritoneum and it may, therefore, be left to heal spontaneously.

Peritoneal toilet
The abdominal pack, if used, is now removed and the abdomen inspected to make sure that all clots and amniotic fluid have been removed. This procedure also allows for a full inspection of the pelvic and abdominal viscera, particularly the ovaries.

Closing the abdomen
The closure is performed as described in Chapter 4.

Cleansing the vagina
This procedure is important following caesarean section as the surgeon must know that the vagina was empty at the end of the procedure in order that he can assess any blood loss that may occur in the postoperative period. The vagina should be mopped out using a swab either on a sponge holder or on the surgeon's finger. The uterine fundus should also be gently pressed to be certain that it is contracting and

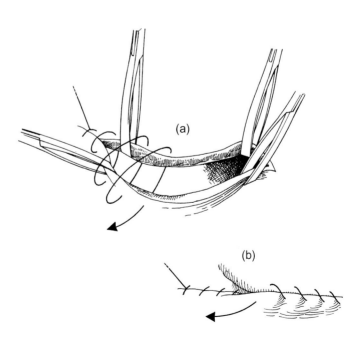

Figure 15.6 (a and b) Suturing the lower segment in two layers.

also to remove any retained clots, which are then cleared from the vagina.

Complications and dangers of lower segment caesarean section

Injury to the bladder

If the surgeon finds difficulty in identifying the uterovesical junction, then there is considerable danger of entering the bladder. The simplest safeguard that can be taken is to be certain that the bladder is emptied immediately before the operation and to follow the recommendations for identifying the loose uterovesical fold as described earlier. Rarely, a part of the bladder may become loculated owing to pressure of the presenting part obstructing proper drainage; this is unusual and should be recognized as the abdomen is opened.

Damaging the uterine artery and veins

If the lower segment incision is made too large and particularly if the incision is extended not with the fingers but with scissors, there is a danger of rupturing the uterine vessels, producing heavy loss of blood. Experience and practice will allow the surgeon to judge the ideal length of incision for the average fetus; occasionally, problems will arise if the presenting part is unusually large. In these circumstances, the surgeon must carefully extend the incision to an appropriate size.

Excessive haemorrhage

In most circumstances, a lower segment incision in labour will be virtually bloodless. However, occasionally haemorrhage can be torrential and life-threatening. Even small amounts of bleeding can impede the surgeon's view and increase risks of damage to the surrounding viscera and the fetus. If the surgeon operates smoothly and rapidly, using broad haemostatic clamps such as the Green Armytage and takes care not to damage large vessels by clumsy technique, haemorrhage can be kept to an acceptable level. If large single bleeding vessels are isolated, the use of mattress sutures is recommended as these do not cut out and will be a more certain way of stopping haemorrhage than single sutures or attempted ties.

The most dangerous areas when dealing with haemorrhage are the angles of the incision; blind suturing at these points will greatly endanger the ureters. It is for this reason that the editors recommend early identification of the angles and clamping with the haemostatic Green Armytage clamps.

Damage to the fetus

This usually takes the form of accidentally incising the skin of the scalp when the lower segment is opened; the surgeon must be cautious, cutting the lower segment over a short distance only and then extending the incision with the fingers.

Classical caesarean section

There are few indications for the use of this technique; they include:

• transverse lie with the fetal back presenting over the pelvis
• as a preliminary to caesarean hysterectomy
• as a preliminary to treating carcinoma of the cervix, whether by surgery or by radiotherapy
• when there has been a previous classical section and the scar is dangerously thinned and would be best treated by resection of the scar and resuture
• when a cervical fibroid obstructs access to the lower segment
• when the surgeon, through inexperience, is unhappy about coping with a placenta praevia with large lower segment vessels.

Preparation, anaesthesia, Syntocinon, instruments and position of the patient are as for the lower segment procedure. However, it may, depending on the circumstances, be sensible to have cross-matched blood arranged.

The operation

Opening the abdomen

A vertical midline subumbilical incision is used; care should be taken to avoid the bladder, which may frequently be drawn well up the abdominal wall. Opening the peritoneum in the upper part of the incision will avoid this problem.

The incision

The uterus is carefully checked to be certain that it is not rotated, a large gauze abdominal pack can be inserted on either side and the tapes marked with a clip. An incision approximately 10 cm long is now made in the anterior surface of the uterus, which may extend into the lower segment. The incision should be made quickly as considerable haemorrhage may occur from the uterine muscle. However, care should also be exercised as the risk of cutting the fetus is greater in this procedure.

Bleeding may be further enhanced if the placental site lies beneath the incision; a careful estimate of the blood loss must be made and replaced if excessive.

Delivery of the fetus
The leg of the fetus is grasped and delivered, enabling the body and then the head to be delivered; the umbilical cord is clamped and cut between pressure forceps.

Extraction of the uterus
It may be valuable to draw the uterus out of the abdomen to lie above the level of the abdominal wound although this should not be performed as a matter of routine. This is easily done by hooking the index finger into the cavity of the uterus and elevating it out of the wound. The packs placed alongside the uterus will control the bowel, although if the abdominal wound has been made an appropriate size it will fit snugly around the uterus.

Removal of the placenta
This is removed as described in the lower segment procedure.

Suturing the uterus
As the uterus has contracted down after delivery of the fetus and under the influence of the Syntocinon bleeding will have reduced. The uterine wound is now closed using a single layer of interrupted sutures followed by a layer of continuous suture using Dexon or Vicryl. Occasionally, oozing continues from the needle holes even when modern atraumatic needles are used; this problem is best dealt with by applying either pressure for a few minutes or a hot pack to the bleeding site.

Peritoneal toilet
The packs are removed and the uterus returned to the abdomen; any clots or amniotic fluid are carefully removed, and the abdomen inspected as described under lower segment caesarean section.

Closure of the abdomen
This is as described in Chapter 4.

Emptying the vagina
The vagina is carefully cleansed at the end of the procedure as described in the lower segment procedure.

General complications of caesarean section

Haemorrhage

In general, haemorrhage is much reduced as soon as the uterine musculature begins to contract; thus, it is important to deliver the fetus expeditiously so that contraction of the uterine muscle may occur. Occasionally, bleeding will occur from the uterine wound as isolated spurting vessels; these should be underrun with single mattress sutures or lightly clamped with the Green Armytage forceps until the edge can be sutured. Usually, suturing the wound is all that is required to control all haemorrhage.

If bleeding persists from the placental site, the uterus should be massaged and a second injection of Syntocinon (5 units) given.

In some departments, 'cell salvage' is used routinely for all elective caesarean sections as the disposables are inexpensive and heterologous transfusions avoided.

Infection

There is always a risk of infection in any abdominal procedure; if the operation is performed under emergency circumstances, the risk increases. A further complicating factor is the length of time the patient has been in labour; it is not unusual for a caesarean section to be the culmination of a long and stressful labour. The tissues are congested and bruised, there have been many vaginal examinations, the bladder has been catheterized, and the membranes have been ruptured for a long period of time. Thus, it is not surprising that infectious morbidity is a common postoperative development.

Intraoperative antibiotic prophylactic antibiotics should be standard in all caesarean sections.

The surgeon must also remember that, in spite of the need for speed in an emergency, his attention should not be taken away from the need to observe the strictest aseptic techniques in both the preparation for and the carrying out of the procedure.

Rupture of a previous uterine scar

This rare complication occurs most frequently in patients who have had previous caesarean sections, but it can also occur in those patients who have had a hysterotomy, plastic procedures on the uterus or previous myomectomy.

There is no doubt that the risk is much greater following a classical caesarean section, the relative rarity of this procedure accounting for the marked rarity of rupture at the present time.

Rupture may be acute and catastrophic, presenting with a moribund patient and a dead fetus; more commonly, rupture may be relatively silent, being discovered at second or subsequent section as a 'windowing' of the previous scar with the membranes ballooning through the gap. The scar is usually avascular, so bleeding is often not a problem.

Pain during the pregnancy or in labour is an ominous sign and should not be ignored. Pain during labour that is becoming resistant to a previously effective epidural anaesthetic is particularly ominous, and should warn the obstetrician that there may be danger in persisting for a vaginal delivery.

Surgical techniques for massive postpartum haemorrhage

CEMACH reports consistently warn of the dangers of massive postpartum haemorrhage and the need for prevention, early detection and prompt and effective management before the patient becomes moribund through excessive blood loss. Delivery suites should have well-rehearsed protocols and procedures in place to deal with these life-endangering emergencies. A number of surgical and non-surgical techniques have become invaluable in such circumstances and the attendant surgeon should be proficient with all available options including use of bimanual compression and uterotonics such as ergometrine and prostaglandins.

The use of hysterectomy to control massive haemorrhage should be a last resort, but should not be delayed to the point of desperation when culminating disseminated intravascular coagulation has superseded all reasonable options. It is imperative that the anaesthetist is experienced and alert and should be allowed sufficient time to order blood and blood products, including fresh frozen plasma, platelets, cryoprecipitate and factor VIIa, by the use of holding measures to control blood loss, including bimanual compression in order to maintain adequate circulation and clotting for the subsequent performance of the techniques described below.

Despite a lack of randomized controlled trials, a recent meta-analysis has shown excellent outcomes following massive postpartum haemorrhage with the use of uterine balloon tamponade; uterine compression sutures, including the B-Lynch suture; and pelvic devascularization methods, including internal iliac artery ligation, arterial embolization and arterial balloon occlusion.

Other than the B-Lynch suture and internal iliac ligation, these techniques will not be described further within this text; trainees and specialists are advised to familiarize themselves with these methods and, in particular, ensure a collaborative working relationship with the interventional radiologist for when such circumstances arise.

The B-Lynch suture was described by Christopher B-Lynch in 1997 and the technique is briefly described here; readers are referred to the original publication for a more detailed description.

The B-Lynch suture

With uncontrolled bleeding at caesarean section the uterus is evacuated of its contents and bimanual compression is performed to assess the potential success of insertion of the bracing suture. A firm Vicryl suture with a round-bodied needle is used to enter the uterus from 3–4 cm below and lateral to the right edge of the lower segment incision. The needle then emerges 3–4 cm above and lateral to the right edge of the incision and then travels over the uterine fundus 3–4 cm from the uterine cornua. The needle is reinserted into the uterine cavity from the posterior uterine wall on the right side at a level corresponding with where it emerged from the uterine cavity anteriorly. The stitch then re-emerges from the uterine cavity via the posterior wall at a corresponding level on the left side, from where it travels over the uterine fundus on the left side and reinserts into the left side of the uterus and out again mimicking the path of the suture on the right side. The stitch is then tightened anteriorly below the uterine incision, aided by manual compression of the uterus to prevent injury to the uterus by the suture length. The uterine incision is then repaired.

Additional sutures can be placed into the uterine bed as required to deal with individual vessels prior to tightening of the B-Lynch suture.

Internal iliac ligation

The pelvic pulse pressure can be reduced by up to 85% with bilateral internal iliac ligation. Access to the internal iliac arteries is described elsewhere in the text (see Chapter 21). Either the internal iliac artery or preferably its anterior division can be ligated at the pelvic sidewall. Caution needs to be exercised as the space behind the artery is developed because the iliac veins lie in close proximity. The space is developed either with Monaghan scissors or Meigs–Navratil forceps using an opening and closing technique as it is gently pushed through to develop the space. A Vicryl tie is then placed into the open ends of the Meigs forceps and pulled through and around the iliac artery from where it can be tied. The manoeuvre is repeated on the contralateral side.

The technique is rarely associated with pelvic pain and buttock ischaemia.

Further reading

B-Lynch C, Coker A, Lawal AH, *et al*. The B-Lynch surgical technique for the control of massive postpartum haemorrhage: an alternative to hysterectomy? Five cases reported. *Br J Obstet Gynaecol* 1997;104:372–375.

Lewis G (ed.). The Confidential Enquiry into Maternal and Child Health (CEMACH). *Saving Mothers' Lives: Reviewing Maternal Deaths to make Motherhood Safer – 2003–2005*. The Seventh Report on Confidential Enquiries into Maternal Deaths in the United Kingdom. London: CEMACH, 2007

National Collaborating Centre for Women's and Children's Health. *Caesarean Section*. Commissioned by the National Institute for Health and Clinical Excellence. NICE guideline no. 13. London: NICE, 2004.

Part 3: Condition

Recognition of surgical special interest and subspecialties

Urinary/pelvic floor

16

Operations for pelvic organ prolapse

Gillian E. Fowler and David H. Richmond

Pelvic organ prolapse (POP) is a common condition affecting millions of women around the world.

The aetiology of POP is multifactorial. Vaginal childbirth, advancing age and obesity are among the most frequently reported risk factors. As our population ages, the prevalence of POP and the demand for surgical intervention will increase further.

The different types of prolapse include:
• upper vaginal prolapse, i.e. uterus, vaginal vault
• anterior vaginal wall prolapse, i.e. cystocoele, urethrocoele, paravaginal defect
• posterior vaginal wall prolapse, i.e. enterocoele, rectocoele, perineal deficiency.

Women can present with prolapse of one or more of these sites. Symptoms reported relate to the prolapse (lump, vaginal bulge) together with a variety of urinary, bowel and sexual symptoms.

In addition to restoring normal vaginal anatomy, the challenge in POP surgery is to restore normal bladder, bowel and sexual functions. The choice of operation depends on a number of different factors, which include the nature, site and severity of prolapse, whether there are additional symptoms affecting urinary, bowel or sexual function, general health of the woman and surgeon preference and capability.

Bonney's Gynaecological Surgery, 11th edition.
© Tito Lopes, Nick Spirtos, Raj Naik, John Monaghan.
Published 2011 by Blackwell Publishing Ltd.

Anterior colporrhaphy

The operation is performed for cystocoele or a combination of cystocoele and urethrocoele. The principle of repair is to separate the vaginal skin from the underlying bladder and support the prolapsed bladder by approximating the weakened pubocervical fascia with the use of buttress sutures. The redundant stretched vaginal skin is removed.

There is no evidence that anterior colporrhaphy provides long-term improvement in stress urinary incontinence symptoms. In the presence of urodynamic stress incontinence, additional stress incontinence surgery can be considered at the same time. The reader should refer to the recommendations in Chapter 17.

Anaesthesia

The procedure is generally quick and straightforward, suited to regional or general anaesthesia.

Patient preparation

The normal lithotomy position is used with emphasis made on correctly placing the buttocks on the end of the table. A minor degree of head-down tilt often helps to improve access to the anterior vaginal wall as well as allowing optimum direction of the operating light. Intraoperative antibiotics to cover bacteroides organisms are advisable. Following vaginal and perineal cleansing, the bladder is emptied. Bimanual

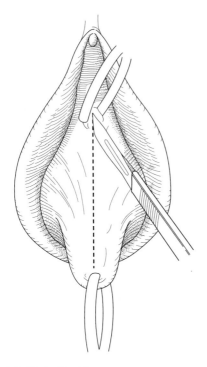

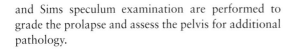

Figure 16.1 Vaginal incision.

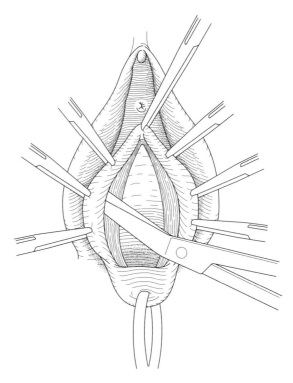

Figure 16.2 Separation of the vaginal skin.

and Sims speculum examination are performed to grade the prolapse and assess the pelvis for additional pathology.

Instruments

The gynaecological general set shown in Chapter 3 is used.

The operation

• *The incision.* Littlewood tissue forceps are placed on the anterior vaginal wall; one close to the cervix at the apex of the cystocoele, and a second at the midurethra to delineate the prolapse. The injection of local anaesthetic and epinephrine (0.5% bupivacaine with epinephrine 1:200 000) into the subepithelial space can be helpful in delineating the tissue planes and reducing bleeding. A midline incision is made along the anterior vaginal wall between the Littlewood tissue forceps (Fig. 16.1).

• *Separation of the vaginal skin from the bladder and the pubocervical fascia.* Kocher forceps are placed at two or three points along the edges of the vaginal incision. The assistant separates the Kocher forceps on the right-hand side of the incision, applying gentle traction. The subepithelial plane is developed on the right-hand side of the cystocoele, with sharp dissection using Monaghan scissors. The pubocervical fascia remains on the bladder. This plane is relatively avascular, and bleeding generally occurs only if the plane is breached or if the woman has undergone a previous repair. The dissection continues until the lateral aspects of the cystocoele are reached. The process is repeated on the woman's left side. The plane is developed under the Littlewood tissue forceps, which are then moved onto the free vaginal edge at the top and bottom of the incision (Fig. 16.2).

• *The repair.* Interrupted sutures are placed into the pubocervical fascia to reduce the cystocoele (Fig. 16.3). The authors use Vicryl sutures routinely,

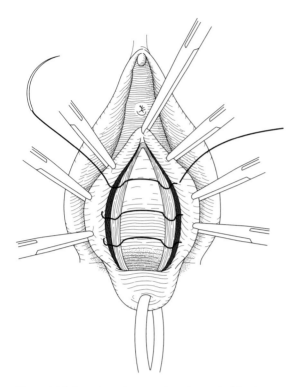

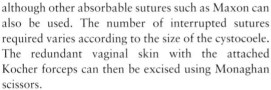

Figure 16.3 Insertion of sutures in pubocervical fascia.

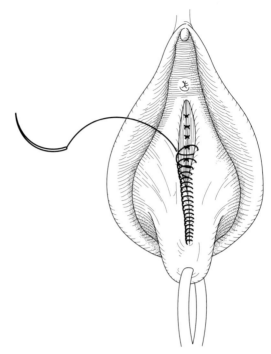

Figure 16.4 Insertion of vaginal sutures.

although other absorbable sutures such as Maxon can also be used. The number of interrupted sutures required varies according to the size of the cystocoele. The redundant vaginal skin with the attached Kocher forceps can then be excised using Monaghan scissors.

• *Closing.* The skin edges of the vagina are then approximated commencing at the cervical end (Fig. 16.4). A series of interrupted or continuous locking Vicryl sutures are used. The authors prefer interrupted sutures as these may avoid haematoma formation by allowing blood to drain into the vagina, but, above all, should one suture give way/pull out the repair is likely to retain its integrity.

• *Postoperative care.* An indwelling urethral urinary catheter is inserted. There is no evidence to support the routine use of a vaginal pack. Therefore, a vaginal pack is inserted by the authors only in difficult cases which are complicated by bleeding or when the procedure is carried out in combination with other POP surgery.

Alternative techniques

Another technique is to identify and excise the vaginal skin to be removed at the onset of the operation by demarcating the edges and excising the redundant skin from the underlying pubocervical ligament and bladder, as shown in Fig. 16.5. Alternatively, the procedure can start by making a 1-cm transverse incision at the cervix. The flap is then grasped using Kocher forceps and a midline subepithelial incision developed using Monaghan scissors (Fig. 16.6). The authors' technique avoids the error of removing too little or too much vaginal skin while ensuring accurate entry into the subepithelial plane.

Posterior colporrhaphy

The operation is performed for a rectocoele. It can be combined with repair of enterocoele or perineorraphy in women with a deficient perineum. The principles are to dissect the vaginal skin off the rectovaginal fascia. The rectocoele is reduced and supported by

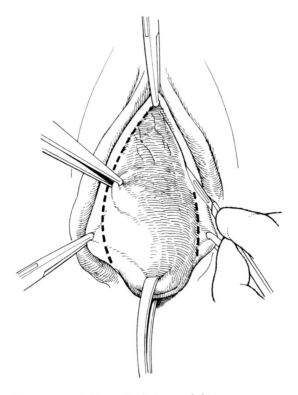

Figure 16.5 Excising redundant vaginal skin.

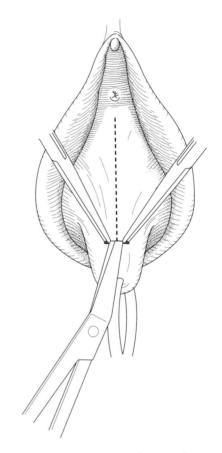

Figure 16.6 Alternative technique for vaginal incision.

sutures in the rectovaginal fascia and redundant posterior vaginal skin is excised. Special care is required when performing this procedure, as poor surgical technique or surgical misjudgement can result in considerable dyspareunia and even apareunia for the patient. The so-called 'registrar constriction ring' is seen to occur just as commonly after the operation has been performed by a consultant.

Anaesthesia, patient preparation and instruments

The comments for anterior colporrhaphy should be noted, with the avoidance of a head-down tilt to the operating table.

Instruments

The instruments required are those in the gynaecological general set shown in Chapter 3.

The operation

• *The incision*. Before beginning the repair it is imperative that the surgeon estimates the severity of the perineal defect as well as the rectocoele. Care should be taken not to constrict the vagina and after completion of the operation the vagina should easily admit two or three finger breadths. Placing Littlewood (or Kocher) forceps bilaterally on the hymenal remnants and approximating them in the midline can help gauge the ultimate size of the vaginal opening and ensure that it is adequate. A Littlewood forceps is used to mark the apex of the rectocoele. The injection of local anaesthetic and epinephrine (0.5% bupivacaine with epinephrine 1:200 000) into the subepithelial space can be helpful in delineating the tissue planes and reduce bleeding. A transverse incision should be

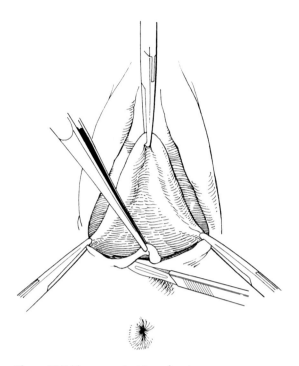

Figure 16.7 Transverse incision of perineum.

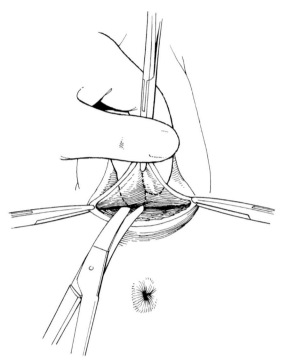

Figure 16.8 Exposing the plane between vagina and rectum.

made between the two lateral Littlewood forceps using a scalpel (or scissors) (Fig. 16.7).

• *Separation of the vagina from the rectum.* The operator now retracts the distal vagina downwards with toothed forceps or a Kocher forceps. The subepithelial plane is developed using Monaghan scissors (Fig. 16.8). A midline incision is made using Monaghan scissors (Fig. 16.9). Kocher forceps are placed along the edges of the incision bilaterally to assist in downwards traction of the free vaginal edges. The dissection with Monaghan scissors continues until it reaches the apical Littlewood forceps. The assistant separates and applies gentle traction to the Kocher forceps on one side of the incision. Using Monaghan scissors, the vaginal subepithelial plane is developed laterally to the edge of the rectocoele. If the correct plane has been found, dissection of the rectum from the posterior vaginal wall is easy, but is more vascular than the anterior vaginal wall. The procedure is repeated on the opposite side.

• *The repair.* Interrupted sutures are placed in the lateral rectovaginal fascia after reduction of the

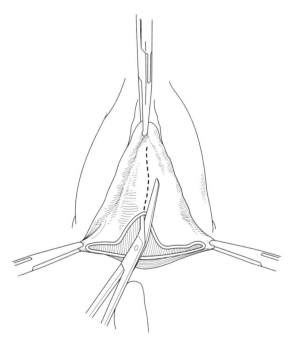

Figure 16.9 Midline incision of vagina.

rectocoele. Care should be taken not to excessively narrow the vagina and to avoid a constriction ring, which commonly occurs at the junction of the upper third and lower two-thirds of the vagina. The authors prefer to use Vicryl sutures but other absorbable suture materials such as Maxon can be used. The redundant vaginal skin with the attached Kocher forceps can then be excised using Monaghan scissors.

• *Closure.* The posterior vaginal wall is closed, starting at the apex. A series of interrupted or continuous locking Vicryl sutures are used. The authors prefer interrupted sutures, as described earlier.

• *Postoperative care.* An indwelling urethral urinary catheter is inserted. There is no evidence to support the routine use of a vaginal pack. Therefore, a vaginal pack is inserted by the authors only in difficult cases which are complicated by bleeding or when the procedure is carried out in combination with other POP surgery.

Perineorrhaphy

The operation is performed in women with a deficient perineal body which can occur as a result of vaginal childbirth. It is associated with an increased rate of superficial dyspareunia. It should, therefore, be used only for women with symptoms related to gaping at the introitus, rather than as a routine part of posterior colporrhaphy. The incision and dissection are similar to the initial steps taken in a posterior repair.

The operation

• *The incision.* Two Littlewood forceps bilaterally on the hymenal remnants at the posterior fourchette. The injection of local anaesthetic and epinephrine (0.5% bupivacaine with epinephrine 1:200 000) into the subepithelial space can be helpful in delineating the tissues planes and reduce bleeding. A transverse incision should be made between the Littlewood forceps using a scalpel.

• *The dissection.* A diamond-shaped piece of vaginal mucosa and perineal skin is marked with Littlewood forceps and excised using sharp dissection. The vaginal epithelium is then dissected off the bulbocavernous and transverse perineal muscles.

• *Reformation of the perineal body.* Deep Vicryl interrupted sutures are inserted to oppose the perineal muscles. Care should be taken to avoid a constriction ring. Minimal vaginal skin trimming is required.

• *Closure.* The perineum is closed using a subcuticular absorbable suture.

Posterior colporraphy with enterocoele repair

The previously described posterior colporrhaphy procedure is followed. The enterocoele is encountered high on the posterior wall, above the rectum. *Per rectum* examination is helpful is deciphering enterocoele from rectocoele. Once identified, the enterocoele sac is mobilized using a combination of sharp and blunt dissection and dissected off the vaginal skin. Incising the peritoneum opens the enterocoele sac. At this point, it is important to avoid injury to the small bowel, which may be lying within the sac. A minor degree of head-down tilt to the operating table can be helpful in emptying the sac. The remaining small bowel contents are then pushed out of the enterocoele sac by use of a small swab wrapped and held by a sponge holder. The redundant peritoneum is then excised up to the neck of the hernial sac, and the new peritoneal edges closed using a purse-string suture using Vicryl. The remainder of the procedure is as described for the posterior colporrhaphy.

Vaginal hysterectomy combined with pelvic floor repair

Pelvic organ prolapse is the most common reason for hysterectomy in postmenopausal women. POP frequently occurs in more than one compartment and, therefore, vaginal hysterectomy is often performed in combination with anterior and/or posterior vaginal repair and/or sacrospinous fixation.

The technique for vaginal hysterectomy is described in detail in Chapter 11. When combining vaginal hysterectomy and anterior repair, the authors' preference is to perform the vaginal hysterectomy first. The technique of combining vaginal hysterectomy and anterior colporrhaphy is described below. Posterior colporrhaphy can then be undertaken if necessary. The logic behind this being that performing the posterior repair first can prevent adequate access to the upper vagina and the anterior vaginal wall. In addition, after dealing with the uterine and anterior vaginal wall prolapse, it often becomes apparent that it is unnecessary to perform the posterior repair for a satisfactory end result.

The ovaries and tubes should be inspected for normality as routine at the time of hysterectomy. When an anterior and posterior repair have been carried out, the authors' preference is to insert a vaginal pack for up to 24 hours in an attempt to avoid the development of vaginal adhesions between the anterior and posterior vaginal walls, which normally lie in apposition. Separation of vaginal adhesions may still be required at the first postoperative clinic visit.

Vaginal hysterectomy combined with anterior colporrhaphy

The operation

• *The incision.* The anterior colporrhaphy, following vaginal hysterectomy, is then undertaken prior to closure of the vaginal vault. The apex of the anterior vaginal wall is grasped using two Littlewood forceps placed side by side. A third Littlewood is placed at the midurethra. The injection of local anaesthetic and epinephrine (0.5% bupivacaine with epinephrine 1:200 000) into the subepithelial space at this stage can be helpful in delineating the tissue planes and reducing bleeding. Using gentle traction on the apical Littlewood forceps the subepithelial space is developed using Monaghan scissors. A midline incision is made on the anterior vaginal wall. Kocher forceps are placed in the cut edge of the midline incision, which is continued until the third Littlewood forceps is reached.

• *Separation of the vaginal skin from the bladder and pubocervical fascia.* The assistant separates the Kocher forceps on one side of the midline vaginal incision, applying gentle traction. The subepithelial plane is developed laterally by sharp dissection using Monaghan scissors. The pubocervical fascia remains on the bladder. This plane is relatively avascular, and bleeding generally occurs only if the plane is breached or if the woman has undergone a previous repair. The dissection continues until the lateral aspects of the cystocoele are reached. The process is repeated on the women's other side. The plane is developed under

the Littlewood tissue forceps, which are then moved onto the free vaginal edges.

• *The repair.* Interrupted sutures are placed into the pubocervical fascia to reduce the cystocoele. The authors use Vicryl sutures routinely, although other absorbable sutures such as Maxon can also be used. The number of interrupted sutures required varies according to the size of the cystocoele. The redundant vaginal skin with the attached Kocher forceps can then be excised using Monaghan scissors.

• *Closing.* The vaginal vault can be closed in continuity with the anterior vaginal wall. In theory, this prevents vaginal shortening. Suturing starts at the vault using a series of interrupted or continuous locking Vicryl sutures. The vaginal skin edge at the vault is often inverted, away from the surgeon. Care should be taken to evert the skin edges during closing and to ensure the vaginal angles are secure. The authors prefer interrupted sutures as these may avoid haematoma formation by allowing the blood to drain into the vagina.

• *Postoperative care.* An indwelling urethral urinary catheter is inserted. There is no evidence to support the routine use of a vaginal pack. A dry vaginal pack is inserted by the authors following difficult cases that are complicated by bleeding or when the procedure is being carried out in combination with other POP surgery.

Surgical management of vault prolapse

Vault prolapse can occur after abdominal or vaginal hysterectomy. It has a higher incidence in women who have undergone hysterectomy for prolapse than for other indications. Vault prolapse is often underdiagnosed and inadequately dealt with by the inexperienced gynaecologists. Attempts to deal with it by a combination of anterior or posterior repair will do nothing to reduce the prolapse and will only shorten and constrict the vagina, making coitus virtually impossible and subsequent attempts to deal with the prolapse more difficult.

The surgical approach to vault prolapse is either vaginal or abdominal. Meta-analysis shows that abdominal sacrocolpopexy is associated with a lower rate of recurrent prolapse and dyspareunia than vaginal sacrospinous fixation. These benefits must be balanced against a longer operating time, longer hospital stay and longer time to return to normal daily activities, together with increased costs. The vaginal approach of sacrospinous fixation also allows simultaneous repair of anterior and/or posterior wall prolapse and, of course, it avoids any mesh-related complications.

Sacrospinous fixation

The principle of sacrospinous fixation (SSF) is to use the sacrospinous ligament as an anchoring site for vault suspension. The fixation is most often performed unilaterally, mainly on the right, but may be carried out bilaterally. There is no evidence that bilateral fixation provides better results. The suture should be placed 2–3 cm medial to the ischial spine. Care should be taken to avoid the pudendal artery; the pudendal vein and the sciatic nerve can lie up to 5 mm medial to the ischial spine. Transient unilateral gluteal pain may arise from damage to the small nerves within the ligament. Surgeons should, however, be aware of acute early gluteal pain, which radiates to the posterior surface of the thigh. This may represent an entrapped interosseous branch of the sacral nerve, requiring immediate operation to release the entrapped nerve by removing and repositioning the suture more medially.

Anaesthesia, patient preparation and instruments

The comments made previously should be noted, with the avoidance of a head-down tilt to the operating table.

The operation

• *The incision.* SSF can be combined with a posterior repair, using the same incision described above. The incision is continued up to the vaginal vault. In cases when a posterior repair is not required, entry can be via a midline incision made in the upper aspect of the posterior vagina wall (Fig. 16.10).
• *Identification of the sacrospinous ligament.* The right ischial spine is palpated. The right pararectal space is bluntly dissected, by introducing the index finger at the 10 o'clock position in the upper aspect of the incision. Using lateral sweeping movements

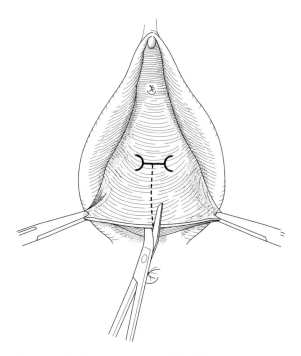

Figure 16.10 Posterior vaginal wall incision up to vaginal vault.

down towards the rectum, the sacrospinous ligament will eventually be both palpated and visualized. The authors' preference is to use two Breisky retractors, one is placed laterally on the right ischial spine with moderate traction in an anterior–lateral direction. The second Breisky retracts the rectum medially and a Sims speculum is placed between the two retractors in the posterior vagina. This allows direct visualization of the right sacrospinous ligament (Fig. 16.11). An alternative technique is to directly palpate the ligament.
• *Insertion of the sacrospinous stitch.* Using a long-handled needle holder, a J-shaped Ethibond suture is placed 2–3 cm medial to the right ischial spine. The stitch should be placed through and not around the ligament. The application of firm traction to the suture length will test the correctness of its placement. A second suture is inserted for additional support. Alternative surgical instruments for placement of the suture include the Miya hook and speculum and the Deschamps ligature carrier (Fig. 16.12). *Per rectum* examination should be undertaken to check for misplaced sutures.

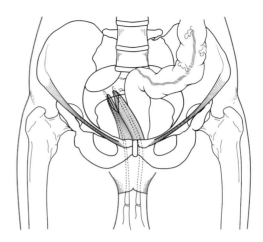

Figure 16.13 Suspension of the vaginal vault to the sacrospinous ligament.

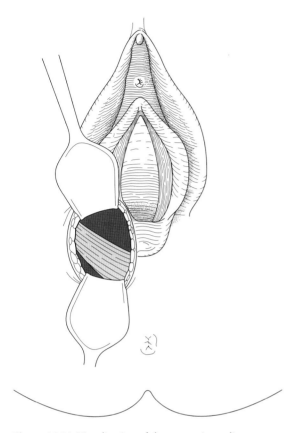

Figure 16.11 Visualization of the sacrospinous ligament.

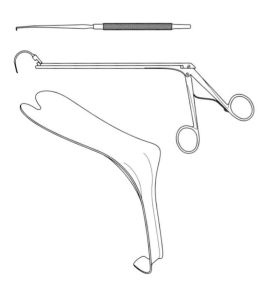

Figure 16.12 The Miya notched speculum, needle and retrieval set.

• *Attachment of the sutures to the vagina.* The two sutures are then secured to the upper posterior aspect of the vaginal skin, creating a pulley system with each suture (Fig. 16.13). Non-absorbable sutures such as Ethibond must be buried beneath the vaginal epithelium to prevent erosion and discharge. An alternative would be a slowly dissolving material such as polydioxanone (PDS) on a J-shaped needle again using a locking technique. These sutures do not need to be buried.

• *Closure and completion of the posterior repair.* The posterior repair is then undertaken, as previously described, including closure of the vagina. The sacrospinous sutures are then tied after pushing the vaginal vault onto the ligament.

• *Postoperative care.* An indwelling urethral urinary catheter and dry vaginal pack is advisable.

Abdominal sacrocolpopexy

The principle of abdominal sacrocolpopexy is to restore the vaginal axis using the anterior sacral ligament as the posterior anchoring site by the attachment of mesh. Directing the vagina towards the sacral promontory is thought to protect the cul-de-sac from enterocoele formation.

Anaesthesia

Regional or general anaesthesia is suitable for this abdominal procedure.

157

Patient preparation

The patient should be put in the lithotomy Trendelenburg position with legs in the stirrups slightly apart and flexed so that an assistant can stand comfortably between them. Care should be taken to avoid pressure points and particularly the peroneal nerve. Preparation should be made as for any abdominal procedure. In addition, the vagina should be cleansed and an indwelling urethral urinary catheter inserted. The degree of prolapse should be assessed to determine the need for concomitant anterior or posterior repairs. The authors' preference is to insert a 'rectal sizer' into the vagina, which can be used to manipulate the vault during the procedure and aid dissection of the rectum and bladder from the vaginal vault.

Instruments

The gynaecological general set shown in Chapter 3 is used. A rectal sizer or probe is required to manipulate the vaginal vault.

The operation

- *The incision.* Entry through a Pfannenstiel incision is preferred; however, in short, obese women the best access is obtained via a subumbilical midline incision.
- *Preparation of the vaginal vault.* The rectal sizer is palpated within the vagina and, using gentle pressure, the inverted vagina is repositioned. The peritoneum overlying the vaginal vault is incised taking care to exclude the possibility that the bladder may be lying within the intervening space. Once the edges of the vaginal vault are identified and exposed, the plane between the posterior vaginal wall and rectum is developed as much as is necessary. The bladder base is then dissected off the superior aspects of the anterior vaginal wall. Sharp dissection is usually required as a result of previous surgical intervention.
- *Preparation of the sacral promontory.* The sigmoid colon is pushed over to the left side. The peritoneum is incised over the sacral promontory, exposing the sacral longitudinal ligaments at the level of S1–S2. Care should be taken to avoid the sacral vessels. The retroperitoneum is then opened from the level of the vagina up to the sacral incision. Alternatively, a

tunnel can be created beneath the peritoneum between the sacral and vaginal incisions.
- *Placement of the mesh.* The appropriate length of mesh is measured in order to reach the sacral promontory without tension and allowing for 20% shrinkage. Commencing at the lower aspects of the posterior vaginal wall and aiming towards the vault, the mesh is sutured to the vaginal tissues using interrupted non-absorbable sutures (absorbable sutures are used by some surgeons). The extent to which the mesh extends down the posterior vaginal wall will depend on the clinical evaluation at the time. The mesh is attached to the vaginal vault and onto the upper aspect of the anterior vaginal wall. Extension of the mesh down the anterior wall is avoided owing to the increased risk of mesh erosion. If required, anterior repair can be undertaken on completion of the sacrocolpopexy. The mesh is then reflected towards the sacrum. The length of mesh used is gauged whereby it adequately holds the vagina in an elevated position, while lying within the hollow of the sacrum, without tension. It is attached using several interrupted non-absorbable sutures to the anterior sacral ligaments (Fig. 16.14).

Any excess mesh length is excised and discarded. The peritoneum is then closed over the entire area.
- *Closure of the abdominal wall.* This is as described in Chapter 4. Vaginal examination is undertaken to assess the need for anterior wall repair. Posterior repair is avoided at the same time owing to the increased risk of mesh erosion.

Laparoscopic sacrocolpopexy

Abdominal sacrocolpopexy can also be undertaken laparoscopically or indeed robotically, offering a minimal access approach to vault suspension. It combines the advantages of long-term success of an abdominal approach with a shorter recovery and hospital stay for the patient. A laparoscopic approach allows better visualization of the pelvic floor. The outcomes of open versus laparoscopic approach are equivalent. The disadvantage of laparoscopic surgery being a longer operating time and increased cost. The procedure itself follows the same steps as for open sacrocolpopexy; however, screws are often used to attach the mesh to the sacrum.

however, there is no evidence to support routine sacro-hysteropexy or sacrospinous fixation to the cervix.

Transvaginal insertion of mesh

The surgical treatment of pelvic organ prolapse is associated with a high risk of recurrence and reoperation. The use of mesh to augment surgical repair has been successful in other areas of medicine; however, there are particular issues with its use in the vagina in terms of sexual, bladder and bowel function. In addition, there is the concern about mesh erosion or infection. Recently, a new generation of mesh kits have been developed. These are based on the concept of transvaginal placement of tension-free mesh and consist of three parts: an anterior part to support the anterior wall, an intermediate part to support the vault, and a posterior part to support the rectum. According to the type and degree of the POP, the whole mesh or only part can be inserted.

The use of mesh for sacrocolpopexy for prolapse, and suburethral tapes for stress incontinence, is supported by evidence from good quality randomized controlled trials. Evidence to support the routine use of transvaginal mesh, however, is limited. Indeed, mesh erosion remains a major concern. Currently, the use of transvaginal mesh kits should be restricted to women with recurrent prolapse and then the surgery should be undertaken by specialists in pelvic floor surgery, ideally as part of a clinical trial.

Obliterative techniques

The aim of POP surgery is to reconstruct the vagina. In a few, rare occasions an obliterative approach involving vaginal closure or colpocleisis may be considered. Closing the vagina can impair body image and function. It may be appropriate for very old, frail women in order to avoid the risks of anaesthesia and major surgery.

Further reading

Pelvic floor surgery is a complex and expanding field. This chapter describes the most common surgical techniques for

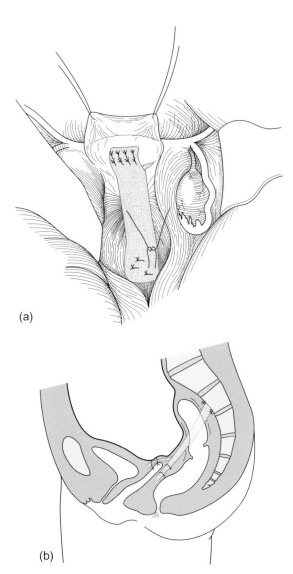

(a)

(b)

Figure 16.14 (a and b) Placement of the sacral colpoplexy mesh.

Uterine-sparing prolapse surgery

There has been a recent revival of prolapse procedures that preserve the uterus. There is no doubt that uterine prolapse is the result, rather than the cause, of POP. Some women may wish to retain their uterus for fertility and the techniques of sacrocolpopexy and sacrospinous fixation have been modified to allow preservation of the uterus. At the time of writing, the management of POP. There are many textbooks available for those trainees with an interest in the assessment, management and outcome of pelvic floor surgical techniques. As highlighted in this chapter, evidence to support the newer surgical techniques is lacking. Up-to-date analysis of evidence is, however, available via the Cochrane Library (www.thecochranelibrary.com) and the National Institute for Health and Clinical Excellence (NICE) (www.nice.org.uk) websites.

17 Operations for urinary incontinence

David H. Richmond

Urogynaecology surgery includes operations for the control of incontinence, whether due to urinary stress incontinence (USI), detrusor overactivity (DO) or fistula. There are over 100 operations to correct USI and the author will review here those that are currently used and of proven value. Fistulae will not be discussed as this is covered in Chapter 18.

Operations for urinary stress incontinence

There is still controversy about the most effective procedure to correct USI. Many gynaecologists, including the author, now favour a suburethral tape approach. The principle 'do the best operation first' is fundamental. The choice of which of the many operations depends upon clinical and urodynamic factors such as mobility and capacity of the vagina, surgical training and expertise. In addition, with appropriate consenting, patients may elect for one of the many vaginal tape procedures or the older and more traditional Burch colposuspension performed suprapubically. Additional factors include the patient's physical health, her weight and her age. Conditions such as detrusor overactivity, reduced bladder capacity and voiding disorder are frequently aggravated by stress incontinence surgery and need

consideration. Finally, additional gynaecological surgery may be required, e.g. hysterectomy for menorrhagia or anterior and/or posterior colporrhaphy for prolapse.

Role of urodynamic assessment

The need to confirm the cause of incontinence before proceeding with surgery for its correction is becoming increasingly evident. Failure to demonstrate stress incontinence by clinical means should be followed by one of several urodynamic procedures to confirm incontinence before surgery is attempted.

When the patient's sole symptom is stress incontinence, there is a 90% chance that this is due to uncomplicated USI and urodynamic investigation may not be required. It is the author's preference, however, to have a low threshold for testing.

Indications for urodynamic assessment

- There are symptoms of urgency, urge incontinence, frequency, nocturnal enuresis (suggesting detrusor overactivity) or symptoms of poor stream, incomplete emptying or straining to a void, which may indicate voiding difficulty.
- There has been a previous attempt to correct stress incontinence.
- Overt or occult neuropathy is present or suspected.

Urodynamic studies include midstream specimen of urine (MSU) for culture and drug sensitivity, subtracted cystometry (CMG) and uroflowmetry. Ultrasound is preferable to catheterization (unless in the course of cystometry) to detect residual urine.

Bonney's Gynaecological Surgery, 11th edition.
© Tito Lopes, Nick Spirtos, Raj Naik, John Monaghan.
Published 2011 by Blackwell Publishing Ltd.

Indications for cystoscopy

• To investigate bladder pain, microscopic haematuria, urgency and frequency.
• Under general anaesthesia, to confirm or refute a small capacity bladder already found on cystometry.
• To detect intravesical pathology such as a non-absorbable suture or tape after previous continence surgery, stone or tumour.

The author finds no use for Q-tip testing. Dynamic urethral pressure measurement is subject to wide variation, and significant artefacts due to catheter stiffness have been found, especially when there has been previous bladder neck surgery. It has clinical and research applications, for example to study the effects of drugs on the sphincteric mechanism.

Bladder drainage

In the majority of procedures now for USI (i.e. the suburethral tapes) postoperative catheterization is not required. However, when coupled with additional vaginal surgery urethral drainage may be beneficial for 24–36 hours. It is advisable to drain the bladder after most suprapubic operations for incontinence. A suprapubic rather than a urethral catheter is preferred, as, with the former, it is easier to initiate voiding and the patient is more comfortable and less prone to urinary tract infection. A Bonanno, Stamey or Foley catheter may be used. The regimen is as follows. A fluid intake of 2–2.5 litres per day is encouraged and a strict fluid chart maintained. The catheter is clamped at about 22:00 hours on the second postoperative day and is released after each void or 8 hours. Obviously, this can be earlier if the patient is in pain or has failed to void. A residual urine is measured by allowing the suprapubic catheter to drain for half an hour. Once the patient is voiding more than 200 mL of urine at a time and the residual is less than 150 mL, ideally on two separate occasions, the catheter can be removed. Antimicrobial therapy is not routinely used but regular specimens of urine should be tested for infection.

Classification of operations

The route of access can be used to classify the various surgical procedures: vaginal; vaginal and suprapubic; or suprapubic alone. Each procedure has its clinical and urodynamic indications.

Vaginal (anterior colporrhaphy)

The use of the anterior colporrhaphy or repair to correct anterior vaginal wall prolapse is well established. It is not the author's operation of choice for the management of USI. Comparison with a colposuspension and the suburethral tapes indicates that both of the latter have a significantly higher cure rate. However, undoubtedly, it does result in some patients with incontinence becoming continent when bladder neck plication is performed. In these circumstances, emphasis is placed on elevating and supporting the bladder neck by deep sutures placed and tied either side of it. The sutures are either inserted as Kelly has described, into bladder muscle, or placed in paraurethral fascia. Consequently, the anterior repair may be appropriate when a shorter operating time with less blood loss, postoperative pain and postoperative morbidity are desirable, e.g. in the elderly or physically frail, and in the situation when there is a cystocoele.

Instruments

The gynaecological general set described in Chapter 3 is required.

Anaesthesia

A general anaesthetic is required, but if the patient is frail or elderly an epidural or spinal anaesthetic has advantages. Perioperative broad-spectrum antibiotics are given and appropriate antiembolic precautions taken depending upon hospital policy.

The operation

A 3- to 4-cm vertical incision is made on the anterior vaginal wall, starting about 0.5 cm below the external urethral meatus. The precise length will depend on the extent of anterior vaginal wall prolapse. The proximal urethra, bladder neck and bladder base are exposed. The dissection is carried out such that the pubocervical fascia is left behind on the anterior vaginal wallflaps. Two absorbable sutures (no. 1 Vicryl) are inserted at the bladder neck region: the

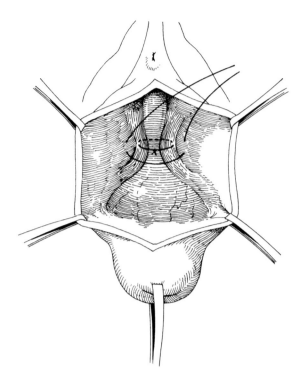

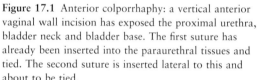

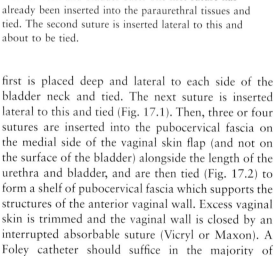

Figure 17.1 Anterior colporrhaphy: a vertical anterior vaginal wall incision has exposed the proximal urethra, bladder neck and bladder base. The first suture has already been inserted into the paraurethral tissues and tied. The second suture is inserted lateral to this and about to be tied.

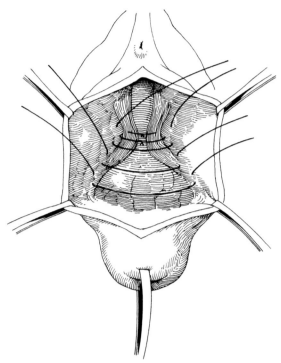

Figure 17.2 Anterior colporrhaphy: bladder neck suture is tied and three sutures inserted into the pubocervical fascia (and on the underside of the anterior vaginal wall flap).

first is placed deep and lateral to each side of the bladder neck and tied. The next suture is inserted lateral to this and tied (Fig. 17.1). Then, three or four sutures are inserted into the pubocervical fascia on the medial side of the vaginal skin flap (and not on the surface of the bladder) alongside the length of the urethra and bladder, and are then tied (Fig. 17.2) to form a shelf of pubocervical fascia which supports the structures of the anterior vaginal wall. Excess vaginal skin is trimmed and the vaginal wall is closed by an interrupted absorbable suture (Vicryl or Maxon). A Foley catheter should suffice in the majority of circumstances.

Variations in techniques

Some gynaecologists believe that pubocervical fascia is found adherent to the bladder, and consequently

their sutures are placed on the bladder surface as opposed to the lateral vaginal skin flap.

The anterior vaginal wall can of course be closed with a continuous suture if a locking stitch is required, but this then carries excess risk of recurrence should one or two bites of tissue give way.

Major complications

Occasionally, a urethral diverticulum is found and the urethra may be entered during the course of dissection. The urethra should be closed with interrupted sutures of 3.0 Vicryl without tension and the bladder drained for 7 days.

Both venous and arterial haemorrhage can occur. Using diathermy and oversewing, haemostasis should be achieved during the operation, and a vaginal pack can be left in place for 24 hours.

Postoperative care

Mobilization of the patient starts on the first postoperative day and is gradually increased until the patient is fit to be discharged home on the second or third day. Intercourse should be avoided until after the follow-up appointment. Heavy lifting is preferably eschewed in the immediate 6 weeks following surgery. Vaginal examination should be performed at follow-up to exclude adhesion formation, which can then be easily separated, and granulation tissue, which can develop, can then be easily dealt with using silver nitrate sticks.

The suburethral vaginal approach using tapes

The TVT or tension-free vaginal tape

This was described by Ulmsten *et al.* in 1996. Overnight, the operation transformed the approach and thought processes for the surgical management of stress incontinence of urine. It has been the subject of considerable scientific scrutiny, randomized controlled trials and comparative studies; suffice to say it is now the most widely used operation for stress urinary incontinence. It can be performed as a day-case procedure in selected cases and can be performed with a range of anaesthetic techniques from the original local anaesthetic method with sedation to general anaesthesia. The clinical outcomes are similar for those of the more traditional Burch colposuspension described later.

Technique
The method involves making two 1-cm-long incisions approximately 6 cm apart just above the superior border of the symphysis pubis. Vaginally 10–20 mL of lidocaine with epinephrine (1 : 200 000) is injected into the vaginal wall and paraurethrally. A single 1.0- to 1.5-cm incision is made longitudinally in the vaginal wall starting 0.5 cm from the external urethral meatus. It should not extend to the bladder neck. From this incision, a lateral tunnel 0.5–1.0 cm long is created to enable the tip of the needle bearing the tape to be placed. With a straight introducer placed along the lumen of a Foley catheter the balloon is inflated. The TVT tape is now ready for insertion. The handle with TVT tape attached is placed on the right side of the urethra in the paraurethral space created earlier by dissection. The hand holding the Foley along with the introducer is angled upwards and to the same side as the needle placement, at the same time pushing the bladder away from the path of the TVT needle insertion. The urogenital diaphragm is perforated and the needle brought to the right-sided skin incision. The handle is then disconnected and reapplied to the other remaining needle for placement on the left side of the urethra in the tunnel created earlier. The Foley is repositioned this time on the left side, angling the Foley tip and balloon backwards and downwards to push the bladder away from the left-sided TVT needle insertion. Now that the TVT tape is in a 'U' shape around the urethra, the Foley is removed for cystoscopy to occur. This enables the surgeon to view the bladder and urethra to exclude perforation and to view ureteric position and possibly function.

If the patient is awake at this stage, either with a local or regional anaesthetic, the patient can be asked to cough to establish the required tightness of the tape to prevent incontinence. The author has found this practice of little value and in recent times has moved to a general anaesthetic technique without any deterioration in outcome or experience for both the surgeon and patient. Under general anaesthesia, the author utilizes a size 6 Hegar dilator placed between the tape and the Foley catheter to reduce untoward tension as the plastic sleeve is gently withdrawn. Remember that the TVT stands for 'tension-free' vaginal tape. The abdominal spare ends of the tape can be cut and the wounds repaired with an absorbable suture. The Foley catheter is removed. Instructions must be given to observe urine output over the next 6–8 hours to reduce the risk of retention of urine.

The 'outside in' transobturator midurethral tape

This was developed in 2001. A vertical midline vaginal incision is made in the middle third of the urethra passing through the whole thickness of the vaginal wall. Starting at the incision, the vagina is released laterally on either side of the urethra with Mayo scissors over a width of approximately 1.5 cm. The dissection stops against the ischiopubic ramus. The dissection must be in the deep tissue layer between the vesicovaginal fascia and the urethra, and not too superficially between the vesicovaginal fascia and the vaginal skin.

Technique

The lateral margin of the ischiopubic ramus is identified between an index finger placed in the lateral vaginal fornix and thumb placed in front of the obturator foramen. A puncture incision is made 15 mm lateral to the ischiopubic ramus on a horizontal line level with the clitoris. The tunneller is held in the same hand as the side on which the operator is working. The tunneller is held vertically with the handle downwards; it is then introduced through the skin incision and crosses the obturator membrane. As the membrane is crossed, a specific resistance is felt which is easily recognized.

The tunneller is then turned to a horizontal position, with the handle pointing medially. The tip of the tunneller is led medially towards the urethra, aiming above the urethral meatus and underneath the symphysis pubis. The safest method is to lead the tunneller round the ischiopubic ramus while remaining in contact with it. The aim of this procedure is to trace a perineal route with the instrument below the superior fascia of levator ani. A finger is placed in the incision to check that the tunneller is not piercing the vagina and is passing well above the lateral vaginal fornix some way away from it. The index finger is introduced into the vaginal incision to fold the urethra upwards and protect it from the needle. The finger will then make contact with the tip of the tunneller laterally underneath the symphysis pubis. The tunneller is then guided by the finger into the vaginal incision.

Once this procedure has been completed, it is prudent to check that the vagina and urethra have not been pierced by the tunneller. The end of the tape is introduced into the eye of the needle and then pulled through to place it in position. The texture of the tape allows the tape to be pulled hard without risk of breaking. The tape is inserted tension-free behind the urethra. The low elasticity of thermally bonded polypropylene makes it possible to adjust the position of the tape very precisely. There are two important points to remember during this adjustment to reduce the risk of compressing the urethra, which causes voiding disorders:

1 Leave a visible space between the tape and the urethra (a few millimetres).
2 Avoid adjusting the tape with the patient in the Trendelenburg position, as the cervical and urethral region is at its highest in this position. It is therefore better to put the patient horizontal.

The tape is positioned so that the silicon-coated surface is facing the urethra and the black line is facing the vagina. After any excess tape has been trimmed, the skin over the incision is moved away from the end of the tape and then sutured with an absorbable suture. The vaginal incision is closed with a few interrupted sutures using absorbable suture thread. The Foley catheter inserted during the procedure is removed on the first postoperative day and post-void residual urine is measured by catheterization.

There are many modifications of both the retropubic tape and also the transobturator approach. Surgical preference for the outside in or inside out method is an individual decision with no scientific evidence to support one technique over the other.

In 2006 a mini-tape procedure was described with only the suburethral incision, consequently potentially reducing further the more common complications of the retropubic and obturator approaches. Further long-term studies are awaited.

Suprapubic

Marshall–Marchetti–Krantz operation

This was first described in 1949. It is rarely if ever performed now. It was superseded by the introduction of the Burch colposuspension in 1961 and more recently by the tapes described earlier.

Burch colposuspension

Burch described this procedure in 1961 and, for 35 years, it has remained the procedure of choice for many gynaecologists and urologists on both sides of the Atlantic.

Indications

The colposuspension will cure incontinence and elevate not only the bladder neck but also the bladder base (properties hitherto unique to the anterior colporrhaphy), which makes it a very suitable choice when urethral sphincter incompetence and anterior vaginal wall prolapse coexist. It does, however, require normal vaginal capacity and mobility for satisfactory elevation of the lateral vaginal fornices. It is contraindicated if elevation is restricted by scarring due to previous surgery or menopausal atrophy.

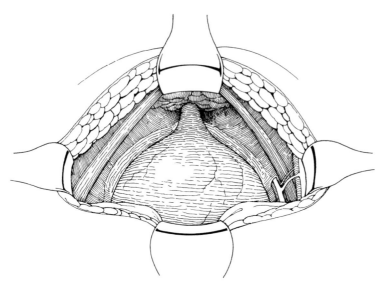

Figure 17.3 Colposuspension operation: diagrammatic representation of anatomy via a Pfannenstiel incision.

Instruments

As well as the gynaecological set described in Chapter 3, the following are required. The author prefers to use a non-absorbable suture no. 1 Ethibond inserted on a heavy, round-bodied J needle size 30 mm. A Lahey swab mounted on a curved Robert forceps is ideal for blunt dissection.

Anaesthesia

A general anaesthetic is required, prophylactic antibiotics are given and antiembolic precautions taken.

The operation

The patient is placed in the horizontal lithotomy position with legs abducted and in Lloyd-Davies stirrups. The lower abdomen and vagina are prepared. Draping must allow access to vagina and abdomen simultaneously. A 14–18 gauge Foley is inserted and allowed to drain freely. The balloon is filled with 30 mL, which can then act as a landmark during suture placement.
• *The incision.* This should be a low Pfannenstiel incision wide enough for access but at the same time may be only 6–8 cm in length.
• *Opening the retropubic space.* A plan of the anatomy is shown in Fig. 17.3. The bladder and urethra are separated gently from the symphysis and

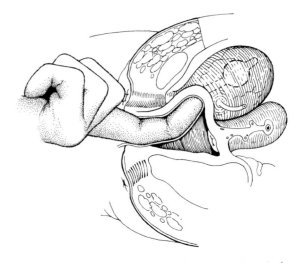

Figure 17.4 Colposuspension operation: surgeon's vaginal finger elevates one or other of the lateral vaginal fornices prior to dissection of the bladder base from the paravaginal fascia.

the retropubic space is exposed. With the finger of the surgeon's left hand in the vagina, pressure is exerted upwards in one or other lateral vaginal fornix (Fig. 17.4).
• *Identifying the paravaginal fascia.* The lateral edge of the bladder base is dissected medially off the paravaginal fascia (Fig. 17.5), which shows as a whitened

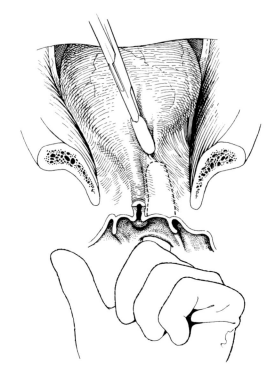

Figure 17.5 Colposuspension operation: start of dissection of the bladder base off the paravaginal fascia in a medial direction.

sheet. Large veins are either cautiously avoided or oversewn – diathermy may exacerbate bleeding. When there is adequate exposure of the fascia, two or three sutures of no. 1 Ethibond are inserted from the highest (most cephalad) point of the lateral fornix, parallel to the bladder base. Subsequent sutures are inserted caudally but not below the bladder neck, as these will lead to delay in spontaneous micturition and possibly to postoperative voiding difficulties.

• *Tying the sutures.* The author's preference is to perform cystoscopy at this stage to exclude sutures passing through the bladder wall (which can then be easily removed) but also other vesical pathology. Each suture is then anchored to the corresponding part of the ipsilateral ileopectineal ligament (Fig. 17.6). This is repeated on the other side. When all the sutures are in place, they are tied alternately, starting from the most caudal suture and moving proximally. Approximation of the vaginal fascia with the ileopectineal ligament is no longer recommended with the emphasis upon support rather than elevation. Bow stringing of sutures will be common but does not detract from the outcome. Passage of a non-absorbable suture completely through the vaginal skin does not seem to be disadvantageous.

• *Haemostasis and wound drainage.* After haemostasis has been completed, the wound is closed routinely

Figure 17.6 Colposuspension operation: two sutures inserted into the paravaginal fascia and ipsilateral ileopectineal ligament. Note the most distal (caudal) suture is never lower than the bladder neck. The sutures are tied initially on the vaginal fascia prior to passage through the ileopectineal ligament.

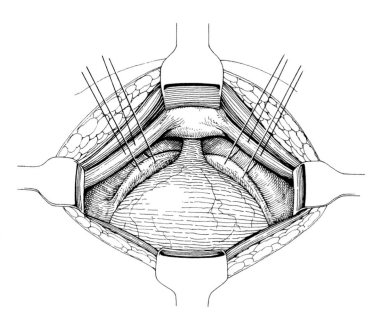

and a vacuum drain placed in the retropubic space. A suprapubic catheter is then inserted.

Should a hysterectomy be required, this may be performed first of all as an abdominal procedure. If an enterocoele is present, this should be corrected irrespective of symptoms, as a colposuspension tends to make it larger. This is carried out prior to the colposuspension using a Moschcowitz closure of the pouch of Douglas. A non-absorbable suture material should be used to encircle the peritoneum and close the hiatus between the uterosacral ligaments (Fig. 17.7a,b). Care should be taken to avoid the pelvic ureter at this stage. If a rectocoele is present, this again is exacerbated by the colposuspension and needs to be repaired; a posterior repair is performed once all the abdominal procedures have been completed.

Variations in technique

Absorbable suture materials such as Dexon, Vicryl or PDS may be used as alternatives, but the author prefers non-absorbable suture material as he feels they offer a more permanent cure rate.

Complications

Bladder and urethral entry and haemorrhage from perivesical veins are the main complications. Methylene blue or milk can be instilled into the bladder to aid its anatomical definition and to disclose where entry has occurred. It is important to recognize trauma to the bladder, which is repaired in the routine way with a single- or double-layer closure. Ureteric ligation has been described. Prompt recognition and treatment are necessary and urological referral may be required.

Postoperative complications include failure to void and detrusor overactivity.

Sling operations

In practice, the suburethral tapes described earlier have superseded the majority of sling procedures. There are numerous variations of sling procedure and material to choose from. Probably the most widely used operation is the Aldridge sling. Slings may be constructed from organic tissue (rectus

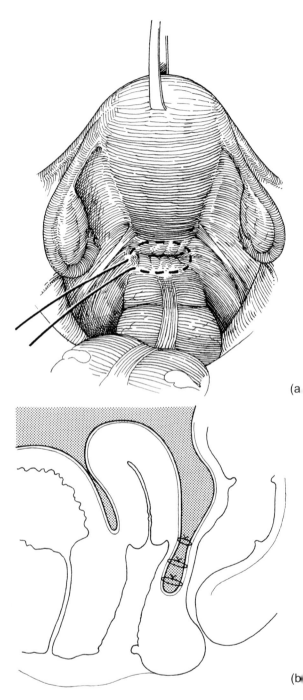

(a

(b

Figure 17.7 Moschcowitz procedure: (a) suture inserted into the pouch of Douglas peritoneum including serosa of the colon and both uterosacral ligaments. (b) Sagittal diagram, showing three successive sutures in place to obliterate the pouch of Douglas.

fascia, fascia lata, lyophilized dura, or porcine skin), which, unless it is heterologous, avoids foreign body reaction and is usually readily available. Its tensile strength may not, however, be consistent or permanent. Inorganic materials are stronger and of consistent strength but may enter into indissoluble fibrosis with bladder neck tissues, making subsequent removal difficult (e.g. nylon, Mersilene, Marlex, Teflon).

Indications

The sling procedures are usually used:
• as a secondary procedure after failed previous surgery
• where there is limited vaginal access or significant reduction of vaginal capacity and mobility (rendering a colposuspension technically impossible)
• where urodynamic studies indicate adequate bladder neck elevation but absence of posterior support to the proximal urethra and bladder neck.

Preoperative preparation

Antibiotic cover and antiembolic precautions as described for the Burch colposuspension procedure are required.

Anaesthesia

A general anaesthetic is required.

The Aldridge procedure

• *The incision.* Two incisions are made: a low Pfannenstiel and a midline anterior vaginal wall incision.
• *Exposure of the rectus abdominis and preparation of the 'sling strips'.* Through the Pfannenstiel incision, the rectus sheath is exposed; two limbs of the sling are cut transversely from the aponeurosis, each about 7–8 cm in length and 1.5 cm wide, starting from the lateral edge and ending 2 cm from the midline where the sling is left attached (Fig. 17.8). If an adequate sling cannot be taken from the rectus fascia, owing to previous scarring, a fascia lata graft, 1 cm wide and 17 cm long, is cut. It is optional at this stage, but probably safer, to carry out a retropubic dissection and display the bladder neck.
• *Exposing the bladder neck from the vaginal incision.* Next, the anterior vaginal wall is infiltrated in the midline with lidocaine 0.5% and epinephrine 1 : 200 000 for haemostasis and definition of anatomical layers. An anterior vaginal wall incision is made from about 1 cm proximal to the external urethral meatus and continuing for about 3 cm proximally to

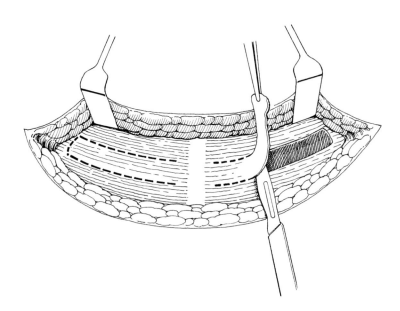

Figure 17.8 The Aldridge procedure: sling flaps cut from the rectus sheath.

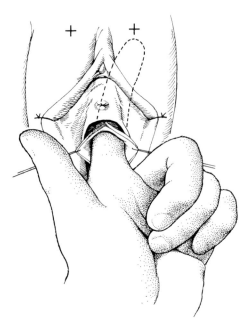

Figure 17.9 The Aldridge procedure: finger being passed via the vaginal dissection, lateral to the bladder and up behind the symphysis pubis.

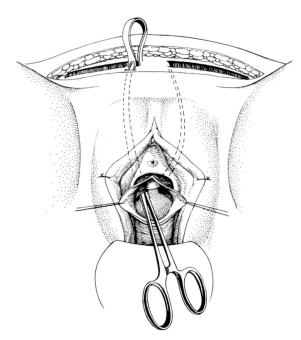

Figure 17.10 The Aldridge procedure: left sling already brought down and attached at the level of the bladder neck; right sling being brought down.

expose the bladder neck area. This is deepened and a plane of dissection is developed laterally between the vaginal sidewall and the bladder neck. A finger is passed into this plane in an upwards direction towards the pubic crest, on either side of the bladder neck (Fig. 17.9).

• *Passing the fascial sling.* A curved clamp is now passed from the vaginal aspect upwards alongside the bladder neck to grasp one of the fascial slings and pull it down to the vaginal dissection; this is repeated on the other side (Fig. 17.10). The slings are then sutured together across the bladder neck with just sufficient tension to slightly elevate it. Excess sling may be sutured together to the base of the bladder to provide extra support.

• *Closure of the incisions.* Excess vaginal skin is trimmed and the vaginal wall closed with interrupted or continuous locking Dexon or Vicryl sutures.

The rectus sheath is closed with Dexon or Vicryl sutures and then the abdominal skin is closed. A suprapubic catheter is inserted and managed in the standard way.

Variations in technique

Other authors have used inorganic materials and their original descriptions should be referred to for details of their techniques. In essence, the sling is shaped beforehand and inserted from the vaginal aspect. The middle portion of the sling is sutured to the bladder neck area and each limb is retrieved in the retropubic area and sutured laterally either to rectus sheath or ileopectineal ligament.

Complications

Injury to the bladder or urethra during the course of dissection is not uncommon and, once recognized, should be repaired in the standard manner and the operation continued. Venous haemorrhage from the paraurethral dissection can be brisk. Urinary retention is common and frequently results from excess sling tension rather than extensive dissection around the bladder neck. It is here that the benefits of suprapubic catheterization are most obvious.

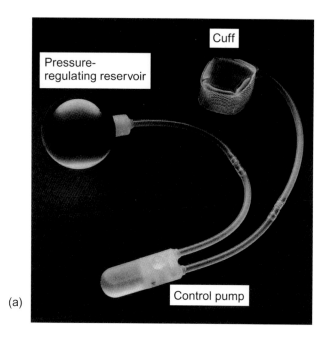

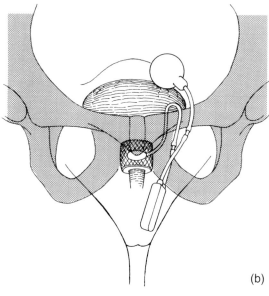

(a)   (b)

Figure 17.11 (a) The artificial urinary sphincter AMS 800; (b) the sphincter in place.

Postoperative care

Postoperative care is similar to previous operations except for the increased incidence of urinary retention. Apart from management by continued suprapubic catheterization, clean intermittent self-catheterization (CISC) may be initiated until the patient voids spontaneously. Resistant cases may require release or removal of the sling. Drug therapy, e.g. bethanechol chloride 25–100 mg four times daily, to stimulate the detrusor or an α-adrenergic blocking agent may be used to reduce urethral resistance.

Artificial urinary sphincter

The artificial urinary sphincter is a fully implantable device, allowing the patient to void *per urethram* under voluntary control with complete urinary continence. In the female, it is used usually for end-stage incontinence or neuropathic causes of incontinence (e.g. myelomeningocoele), or as a preferable alternative to permanent catheterization or urinary diversion. However, the device is expensive, and the insertion can be technically difficult. It should only be per-

formed after careful consideration. In reality, it will only be performed in regional or even national centres. A description of the operation is provided in the previous edition of this book.

The sphincter is made of medical grade silicone rubber. It is hydraulically operated and consists of an occlusive cuff (in different sizes) made of silicone elastomer and is placed circumferentially around the bladder neck (Fig. 17.11a,b). It is linked by silicone tubing to a pressure-regulating balloon placed in the retropubic space, which controls the amount of pressure exerted by the cuff.

Indications

The main indications are resistant incontinence due to urethral sphincter incompetence despite at least two appropriate and well-performed conventional incontinence procedures, where the alternative would be continuous incontinence, permanent catheterization or urinary diversion. It is also indicated for neuropathic causes of incontinence; should there be detrusor hyperreflexia, this should be adequately controlled beforehand by drug therapy. Finally, it may be used for congenital causes of incontinence such as epispadias or bladder extropy, where closure has been obtained but the patient is still incontinent.

Injectable urethral bulking agents

Many injectable substances have been developed and these include collagen, silicone and carbon beads, to name a few. They are injected into the periurethral space under general, local or regional block and can be done blindly by simple injection or via a cystoscope with placement at the level of the bladder neck. Morbidity is low, although hypersensitivity, particle migration and granulomatous development do occur, efficacy tends to be short term and cost high. In the UK, this is not a first-line therapy and the indications appear to be few.

Outcomes

Anterior repair is the least likely of the surgical approaches to be efficacious in the long term and should no longer be considered as an operation for stress incontinence. The needle suspensions (Pereyra and Stamey or modifications thereof) are rarely if ever performed now, particularly with the introduction of the myriad of tapes. Bone anchor techniques have been abandoned.

The Burch colposuspension was the gold standard for the surgical cure of stress urinary incontinence until the introduction of the TVT in 1996 and its numerous modifications since. The subjective and objective cure rates for the Burch colposuspension are quoted as 78% and 85%, respectively. This tends to decline with time and is similar for either open or laparoscopic approaches. Significant intra- and perioperative complications occur in approximately 6% cases, of which 2% need surgery. Voiding difficulty arises in approximately 13% and *de novo* urgency in 7%. Prolapse, mainly enterocoeles, occur in 22% and lower abdominal or pelvic pain in 12% of patients. These are more common than for anterior repair operations or traditional sling procedures. There seems little if any difference in outcome if a laparoscopic approach is undertaken and sutures are used. Similarly, the newer midurethral tapes offer similar success regarding outcome measures with different

complications. The voiding difficulty and urgency are the same as the Burch colposuspension but bladder perforation (3–5%) and tape erosion, depending upon the material used (9–55%), must be borne in mind during the consent process. Perforation is more evident in the retropubic tape approach. Erosion appears more common in the transobturator approach but with reduced bladder trauma. The voiding difficulty and urgency remain the same and overall outcome of the transobturator approach similar to the TVT and also that of the Burch procedure. Longer term data are still awaited. The single troublesome complication from the transobturator approach remains groin pain, which can be persistent.

Traditional suburethral slings have been used for many years. Their cure rates are similar to those of the Burch colposuspension and tapes at around 85% with good long-term datasets. Complications are said to occur in 10%, with 3% requiring surgery. Voiding difficulty is around 10%, with urgency in 17%. The autologous slings have the lowest erosion complication rate at <0.5%, while the synthetic material sling erosion rate is 2.4%. Obviously, the open procedures (Burch colposuspension and suburethral slings) tend to have increased delayed voiding, longer hospital stay and also recovery, and longer use of analgesia.

Which operation?

The author's preference as a first-line approach will be to discuss the advantages and disadvantages of the Burch colposuspension and TVT procedure, highlighting the approximate complication rates as described earlier. The majority of patients (90%) select the tape. Obviously, the obturator approach could easily be substituted.

With concomitant anterior prolapse, an anterior colporrhaphy or abdominal/laparoscopic paravaginal repair can be performed simultaneously, but again the morbidity and length of hospital stay favour the former approach.

In situations with recurrent stress incontinence the surgical options may be more limited and careful thought must be given to the chance of success compared with the risk of complications. In addition, the reason for the recurrence must be ascertained. Is the loss all attributable to stress incontinence or is there an element of detrusor overactivity? What are the voiding parameters and can or could the patient perform intermittent self-catheterization should the need arise? Have the sutures in a Burch procedure simply given way or was the tape placed in the wrong position or inadequately 'tensioned'? Each of these situations must be considered before embarking upon repeat surgery. It behoves each surgeon to know their own outcome measures in such situations before blindly and misguidedly agreeing to further surgery. Adequate consent is fundamental on such occasions.

The use of injectable agents has limited value in such circumstances with low efficacy and short-term duration of any effect.

Operations for detrusor overactivity

Traditionally, surgery has been used only as a last resort for the treatment of intractable detrusor overactivity when every possible conceivable conservative approach has been exhausted. The techniques described include denervation procedures (both chemical and surgical), augmentation (clam caeco-cystoplasty), detrusor myectomy and ileal conduit formation. Studies for each of these are limited to case report series and lack comparative analysis and often long-term follow-up. Most authors describe variable success which, in the past, has merited such an approach in selected patients appropriately counselled. The morbidity with each of the procedures above is significant, and, in particular, with bowel substitution or interposition there is a risk of malignant change with time.

More recently, sacral neuromodulation using an implanted pulse electrode stimulating the S2–4 nerve roots has been introduced. A temporary external stimulator is provided for 1–2 weeks as a trial prior to considering the insertion of the permanent stimulator. A 50% improvement can be expected. The long-term benefit looks promising, but equipment costs initially are high. In addition, botulinum toxin used in the treatment of dystonia and spasticity as well cosmetic surgery has been introduced. It appears effective for up to 12 months before repeat injection needs to be considered. Often, the response time, however, is much shorter. The technique is simple (transvesical cystoscopic injection using a series of aliquots of botulinum into the detrusor muscle). It is at most a day-case

procedure. The morbidity is minimal, although a significant number of patients suffer voiding difficulty often needing self-catheterization.

Conclusion

While the procedure for selecting the correct operation is still crude and sometimes deficient, it is appropriate to restate the dicta 'The first operation has the best chance of success' and 'Do the best operation the first time'. A sound knowledge of the pathophysiology and of the indications and limitations of each operation, together with an application of good surgical technique, are important considerations each time surgery is carried out for incontinence. Urodynamic studies must now be recognized as providing relevant information prior to operations for incontinence and as mandatory if surgery has already been attempted and failed.

Further reading

Textbooks

Cardozo L, Staskin D (eds). *Textbook of Female Urology and Urogynecology*, 2nd edn. Abingdon: Informa Healthcare, 2006.

Chapple CR, Zimmern PE, Brubaker L, Smith ARB, Bø K. *Multidisciplinary Management of Female Pelvic Floor Disorders*. Edinburgh: Churchill Livingstone, 2006.

Dwyer PL. *Atlas of Urogynecological Endoscopy*. Abingdon: Informa Healthcare, 2007.

Journals

For those with an interest in the original articles for the eponymous procedures in gynaecological urology, the editor recommends the following references:

Aldridge A. Transplantation of fascia for the relief of urinary stress incontinence. *Am J Obstet Gynecol* 1942;44: 398–411.

Burch JC. Uretrovaginal fixation to Cooper's ligament for correction of stress incontinence, cystocoele and prolapse. *Am J Obstet Gynecol* 1961;81:281–90.

Kelly H. Incontinence of urine in women. *Urol Cutan Rev* 1913;17:291–293.

Low J. Management of severe anatomic deficiency of urethral sphincter function by a combined procedure with a fascia lata sling. *Am J Obstet Gynecol* 1969;105:149.

Marshall VT, Marchetti AA, Krantz KE. The correction of stress incontinence by simple vesico-urethral suspension. *Surg Gynecol Obstet* 1949;88:509–518.

Millin T. Reported discussion on stress incontinence in micturition. *Proc R Soc Med* 1917;40:361–370.

Pacey K. Pathology and repair of genital prolapse. *J Obstet Gynaecol Br Empire* 1949;56:1–15.

Stamey TA. Endoscopic suspension of the vesical neck for urinary incontinence. *Surg Gynecol Obstet* 1973;136:547–554.

Stanton SL, Brindley G, Holmes D. Silastic sling for urethral incompetence in women. *Br J Obstet Gynaecol* 1985;92:747–750.

Ulmsten U, Henriksson L, Johnson P, Varhos G. An ambulatory surgical procedure under local anesthesia for treatment of female urinary incontinence. *Int Urogynecol J Pelvic Floor Dysfunct* 1996;7:81–5.

18 Operations for the correction of urinary fistulae

David H. Richmond

Urogenital fistulae can be congenital or acquired and the latter occur following parturition, surgery, radiotherapy and in situations in which there is significant pelvic malignancy. On the international stage, 90% of fistulae occur in relation to obstetrics, predominantly due to obstructed labour. In the developed world, the majority occur following pelvic surgery or radiotherapy. In these situations, although a fistula can develop following direct trauma to the urinary tract the majority are due to a suture or clamp compromising the blood supply or tissue viability such that tissue necrosis ensues and a fistula forms. Characteristically, this is 10–14 days after operation. These situations arise when dissection may be difficult; for example, freeing the bladder from the cervix after caesarean section or when suturing the vaginal vault after hysterectomy and the relationship of the bladder base to the vaginal cuff is not clearly defined. Occasionally, this might be secondary to a haematoma that becomes secondarily infected, for example at the vault after hysterectomy. The incidence of fistulae following hysterectomy is in the region of 1 : 1300 operations in the UK.

The most frequent cause of fistula formation after hysterectomy is failure to dissect the bladder free of the cervix and upper vagina. This problem may be caused by previous surgery, especially caesarean section, or by the presence of infection, scarring or

Bonney's Gynaecological Surgery, 11th edition.
© Tito Lopes, Nick Spirtos, Raj Naik, John Monaghan.
Published 2011 by Blackwell Publishing Ltd.

endometriosis. Fibroids may so distort the uterus that the bladder is drawn up and inadvertently entered. The bladder may also be damaged when the vaginal edge is being sutured because the surgeon fails to recognize the bladder wall.

Even when the bladder is not entered, the damage to the bladder wall may result in avascular necrosis and the appearance of the fistula some 1–2 weeks after the operation.

Presentation

This can be variable. The history of constant and substantial loss of fluid *per vagina* makes the diagnosis straightforward. There are, however, situations in which the presentation is less clear-cut and an index of suspicion is essential in making the diagnosis, i.e. could the vaginal loss/secretion be urine? Could the fluid loss from a drain site be urine? These questions will help the clinician in establishing the diagnosis in a timely fashion.

Patient preparation

Prior to any surgical management, the entire urinary tract should be fully assessed. It is important to do so as it is not unusual to find damage to other parts of the tract which may require concurrent or subsequent management.

An intravenous urogram (IVU) should be performed to evaluate the kidneys and the ureters. Although an IVU is essential, it is more to establish the normality of the upper tracts than the diagnosis of the fistula that is important. A cystoscopy is also helpful to determine the relationship of the fistula to the ureteric orifices.

In order to assess the bladder, it should be filled with methylene blue dye in solution via a transurethral Foley catheter. This is commonly called the three-swab test for a urinary fistula. If a tampon is inserted into the vagina, any leakage from the bladder will show up as a blue stain on the tampon; however, if leakage is occurring from a ureter, the tampon will be wetted with clear urine. Rarely, ureteric reflux associated with a low fistula may confuse the picture.

In general, repair of the vesicovaginal fistula should be delayed for 2–3 months; this occasionally results in spontaneous closure but, most importantly, allows infection to settle and the tissue planes to re-establish themselves.

The exception to this policy of waiting is when the fistula is recognized shortly after it occurs, when it is probably best to carry out an immediate repair.

As with most surgical procedures, the first chance of repair is the best one.

Prophylactic antibiotics are recommended in the preoperative period, and if the patient is postmenopausal, and there are no contraindications, she should be given oestrogens to improve the quality of the vaginal skin.

Principles of fistula repair

Bonney described six general principles which should be adhered to when repairing any fistula, whether of the urinary tract, alimentary system or any epithelial surface.

1 The tissues to be repaired must be as healthy as possible. In the case of urinary fistulae, the urine should be rendered sterile and the area free of infection. Sloughs due to irradiation, trauma or infection must have separated to leave clean healing or healed surfaces.

2 There must be an adequate exposure of the affected area and the tissue surfaces surrounding the defect.

3 There must be no tension on the suture lines when the fistula is closed. This applies not only at the time of operation but also in the postoperative period. Therefore, adequate drainage of the bladder must be maintained following the procedure.

4 Meticulous haemostasis is essential throughout the operation to avoid haematoma formation and to facilitate healing.

5 Infection must be guarded against as it will seriously jeopardize healing.

6 The final principle applies when a bladder fistula affects the region of the bladder–urethral junction. This is a vulnerable area in relation to urinary control and, for this reason, it is not only important to close the fistula but also to reinforce the area with adjacent fascia and muscle, including the anterior fibres of the pubococcygeus muscles when necessary, thus reducing the risk of postoperative stress incontinence. A Martius fat pad graft from the labia may also be necessary. Unless these precautions are taken, stress incontinence, even on walking, will make the patient's life a misery. Also, the insertion of this support will obviate the risk of a new fistula developing if a later attempt is made to correct the stress incontinence.

Repair of the postoperative fistula

Instruments

The instruments in the gynaecological general set, shown in Chapter 3, will be required together with vaginal retractors and Sims right-angle skin hooks. Fine dissecting scissors such as McIndoe scissors are of great value.

The operation

The best results for repair of vesicovaginal fistulae are obtained when the patient is operated upon by an expert, i.e. a surgeon who has committed his skills, time and experience to caring for these unfortunate women with this distressing condition. It is not an operation for the part-time enthusiast. This applies to both urologists and gynaecologists. All fistulae, ideally, should be repaired by individuals with appropriate training and, above all, surgical experience. The technique described here relies heavily on the experience of others, particularly Chassar Moir and Sims.

The choice between using a vaginal or abdominal approach will depend to a large extent on the training of the individual: urologists and general surgeons tending to favour the abdominal approach and gynaecologists the vaginal. Occasionally, when the fistula is placed high in the vault, a combined approach will yield the best results.

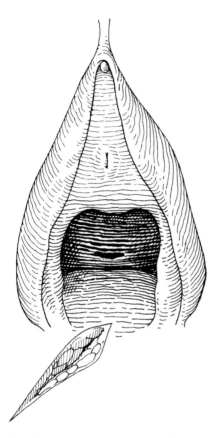

Figure 18.1 The Schuchardt incision for gaining access to a narrowed introitus.

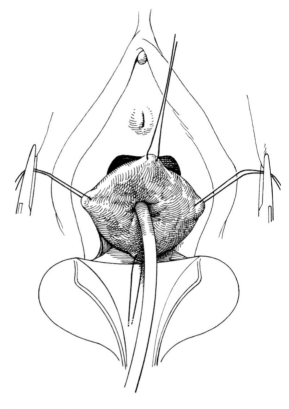

Figure 18.2 Drawing down the fistula using a small Foley catheter.

Exposure

The lithotomy position gives an adequate approach for most vesicovaginal fistulae. The patient's buttocks should be drawn well down the table. Occasionally, the knee–chest position will be needed for an inaccessible fistula behind the pubic arch. A sucker is essential to keep the operative field clear and dry. Tilting the table to lower the patient's head, the so-called lithotomy Trendelenburg position, can be useful.

If the lower vagina is scarred or narrowed, a Schuchardt releasing incision will give considerably improved access (Fig. 18.1).

Excision of the fistula edges

The edges of the fistula may be made prominent by grasping them and everting using Allis tissue forceps;

alternatively, a Foley catheter can be inserted into the fistula and the area drawn down towards the surgeon (Fig. 18.2). The full depth of the fistula edge is now resected through to the bladder in order to remove the full length of the fistula tract. The vaginal wall is first incised, dissected laterally and marked using sutures or tissue forceps (Fig. 18.3).

Dissection of the bladder muscularis

Next, the muscularis is identified and separated from the vaginal wall for approximately 2 cm around the fistula; any remaining scar tissue around the fistula should now be removed. A purse-string suture is placed around the edges of the mucosa using a Vicryl stitch on an atraumatic needle (Fig. 18.4). The needle should be so placed that the stitch does not present on the bladder surface of the mucosa.

177

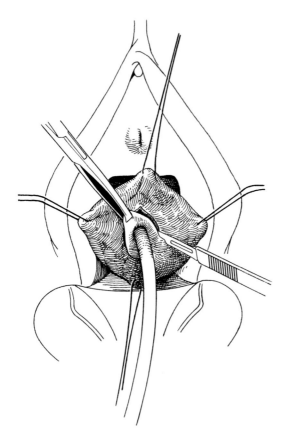

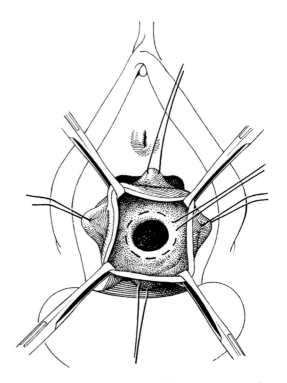

Figure 18.4 Separating the vaginal skin and the muscularis of the bladder and inserting the purse-string suture around the fistula.

Figure 18.3 Incising the vaginal skin around the fistula and removing the scarred tissue throughout the full depth of the defect.

Closure of the fistula and placing of support sutures
The purse-string suture should now be tied, invaginating the mucosa towards the bladder cavity (Fig. 18.5). This manoeuvre may be aided by looping a suture through the edge of the fistula and drawing it out of the urethra; pulling on this loop assists in invaginating the mucosa and the loop can be simply removed by pulling on one end.

The muscularis is now brought together by placing a number of separate sutures across the defect using an invaginating stitch and drawing the muscularis over the defect (Fig. 18.6). It is important to keep these sutures clear of the mucosa.

Closing the vagina
Finally, the vaginal skin is closed longitudinally using interrupted vertical mattress sutures (Fig. 18.7).

Meticulous haemostasis must be maintained throughout the procedure.

Postoperative management

A Foley catheter is inserted into the bladder and a vaginal pack covered with an antiseptic such as acriflavine is inserted into the vagina. The pack is removed 24 hours after operation and the catheter is maintained until there is no evidence of haematuria, but usually for at least 10 days. Prophylactic antibiotics are prescribed and the patient is usually fit to go home after 8–10 days in uncomplicated cases. Occasionally, it may be beneficial to insert suprapubic and urethral catheters for drainage as a precaution. The urethral catheter can be removed with the suprapubic catheter left *in situ* as a reserve during trial voids.

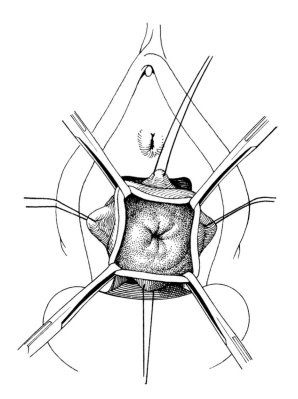

Figure 18.5 Tying the purse-string suture.

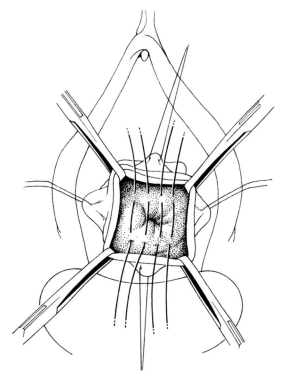

Figure 18.6 Suturing the muscularis with interrupted invaginating sutures.

Repair of the obstetric fistula

This type of fistula presents special problems, mainly because of the large area of bladder that may be lost as a consequence of the avascular necrosis that occurred at the time of the injury. If the defect is large, special techniques have to be used to close the gap without tension.

• *Bladder mobilization* downwards will allow the defect to be bridged by drawing the upper freed part of the bladder down to meet the lower relatively fixed section.

• *Labial fat pads* (Martius grafts) are used to support and improve the blood supply of the large defect.

• *A gracilis muscle* rotation procedure will also add support and improve the blood supply to those fistulae where tension may be present if they were closed in the traditional manner.

• *Omental grafts* are of help if the fistula is approached from within the abdomen; by preserving the gastroepiploic arteries an excellent new blood supply can be brought to the defect and the repair site.

Repair of fistulae developing after pelvic irradiation

Patients presenting with postirradiation fistulae are the most difficult group to manage, calling for great experience and skill from the surgeon.

The fistula may develop at a variable period after the radiotherapy, occasionally occurring up to 25 years after treatment.

The fistula formation rate is dose related and is exacerbated by trauma to the area of irradiation, especially by inappropriate surgery.

If the patient has had successful treatment for a carcinoma invading the bladder, fistula formation is almost a natural consequence of successful treatment.

179

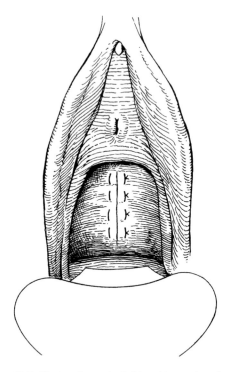

Figure 18.7 Closing the vaginal skin with a series of interrupted vertical mattress sutures.

Not infrequently, the vesicovaginal fistula is associated with other fistulae of the gastrointestinal tract, also caused by the radiotherapy. It is important to be sure that the fistula has not developed as a consequence of tumour recurrence. In these circumstances, the simplest and most effective management may be a diversion of urinary and bowel function using a conduit and/or a colostomy.

The operation

If a repair of an irradiation fistula is to be attempted, there must be no evidence of recurrent cancer, and the principles outlined by Bonney must be adhered to.

The surgeon must also decide whether to retain a functioning vagina or whether, in the interests of simplicity and a more certain result, some form of colpocleisis should be used.

Frequently, the vaginal skin is extremely atrophic with associated radiotherapy changes, including scar-

ring and stenosis, producing grave difficulties with access.

Oestrogens should be used for a short period before surgery is attempted. This will improve the quality of the skin and facilitate healing and the identification of tissue plane.

The use of Martius grafts, gracilis muscle rotation flaps, bulbocavernosus muscle transplant and omental pedicle grafts will all serve to improve the prospects of cure of the fistula by bringing into the area a much improved blood supply and also allowing the fistula to be closed without tension. Occasionally, the fistula is reduced in size without being completely closed; a second attempt will often be successful.

Unfortunately, a high proportion of patients with postirradiation fistulae will require diversionary procedures to solve their problems.

Further reading

Textbooks

Buchsbaum HJ, Schmidt JD (eds) *Gynecologic and Obstetric Urology.* Eastbourne: W.B. Saunders, 1982.
Jewett M (ed.) *Urological Complications of Pelvic Surgery and Radiotherapy.* Oxford: Isis Medical Media, 1995.

Journals

Lawson JB. Vesical fistulae into the vaginal vault. *Br J Urol* 1972;44:623–631. Very few individual gynaecologists have an opportunity to develop a large experience in the management of vesicovaginal fistulae; one who has is J.B. Lawson. In his working lifetime, in both Africa and the UK, he has dealt with hundreds of such operations and his writings are worth searching out and reading.
Turner-Warwick R. The use of pedicle grafts in the repair of urinary tract fistulae. *Br J Urol* 1972;44:644–656. Another master urological surgeon, who should be read when possible.

Other major landmark references include:
Boronow RC, Rutledge F. Vesico-vaginal fistula, radiation and gynecologic cancer. *Am J Obstet Gynecol* 1971;111:85–90.
Martius C. *Gynaecological Operations* [trans. McCall ML, Bolton KA]. London: J & A Churchill, 1957.
Moir JC. Personal experience in the treatment of vesicovaginal fistulas. *Am J Obstet Gynecol* 1956;71:476–491.
Moir JC. Vesico-vaginal fistulae as seen in Britain. *J Obstet Gynaecol Br Commonw* 1973;80:598–602.

Oncology

19 Surgery for carcinoma of the vulva

For many years the accepted management for carcinoma of the vulva was to carry out a radical vulvectomy and groin node dissection as an en bloc procedure or through separate incisions. In the last 30 years, there has been a move to wide excision of the primary tumour rather than full organ extirpation, and there is increasing evidence that sentinel lymph node sampling is an appropriate substitute for systematic lymphadenectomy for early tumours.

This chapter is divided into two sections: lymph node assessment and excision of the vulval tumour. However, the operation described is as in the previous edition as an en bloc dissection using a butterfly skin incision. The reason for this is that, surgically, it is simple to modify the butterfly incision operation into separate incisions for the groins and vulva, but the reverse is difficult if one does not know how to place the incisions. Although it is increasingly rare to use the butterfly en bloc incision, it is still useful for large tumours involving the clitoris and mons pubis and when there are large fungating nodal masses with concern of lymphatic channel involvement between the vulva and groins increasing the risk of skin bridge recurrences if left *in situ*.

The operation should be carried out in departments with a considerable surgical, anaesthetic and nursing experience of the operation; this will result in high operability rates (97% in the Gateshead series) and excellent long-term survivals. In the same series of

over 760 cases, an overall actuarial 5-year survival of 72%, with an operative mortality of 3% was attained. When the groin nodes were negative, the survival rose to 94.7% and fell to 62% when they were positive.

Lymph node assessment

It is not justifiable to dispense with the groin node assessment except when the carcinoma invades for less than 1 mm or in cases of verrucous carcinoma. In these cases, the risk of lymph node involvement is negligible. In vulval melanomas, there is no survival benefit to inguinal lymphadenectomy, and a wide excision with or without sentinel node sampling is all that is necessary.

When performing a systematic lymphadenectomy, the anatomical distinction between different levels of nodes in the groin is unimportant as the aim of the technique is to remove all the groin nodes en bloc.

There is no evidence that direct extension of vulval carcinoma to the pelvic nodes occurs without first passing through the groin nodes. Pelvic node dissection should be dissected only when nodal disease is seen to extend into the femoral canal (involvement of Cloquet's node).

Sentinel node identification

The concept of there being a single or a small number of sentinel nodes identifiable as the first lymph node group to be involved when cancer spreads from the vulva to the groin nodes has been mooted for many years. DiSaia in 1979 first commented on the possibility of performing a sentinel node dissection in order

Bonney's Gynaecological Surgery, 11th edition.
© Tito Lopes, Nick Spirtos, Raj Naik, John Monaghan.
Published 2011 by Blackwell Publishing Ltd.

to determine the necessity for carrying out a full groin node dissection.

Levenbach and his colleagues in the 1990s used vital blue dyes which, when injected in the leading edge of a cancer of the vulva, would spread by the lymphatics and could be identified in the first lymph node involved in the lymphatic chain close to the medial side of the superficial nodes in the groin. However, there remained a small proportion of patients in whom it was not possible to identify a sentinel node, and therefore the technique's application to most patients with vulval cancer was deemed too inaccurate to be acceptable. Ansink *et al.*, in a multicentre study, reported identification of the sentinel nodes in only 56% of groins dissected.

In more recent times, the use of technetium-99m-labelled nanocolloid injected intradermally around the tumour has demonstrated a very high level of accuracy in the identification of the sentinel node or nodes. Lymphoscintigraphy is performed soon after the injection and the first appearing persistent focal accumulation is considered to be a sentinel node (Fig. 19.1). At surgery 2 mL of patent blue-V is injected at four points around the tumour. The Neoprobe, a handheld gamma-ray detection probe, is used to confirm the lymphoscintigraphy marked area of greatest activity in the groin (Fig. 19.2) and a small skin incision is made at this spot. The sentinel node is identified using the Neoprobe, and is often, though not always, stained blue. Once identified, it is removed, and the area checked for any other activity from other sentinel nodes. The resulting incision is much smaller than the standard groin incision (Fig. 19.3). In a large international study involving 259 women with unifocal early cancer and negative sentinel lymph node and no further groin node dissection, the groin failure rate was 2.3%. In some centres, the technique is already routine, thereby conserving the groin nodes in a high proportion of patients, reducing markedly the dire consequence of leg lymphoedema and discomfort generated following dissection of the groin lymphatics and the associated nerve bundles lying close to the nodal tissues.

Lymphadenectomy

Separate incisions

The standard technique for the groin node dissection is through separate incisions. The traditional Gateshead

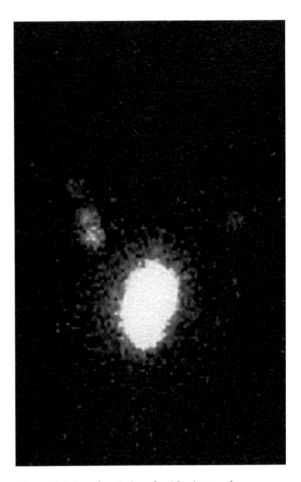

Figure 19.1 Lymphoscintigraphy 15 minutes after injection showing the central hotspot of the vulval tumour and an obvious hotspot of one or two right sentinel lymph nodes.

approach is modified from the butterfly incision, with an elliptical incision from the anterior superior iliac spine to a point about 8 cm below the pubic tubercle. This gives excellent access to the superficial inguinal nodes as well as to the deep femoral nodes. However, the editors' preference is to use a 'crease' incision; a linear incision made through the skin and subcutaneous fat approximately 1 cm below and parallel to the groin crease (Fig. 19.4). Laterally it starts about 2 cm medial to the anterior superior iliac spine and extends to below the pubic tubercle. This again provides good exposure with excellent primary healing. Once the

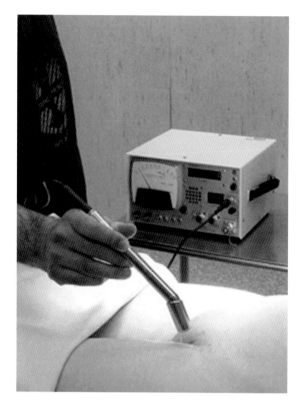

Figure 19.2 Gamma probe used to identify the area of greatest activity prior to surgery.

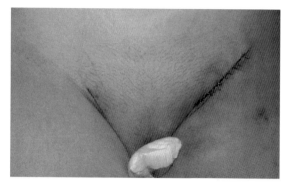

Figure 19.3 Sentinel incision (right) compared with crease incision in the left groin.

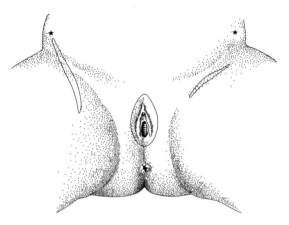

Figure 19.4 The triple incision technique. Traditional Gateshead groin incision (right) and crease incision (left).

skin incision is made, the lymph node dissection is as described below.

Butterfly incision
This approach is rarely used today except for large clitoral tumours extending to the mons pubis or groins where an adequate skin bridge may not exist.

The operation

The patient is positioned lying supine with the feet approximately 25 cm apart and supported by ankle rests to elevate the calves from the table. Some authorities recommend the 'ski' position so that two, or even three, teams can operate simultaneously. This is a recipe for confusion and does not significantly speed up the operation. Slight Trendelenburg is sometimes necessary to facilitate access to the groins, especially if the patient is obese.

Skin incision
An incision curving down towards the groin is made from the anterior superior iliac spine to a midpoint over the symphysis pubis, followed by an incision from the anterior superior iliac spine to a point 8 cm below the public tubercle with a curve towards the groin fold. A third incision is now made from this last point, curving upwards and medially to meet the crural fold (Fig. 19.5). The skin removed from the groin will be minimal, a narrow band less than 0.5 cm wide, with a narrow releasing incision over the line of the upper part of the saphenous vein. The vein is preserved where possible as data suggest that it may reduce wound cellulitis, wound breakdown and chronic lymphoedema.

183

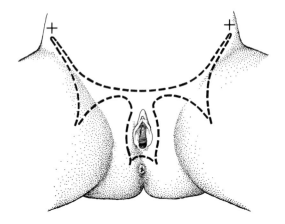

Figure 19.5 Butterfly skin incision.

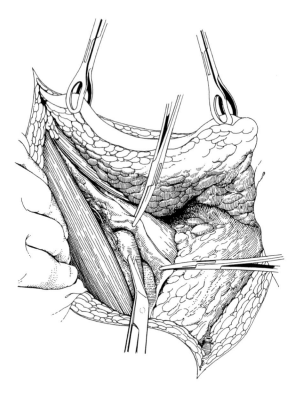

Figure 19.7 Elevating the medial edge of the sartorius fascia and cleaning the femoral artery.

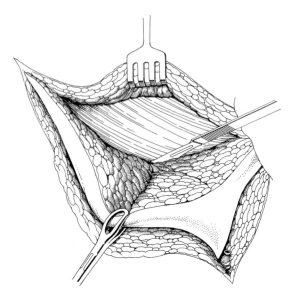

Figure 19.6 Cutting the upper incision down to the external oblique aponeurosis.

Defining the fascial planes
The strip of skin in the groin is picked up using Lane tissue forceps so that the block of tissue in the groin can be manoeuvred during the dissection. By putting slight tension on the upper and lower edges of the skin incisions, undercutting can be achieved down to the aponeurosis of the external oblique muscle above the groin (Fig. 19.6) and to the fascia over the sartorius muscle, which forms the lateral boundary of the

femoral triangle. This fascia is incised from the anterior superior iliac spine to the apex of the femoral triangle. The medial edge of the fascia is now picked up using two small Spencer Wells clips and elevated (Fig. 19.7). The strands of the femoral nerve can now be seen in the soft tissue at the medial side of the sartorius muscle. Some of these fibres are cut as the femoral artery is defined and meticulously cleaned from the apex of the femoral triangle to the inguinal ligament. The condensation of fascia lateral to the artery along the inguinal ligament is separated with scissors to leave the external oblique aponeurosis clean.

Removing the groin nodes from the femoral vessels
On the medial side of the femoral artery the femoral vein can be seen; it is cleaned from the inguinal ligament distally, the saphenous vein is identified as it enters the femoral vein and is either preserved or clamped, cut and ligated and the whole block of

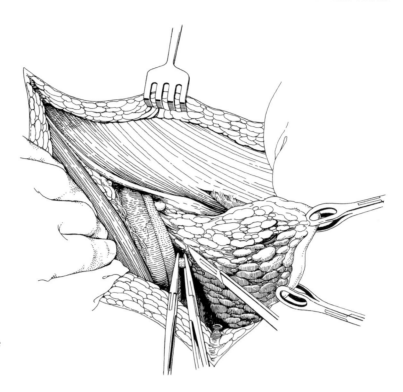

Figure 19.8 Clamping and dividing the saphenous vein below the cribriform fascia.

tissue containing the groin nodes is turned medially (Fig. 19.8). To preserve the saphenous vein, the tip of the scissors is run along the tract of the vein to create a space, and the block of tissue containing the groin nodes is incised to identify and mobilize the vein along its tract. On the medial side of the femoral vein, the fascia over the adductor muscles is incised longitudinally and, having cut through the fat at the apex of the femoral triangle, the fascia is stripped from the adductor muscles as far medially as the gracilis aponeurosis.

With separate incisions, the medial dissection stops here, removing the block of tissue at the point where the round ligament appears from the inguinal canal.

With the butterfly incision, the subfascial dissection is then completed through to the pubic symphysis. The entire groin nodes have been removed en bloc (Fig. 19.9).

Pelvic node dissection
The pelvic nodes are now approached by incising through the external oblique muscle approximately 2 cm above the inguinal ligament, beginning above the femoral canal and extending superolaterally along the direction of the fibres for about 8 cm. The internal oblique muscle is then incised along the line of its fibres, exposing the transversalis fascia and peritoneum. Using the fingers, the peritoneum is swept from the outer pelvis, exposing the external iliac vessels. The exposure is completed by extending the medial end of the wound down to the femoral canal, applying large Spencer Wells clips to Poupart's ligament (Fig. 19.10).

Through this incision, the external iliac vessels can be cleaned of nodes up as far as the common iliac vessels, and in direct continuity with the groin node dissection (Fig. 19.11).

Closure of the abdomen
This is achieved by a continuous Vicryl suture, beginning at the medial end over the femoral canal, travelling laterally, and then returning to the medial end to complete the closure of the external oblique muscles. At this point, the femoral canal is reconstituted by

185

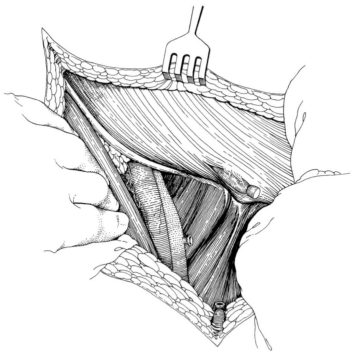

Figure 19.9 The completed groin dissection.

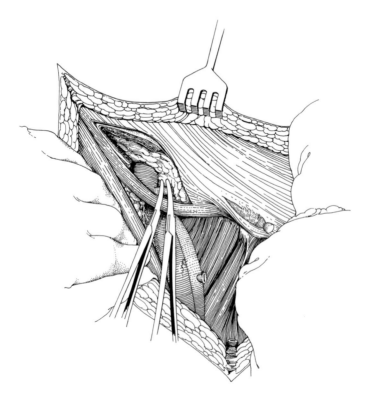

Figure 19.10 Clamping the inferior epigastric artery and Poupart's ligament.

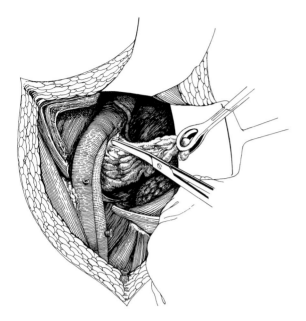

Figure 19.11 Removing the pelvic lymph nodes.

suturing the medial part of the external oblique incision to the fascia of the pectineal line, so that the femoral canal admits a fingertip and pressure is not put on the femoral vein (Fig. 19.12).

Closure of the skin and drainage of the groin
Using the linear and releasing incisions, closure of the skin presents no problems and can be carried out without tension either using interrupted Vicryl suture or skin staples for extra speed. Drainage of the space left in the groin is mandatory as up to 300 mL of fluid can collect on each side per day. Drainage is carried out through narrow diameter suction drains. The practice of sartorius muscle transposition to cover the femoral vessels is not necessary, as the risk of disruption is more theoretical than real.

A similar procedure is now performed on the opposite side.

With separate groin incisions, as there is no releasing incision, the wound is closed in a straight line. The subcutaneous tissue is approximated with a continuous 2/0 Vicryl suture along the length of the incision, and with the crease incision a subcuticular stitch or staples can be used for skin closure.

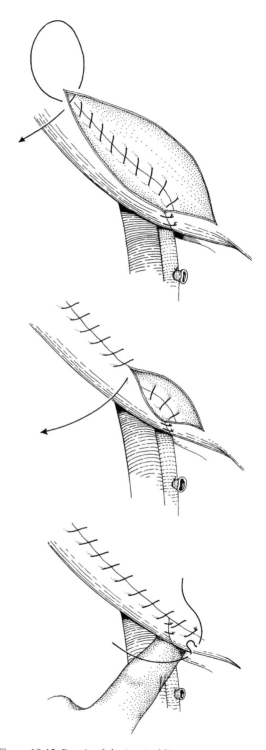

Figure 19.12 Repair of the inguinal ligament.

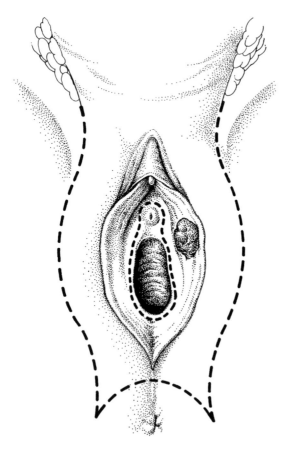

Figure 19.13 The vulval incision.

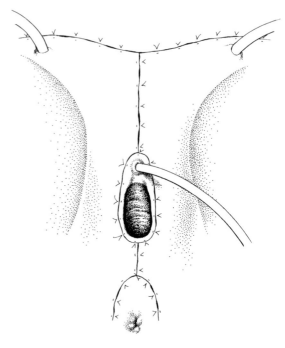

Figure 19.14 Completed repair of the vulval wound.

Excision of the vulval tumour

The patient is now placed in the lithotomy position.

The vulval incision must be varied according to the size and position of the carcinoma. The basic principles of removal are:

• A wide margin of normal skin must surround the carcinoma.

• The margin must be adequate at the deep as well as at the lateral and medial resection margins.

• All dystrophic skin should be removed with the specimen if possible.

The incision that was carried into the crural fold is now extended laterally to the vulva to end alongside the anus, the anus is skirted by a curved incision, and a similar incision is made on the opposite side (Fig. 19.13). The urethra and vagina are now encircled by the inner incision; if the lesion extends close to the urethra, it may be necessary to remove the lower half of the urethra.

The lateral incisions are deepened down to the deep fascia and periosteum and the vulval specimen removed. Free bleeding occurs at this time from three sites in the main: the ends of the two internal pudendal arteries and the vascular tissue around the base of the clitoris. Square mattress sutures are of great value in dealing with these points.

Primary closure of these wounds is easily achieved with interrupted Vicryl sutures and the patient leaves theatre lying flat with suction drains in the groins and a catheter in her bladder (Fig. 19.14).

Postoperative care

The epidural catheter is left *in situ* for 24–48 hours for analgesia and the patient is encouraged to commence active movements at a very early stage.

Primary healing is achieved in the majority of patients, especially with the use of separate incisions.

Complications

Wound breakdown and femoroinguinal lymphocyst formation are the two main postoperative complications. Rarer complications include secondary haemorrhage, thromboembolic disease, hernias and vaginal prolapse.

The recent changes made in the incisions have resulted in an increase in primary healing, rapid mobilization and a shortening of the time spent in hospital.

The major long-term complication is lymphoedema, with the majority of women being symptomatic to varying degrees. Referral to lymphoedema specialists at an early stage will prevent long-term morbidity. There is a suggestion that the prophylactic use of compression stockings for 6 months postoperatively reduces the incidence and severity of lymphoedema.

Further reading

For those readers with an interest in landmark references, the editors recommend the following.

Radical surgery

Taussig FJ. Primary cancer of the vulva, vagina and female urethra: five-year results. *Surg Gynecol Obstet* 1935;60:477.
Taussig FJ. Cancer of the vulva: an analysis of 155 cases. *Am J Obstet Gynecol* 1940;40:764–770.
Way S. The anatomy of the lymphatic drainage of the vulva, and its influence on the radical operation for carcinoma. *Ann R Coll Surg Engl* 1948;3:187.

Saphenous vein preservation

Dardarian TS. Saphenous vein sparing during inguinal lymphadenectomy to reduce morbidity in patients with vulvar carcinoma. *Gynecol Oncol* 2006;101:140–142.

Sentinel node dissection

Ansink AC, Sie-Go DM, van der Velden J, *et al*. Identification of sentinel lymph nodes in vulvar carcinoma patients with the aid of a patent blue V injection: a multicenter study. *Cancer* 1999;86:652–6.
DiSaia PJ, Creasman WT, Rich WM. An alternate approach to early cancer of the vulva. *Am J Obstet Gynecol* 1979;133:825–32.
Levenback C, Coleman RL, Burke TW, *et al*. Intraoperative lymphatic mapping and sentinel node identification with blue dye in patients with vulvar cancer. *Gynecol Oncol* 2001;83:276–81.
Van der Zee AG, Oonk MH, De Hullu JA, *et al*. Sentinel node dissection is safe in the treatment of early-stage vulvar cancer. *J Clin Oncol* 2008;26:884–889.

Lymphoedema

Sawan S, Mugnai R, Lopes Ade B, *et al*. Lower-limb lymphedema and vulval cancer: feasibility of prophylactic compression garments and validation of leg volume measurement. *Int J Gynecol Cancer* 2009;19:1649–1654.

Overview on the management of vulval cancer

Royal College of Obstetricians and Gynaecologists. *Management of Vulval Cancer*. London: RCOG, 2006. See www.rcog.org.uk/files/rcog-corp/uploaded-files/WPRVulvalCancerFull2006.pdf

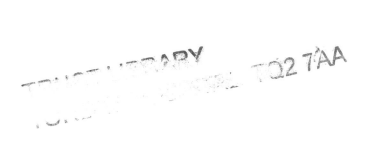

20 Vaginal cancer surgery

Primary vaginal cancer is rare, accounting for less than 2% of gynaecological cancers; however, metastatic cancers to the vagina occur two to three times more commonly. The incidence of primary vaginal cancer increases with age, being most common in women aged 65 and older. The majority are squamous cell carcinomas (80%) associated with human papillomavirus exposure; of the 14% of adenocarcinomas, there are a small number of clear cell carcinomas arising in young women exposed to diethylstilboestrol *in utero*, which occurred in the 1950s and 1960s. Melanomas and sarcomas account for about 7% of primary vaginal tumours.

The majority of women present with abnormal vaginal discharge or bleeding, although about 20% will be asymptomatic.

Treatment

The majority of vaginal cancers are treated by radiotherapy with or without chemotherapy and there are only a small number of centres, including Gateshead, where more than 50% of cases are treated surgically with or without radiotherapy.

Surgery is used predominantly for early cancers or those failing to respond to radiotherapy. The extent of surgery depends on the size, position and extent of the primary lesion.

Wide excision

Small lesions in the lower third of the vagina may on occasion be cured by wide local excision without compromising the nearby urinary or bowel structures. As with vulval cancers, when invasion is greater than 1 mm, an inguinofemoral node dissection or sentinel node sampling should be performed, as described in Chapter 19.

Partial or total vaginectomy

Small lesions in the upper vagina can be treated with a partial upper vaginectomy or radical hysterectomy and upper vaginectomy when the uterus is still present, combined with pelvic lymphadenectomy as described in Chapter 21.

A total vaginectomy is rarely performed and, in the majority of cases, it is for the treatment of vaginal intraepithelial neoplasia (VaIN) rather than invasive cancer. The surgical technique is described in Chapter 8. The surgery is complex, and many of the women will require postoperative radiotherapy such that the use of the procedure should be limited to individualized cases.

Bonney's Gynaecological Surgery, 11th edition.
© Tito Lopes, Nick Spirtos, Raj Naik, John Monaghan.
Published 2011 by Blackwell Publishing Ltd.

Exenteration

The procedure is described in Chapter 24. It may be an option if the primary cancer has extended to involve the bowel or bladder, or if the disease has recurred. Vaginal reconstruction should be considered especially in the younger woman.

Further reading

Tjalma WA, Monaghan JM, de Barros Lopes A, *et al*. The role of surgery in invasive squamous carcinoma of the vagina. *Gynecol Oncol* 2001;81:360–365.

21 Cervical cancer

Carcinoma of the cervix is the second most common female cancer worldwide and remains the most common in some developing countries. Although it is estimated that there are over 555 000 new cases a year worldwide, it has become a rare tumour in both the UK, with only 2800 cases registered in 2006, and the USA, with an estimated 11 000 new cases in 2008. The reason for these low rates in developed countries has been the introduction of national cervical screening programmes.

Persistent infection with high-risk types of human papillomavirus (HPV) has been identified as having a causal role in cervical cancer and HPV DNA can be identified in almost 100% of tumours. Prophylactic vaccines against HPV16 and HPV18 have been licensed in recent years and introduced into vaccination programmes in an increasing number of countries. Smoking and prolonged use of the oral contraceptive pill have also been recognized as risk factors. Immunocompromised women, either as a result of immunosuppressants for organ transplant or women with HIV not on antiretroviral treatment, are also at an increased risk of developing cervical cancer.

Treatment of cervical cancer is with either surgery or chemoradiation; the latter being used to treat most stages of the disease, with radical surgery reserved for stage IB and some IIA disease, especially in younger women. Adjuvant chemoradiation following surgery is used in the 15–30% of surgical cases in which the pelvic lymph nodes are found to contain metastatic disease or when the surgical excision margins of the radical procedure are considered to be inadequate.

The major advantage of surgery over chemoradiotherapy in younger women is the possibility of preserving the ovaries and the avoidance of short- and long-term side-effects associated with external beam radiotherapy and brachytherapy, particularly the reduction in vaginal morbidity. Chemoradiation invariably results in ovarian failure unless pre-treatment oophoropexy has been undertaken, and the vagina is often irreparably damaged with shortening and narrowing.

In the surgical management, nerve-sparing procedures causing less resultant damage to the pelvic nerves supplying the bladder have become fashionable in today's surgical practice. The laparoscopic approach has gained in popularity and has several advantages over the open approach. The short-term morbidity is less and it provides increasing variation in management, including fertility-sparing operations such as radical trachelectomy.

Small volume disease is increasingly being managed by conservative surgical methods, including cone biopsy or simple hysterectomy, often combined with laparoscopic pelvic lymph node dissection.

Radical hysterectomy and pelvic node dissection

History

Radical hysterectomy for the treatment of cervical cancer consists of the removal of the uterus, approxi-

Bonney's Gynaecological Surgery, 11th edition.
© Tito Lopes, Nick Spirtos, Raj Naik, John Monaghan.
Published 2011 by Blackwell Publishing Ltd.

mately the upper one-third of the vagina and the parametrium and paracolpos to the pelvic sidewall. The pelvic lymph nodes are dissected up to and including the common iliac nodes, although in some practices node dissection is extended to include the lower para-aortic lymph nodes up to the renal vessels.

W.A. Freund, in 1879, was the first to advocate abdominal hysterectomy for the treatment of cancer of the uterus, but it is to Reis of Chicago that the honour of developing the radical operation is given. In 1895, he demonstrated by operations on dogs and the human cadaver that it should be possible to remove the uterus, its appendages, the cellular tissue of the pelvis and the lymphatics up as far as the common iliac vessels. Clark, in 1895, put this suggestion into practice on a living woman at the Johns Hopkins Hospital and was quickly followed by others, while Thring of Sydney independently began to practise a similar procedure. The establishment of the radical technique as an accepted procedure was, however, due to Wertheim of Vienna, who performed the first of his extensive series in 1898.

In the first half of the twentieth century the operation was used extensively to treat almost all stages of cancer of the cervix. During this period, however, it became increasingly clear that radiotherapy was superior to surgery in treating all later stage disease and of at least equal potency in treating earlier disease. Also, the risks of surgery, in an era when there was no blood transfusion service and antibiotics were not available, were enormous.

The primary mortality from the operation as performed by Wertheim was initially 30%, later reduced to 10%. Bonney, in his series, produced similar figures, reducing his primary mortality from 20% to 11% in the last 200 of his first 500 cases. Although these figures are horrific by modern-day standards, they must be taken in the context of a time of no antibiotics and no blood transfusions. Nowadays, the emphasis has moved from mortality towards morbidity and great efforts must be made to continually reduce this to the absolute minimum.

Various classifications for the degree of radicality have been devised over the years, with the most well known being the Piver–Rutledge–Smith classification published in 1974. More recently, Querleu and Morrow have recommended a simplified classification.

Preoperative assessment

Before treatment can commence, a histological diagnosis must be made. If an invasive lesion of the cervix is suspected, an adequate biopsy must be performed, under colposcopic guidance if appropriate. Any diagnostic biopsies should be greater than 5 mm in depth or more than 7 mm apart for histology to confirm disease greater than FIGO stage IA disease requiring more radical surgery. A large cone biopsy adds little to the diagnosis, induces a marked inflammatory response and compromises assessment of tumour size by both histology and preoperative MRI. A small diagnostic loop biopsy is ideal and conization should be considered only as a therapeutic option for complete excision of a small lesion. Examination under anaesthesia (EUA) is not essential if pelvic examination assessed while awake is deemed to be adequate. However, one should have a low threshold for performing an EUA if there is any doubt.

FIGO staging remains a clinical procedure based on bimanual examination as the majority of cancers arise in underdeveloped countries where MRI scanning is unavailable and the disease presents at an advanced stage when surgery is not indicated. The tumour is examined to determine its size and any spread within the pelvis. This is achieved by performing a *bimanual examination*. First of all, the vagina is examined using two fingers of the right hand; this gives information about the cervix and the size and shape of the tumour. It also indicates whether there has been any spread to the fornices or into the mid- or lower vagina. The vaginal examination is not of great value in assessing the extent of spread towards the pelvic sidewall. This is best determined by carrying out a bimanual examination with one finger of the right hand in the rectum and the left hand on the abdomen. Using this technique, the rectovaginal septum, the uterosacral ligaments, the parametrium and the pelvic sidewall can be accurately assessed. Some teachers recommend the use of the combined examination, whereby the index finger is inserted into the vagina and the middle finger is inserted into the rectum.

We have found routine cystoscopy singularly uninformative for most small tumours less than 4 cm and reserve it for large tumours and those small tumours encroaching onto the anterior vaginal fornix. Proctosigmoidoscopy should be considered for large tumours with posterior extension. In the USA, for women over age 50 who have not been screened for colon cancer, a proctosigmoidoscopy is frequently performed at the same time as staging. The kidneys should be investigated for hydronephrosis by intravenous urogram (IVU), ultrasound or MRI as ureteric obstruction stages the tumour as at least stage IIIB. However, as with cystoscopy, an abnormal finding is extremely rare with apparent IB1 tumours.

Once the cancer has been staged, the most appropriate form of treatment must be discussed with the patient, accounting for age, stage, co-morbidities and treatment methods available. Surgery may be undertaken via laparotomy or using minimally invasive techniques. Fertility preservation may be possible.

For a radical abdominal hysterectomy the patient should be preassessed and prepared as for a major abdominal procedure.

Anaesthesia

The editors use a technique of epidural or spinal analgesia combined with general anaesthesia and are convinced that there are major advantages in terms of reduced blood loss through peripheral vasodilatation resulting in less intraoperative ooze. The regional anaesthesia also provides a sympathetic block and relaxation of visceral musculature allowing for easier packing of the bowel, resulting in better visualization during surgery. This is particularly true in laparoscopic cases. Where facilities are available, the epidural can be used for effective postoperative analgesia.

Surgery

It is the editors' practice to operate from the right side of the patient, and this should be taken into account when reading the surgical description.

The surgeon undertaking a major operation for a gynaecological cancer must not be compromised by having only one assistant. A second assistant is required as a 'dynamic retractor' that needs to be adjusted at various times during the operation. This is particularly the case with a radical hysterectomy in which the 'third' blade is sited at different points during the operation. In cases in which a second assistant is unavailable, the Martin arm retractor can provide the much needed dynamic retraction.

Instrumentation

A gynaecological general set as described in Chapter 3 is required with the addition of a disposable automatic blood vessel clip ligator. There is no replacement for good surgical techniques using basic instrumentation and sutures with well-thrown and placed knots. However, many new energy sources and stapling devices are currently available that can replace these techniques and these are described in the chapter on instrumentation.

Preparation

The patient is initially placed in the lithotomy position and the vulva and vagina are prepared. The bladder is catheterized with a self-retaining catheter and attached to a drainage device.

A vaginal pack facilitates reflection of the bladder and opening of the rectovaginal space (in laparoscopic surgery this function is duplicated by the use of the Gyne Tube (Paragon Imex Co., Menlo Park, CA, USA). An Amreich retractor is inserted into the vagina and, using a packing forceps, the vagina is firmly packed using a dry vaginal gauze roll (see Fig. 24.2). The patient's legs are then taken down from the lithotomy position. The end of the pack should be left long and placed between the patient's legs, with a forceps attached to the end so that the pack can be easily removed during the procedure.

The abdomen is now prepared and draped appropriately for the incision to be used.

Incision

The editors favour a midline subumbilical incision that can be extended above the umbilicus as necessary. This gives excellent access to the pelvis as well as to the lower para-aortic area. However, in obese women with a short distance between the umbilicus and pubic symphysis and a large pannus, a Cherney or Maylard incision can provide excellent access and may be combined with a panniculectomy. The abdomen is opened as described in Chapter 4.

Inspection

It is essential to fully inspect the pelvis to confirm the operability of the tumour. The parametrium is palpated for infiltration with tumour and the pelvic sidewalls for enlarged lymph nodes. The upper abdomen is inspected for evidence of metastatic disease and para-aortic lymphadenopathy.

Primary tumour (radical hysterectomy)

The editors' preference is to perform the radical hysterectomy first followed by the lymphadenectomy, although many surgeons perform the operation in the reverse order. The choice is based on the surgeon's preference and on the philosophy as to whether one should abandon surgery for the primary if there is obvious metastatic disease in the pelvic lymph nodes that will require adjuvant therapy. Our practice is to remove enlarged involved lymph nodes, as they are more likely to be radio-resistant and abandoning the radical hysterectomy.

Operative position and packing of the intestine

The patient should be placed in a steep Trendelenburg position, allowing the intestines to be easily packed away from the pelvis. This is usually achieved with one large moist pack. It is sometimes necessary to incise the peritoneum along the lateral side of the sigmoid colon at the pelvic brim to mobilize and elevate the sigmoid colon out of the pelvis.

Forceps to uterus

The uterus is grasped with two tissue forceps at the uterine cornu incorporating the round and ovarian ligaments as well as the tubes (see Chapter 11).

Round ligament

The right round ligament is grasped with tissue forceps in its lateral half and cut.

Uterovesical fold

At the same time the first assistant lifts the loose peritoneum over the bladder with a toothed forceps and the surgeon runs the scissors under the uterovesical fold separating the soft fascia. The peritoneum is then incised along the fold across to the left round ligament.

Infundibulopelvic/ovarian ligaments

If the ovaries are to be removed, the pelvic peritoneum lateral and along the ovarian vessels is cut to mobilize the infundibulopelvic ligament. The left index finger now elevates the ovary and tube and thrusts through the thin peritoneum of the posterior

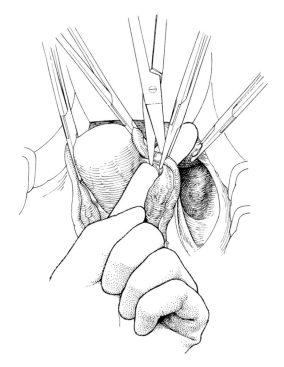

Figure 21.1 Dividing the right ovarian ligament.

leaf of the broad ligament medial or lateral to the ovary depending on whether it is to be preserved or removed. The infundibulopelvic or ovarian ligament is then clamped with a medium tissue forceps with the tip in the defect created by the index finger. Prior to cutting the ligament it may be appropriate to adjust the uterine clamp with its tip in the peritoneal defect to prevent a back flow of blood. The ligament can now be cut, stapled or cauterized (Fig. 21.1).

The round and infundibulopelvic/ovarian ligaments are tied or may remain held by the clamps until the end of the operation to facilitate the maintenance of tension on the tissues. However, using this technique often requires one or other of the assistants to be constantly holding the clamps to prevent them entering the pelvis.

The same procedure is now performed on the left side.

Identification of ureter, identification and ligation of uterine artery

The uterine clamps are now handed to the first assistant, who draws the uterus over towards him- or herself. The second assistant controls the clamps on the round and infundibulopelvic ligaments (if used), and maintains traction on the Morris retractor. If the assistants maintain this slight tension, the space alongside the uterus is immediately available.

The surgeon now separates the soft areolar tissue of the opened broad ligament down to the level at which the anterior division of the internal iliac artery becomes visible. Using the Monaghan scissors, the ureter, uterine artery and the obliterated hypogastric artery are readily identified. The uterine artery is cleared in front and behind so that it is completely separated from the ureter which it overlies (Fig. 21.2). The ureter is separated from the peritoneum for a short distance and a Meigs forceps is inserted below the uterine artery. This forceps is then lifted up, gently putting the artery on the stretch. If the forceps is opened, all the areolar tissue below the artery is separated and the ureter can be seen to be completely clear. A straight tissue forceps is now placed between the open jaws of the Meigs forceps and the artery clamped (Fig. 21.3). The Meigs forceps is now

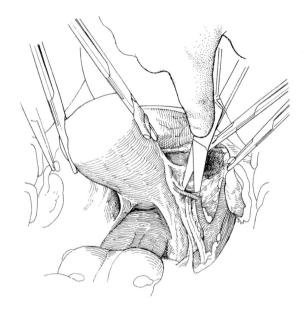

Figure 21.2 Identifying the uterine artery close to the pelvic sidewall.

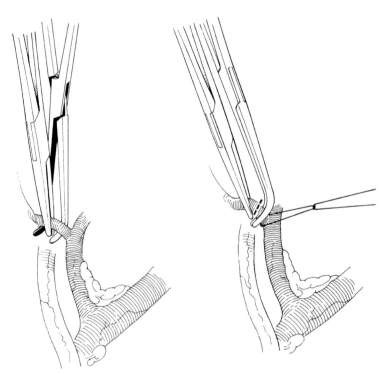

Figure 21.3 Dividing the right uterine artery at its origin.

removed and, using the straight forceps to elevate the artery, the vessel can be accurately clamped close to its origin at the internal iliac artery. The vessel is now cut close to the Meigs forceps and ligated. It is here that the Meigs forceps are of such enormous value: they are long, the tip or the heel can be used to loop the tie around, yet they are delicate enough not to leave a large mass of tissue behind in the ligated pedicle. This dissection can be facilitated by the use of hydrodissection and the vessels can also be stapled, cauterized or otherwise sealed.

The same procedure is performed on the opposite side.

In obese women with a deep pelvis in whom access may be limited, it is sometimes easier to ligate the uterine artery using the arterial Ligaclips (Ethicon Endo-Surgery Inc., Cincinnati, OH, USA) rather than applying a Meigs forceps and tying around it. The medial end of the uterine artery can still be held with a straight tissue forceps, which provides traction while dissecting the ureteric tunnel.

Occasionally, small veins close to the ureter or the artery bleed; this can produce a confusing picture to the trainee surgeon. It is important not to clamp any structure in this area until it is clearly identified; therefore, the editors would recommend the insertion of a swab into the space to stem oozing and to return to the area after a few minutes. Soaking the swab with epinephrine or thrombin enhances haemostasis. (The scrub nurse must be informed that a swab has been inserted and the fact marked on the count board.) Upon returning to the area it will be found that the structures are easily identified and the dissection can be proceeded with.

Reflection of bladder

It is recommended leaving this stage until after the ureters and the uterine artery have been isolated, as there is frequently troublesome bleeding from small vessels which are injured. Separation is easily achieved by pushing down the uterovesical fold with a swab folded over the finger. The smooth surface of the packed upper vagina is readily recognized and small fibres of tissue can be divided. If there is difficulty in finding this tissue plane, a light stroke with a knife across the width of the upper vagina with traction on the bladder and uterus will reveal the correct level. Frequently, engorged veins are found lying in the lateral part of this dissection. These should be handled

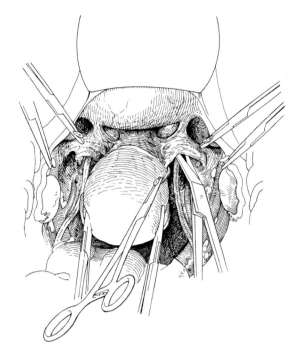

Figure 21.4 Identifying the ureteric tunnel.

gently; otherwise, profuse haemorrhage can occur and cause problems in the next steps.

If the finger or the back of the closed Monaghan scissors is pushed into the lateral part of this dissection, the ridge of tissue which is formed gives a clear indication of the site of the ureteric tunnel; occasionally, the ureter in the last 2 cm of its course is visible at the bottom of this dissection.

The lateral dissection should be performed one side at a time because of potential for venous bleeding.

Development and incision of the roof or the ureteric tunnel

The roof of the ureteric tunnel can often be well demarcated by placing the Morris retractor centrally and applying an upward pull countered by the uterus being gently pulled cranially.

The tissue forceps on the uterine artery is drawn medially over the top of the ureter, and Monaghan scissors are inserted over the top of the ureter along its track to open out the ureteric tunnel (Fig. 21.4). If the opened scissors are elevated, the ureter can be seen along its tract, completely separated from the

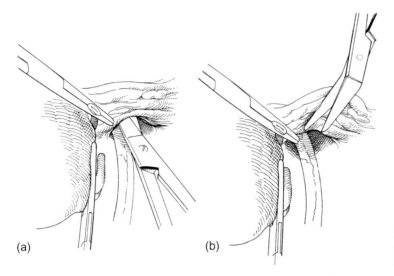

Figure 21.5 (a and b) Separating the ureter from the roof of the ureteric tunnel.

(a)

(b)

roof of the tunnel (Fig. 21.5a,b). With the scissors protecting the ureter, a straight tissue forceps is placed along the tunnel roof and clamped. The roof is cut medial to the forceps, exposing the ureter as it enters the bladder. The pedicle is now firmly tied. Use of hydrodissection into the tunnel can help create and enlarge the ureteric tunnel.

The division of the left ureteric tunnel can be facilitated by performing some of the dissection from the medial aspect of the tunnel.

Separation of the ureter from the upper vagina
Using Monaghan scissors, the ureter is separated from the upper vagina and dislocated laterally; this reveals the cardinal ligament passing downwards and laterally. The ureter is completely separated from the peritoneum in the lower part of the pelvis but remains in contact in the upper part. It is not necessary to strip the ureter to its full length in the pelvis.

Opening of the rectovaginal space
This step can be performed prior to the dissection of the ureteric tunnels as bleeding from the vaginal veins during the preparation and dissection of the tunnels may be difficult to control while the uterus is *in situ*. As a result the surgeon may often rush this step of the operation in a hurry to remove the uterus. In contrast, the opening of the rectovaginal space is bloodless and the reflection of the rectum off

the vagina and the development of the uterosacral ligaments can be performed precisely and at ease before proceeding to the ureteric tunnels.

The Morris retractor is now removed and the uterine clamps are handed to the second assistant, who elevates the uterus at the front of the abdominal incision. This brings into view the whole of the pouch of Douglas and makes the uterosacral ligaments prominent. The peritoneum immediately below the cervix is grasped with a pair of toothed dissectors held in the left hand and the surface is cut with Bonney scissors. The scissors are then introduced into the space and opened, revealing the soft areolar tissue running down between vagina and rectum (Fig. 21.6). This incision across the peritoneum is completed posteriorly in a transverse manner, keeping the ureter under direct vision at all times. The incision runs over the surface of the uterosacral ligaments; it is important not to cut into these ligaments but to merely separate the peritoneum from their surface.

Placing a swab over the first three fingers of the left hand, the rectum is swept from the vagina using an extension movement of the hand; at the same time, the peritoneum is separated from the uterosacral ligaments, revealing them as an arched structure (Fig. 21.7).

Sharp dissection can also be used to identify and skeletonize the uterosacral ligaments further.

198

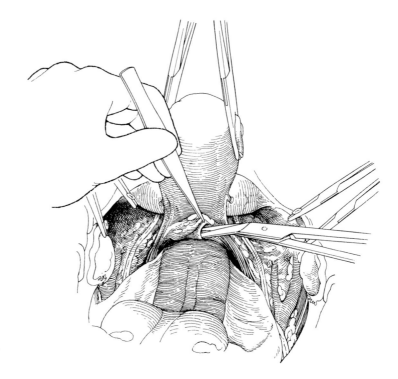

Figure 21.6 Opening the space between the rectum and the vagina.

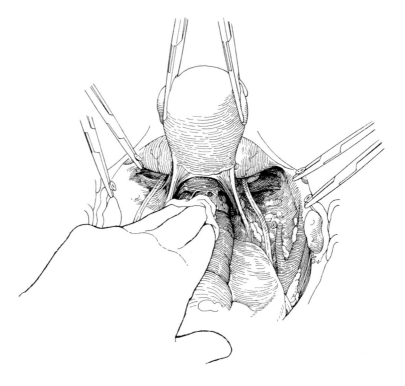

Figure 21.7 The rectum separated from the vagina, showing the arch of the uterosacral ligaments.

Placement of clamps, and incision

At this point in the dissection, the surgeon can put the final touches to this part of the procedure by checking that the ureters are free from the vagina and cardinal ligaments and that the bladder is reflected down far enough to expose the requisite length of vagina.

The uterosacral ligaments run posteriolaterally from the cervix. They can be palpated by hooking the index finger around them. The hysterectomy tissue forceps are now placed midway along the ligaments, which are divided using the scissors. It is unnecessary to place the clamps as far laterally as possible except when dealing with a large primary tumour.

A second set of hysterectomy clamps are placed on the cardinal ligaments; again, the lateral extent being based on the size of the primary lesion. The ligaments are divided and the vaginal pack is removed and a third set of clamps, more angled than the previous, is placed on the paracolpos, which are excised (Fig. 21.8).

Increasingly, surgeons are using staplers or a variety of energy sources such as the Harmonic Scalpel (Ethicon Endo-Surgery Inc.), PlasmaKinetic (Gyrus PK; Gyrus ACMI, Southborough, MA, USA) or Ligasure (Covidien Inc., Boulder, CO, USA) to transect the ligaments.

Incision of vagina

The anterior wall of the vagina is incised with a scalpel and the incision is extended through the posterior wall while lifting the uterus upwards and cranially to protect the rectum from injury.

Ligation of pedicles

Some bleeding occurs as the vagina is incised and a small swab can be pressed against the incised edge while the hysterectomy clamps are individually stitch ligatured. Great care is taken to have the ureter fully visible at this time. Some authorities recommend pulling the ureters away from the field with coloured vascular loops, but the editors do not recommend this, preferring the ureter to lie naturally within the operation field.

Oversewing vaginal edge

After the pedicles are secured with a Vicryl stitch, the rim of the vagina is sutured using a continuous stitch as a haemostat. This should be locked on the posterior edge and run continuously on the anterior edge to help evert the rim, making the taking of the next 'bite' easier. The surgeon should hold the thread of the suture him- or herself to provide the correct tension required.

Once all bleeding is controlled the pelvis can be left and the node dissection carried out.

Lymphadenectomy

The extent of the node dissection varies between different surgeons, but should consist of the removal of all visible pelvic lymph nodes from the bifurcation of the common iliac artery caudally. If there are any enlarged nodes identified during the procedure, dissection should extend cranially to include the common iliac lymph nodes. Any enlarged common iliac or para-aortic nodes should be removed.

The second assistant places a Morris retractor under the lateral aspect of the round ligament and retracts caudally, exposing the iliac vessels. A second Morris retractor is placed under the peritoneal fold at the point where the ovarian or the infundibulopel-

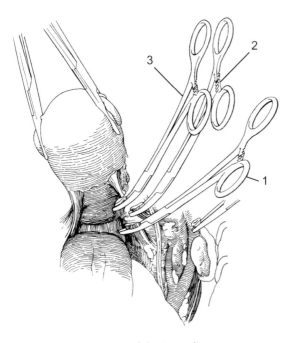

Figure 21.8 The position of the tissue clamps on the uterosacral (1) and cardinal (2) ligaments and the paracolpos (3).

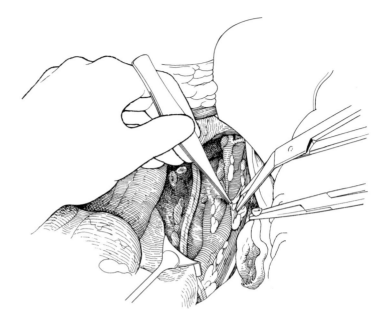

Figure 21.9 Beginning of the pelvic node dissection.

vic ligament was cut and is retracted cranially by the first assistant, exposing the common iliac vessels and displacing the ureter medially. The fascia over the iliopsoas muscle is now picked up in toothed dissectors and incised along the line of the artery (Fig. 21.9), taking care not to damage the genitofemoral nerve. This incision is carried up to the retractor, and the lateral external iliac nodes lying under the inguinal ligament are drawn down across the vessels. Individual lymphatic channels are meticulously diathermied or clipped using small metal clips (Auto Suture Ligaclips); occasionally, small blood vessels are severed and should also be clipped (Fig. 21.10).

The line of dissection now continues along the length of the external iliac artery, developing a sheet of fascia and nodal tissue, which will leave the arteries clean from the bifurcation of the common iliac artery to the inguinal ligament. If tension is maintained on this fascia with the left hand, and separation and dissection performed using the Monaghan scissors in the right, it is possible to roll the vessels round so that all nodal tissue is removed en bloc. The artery is then retracted laterally gently with the Cushing vessel retractor and the dissection is repeated along the external iliac vein. At the upper end of the dissection, the sheet of tissue separated is continued down the internal iliac artery (Fig. 21.11), taking great care to

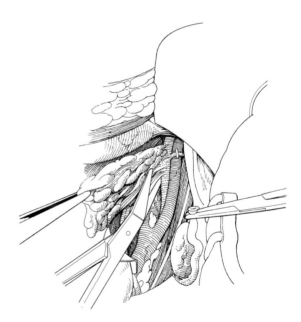

Figure 21.10 The complete block of lymph nodes being removed from the external iliac vessels.

keep an eye on the ureter. Finally, this dissection dips below the external iliac vein so that the obturator fossa can be emptied of all nodal material, resulting in a block of tissue lying close to the tied uterine

201

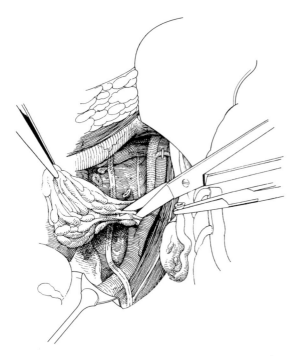

Figure 21.11 Completing the pelvic node dissection in the obturator fossa.

artery. Retracting the external iliac vein and artery laterally with the Cushing vessel retractor exposes the obturator fossa, facilitating the dissection. The mass is lifted out and may be separated into its constituent parts. Bleeding is surprisingly little, especially if small vessels and lymphatics are clipped with the metal clips as the dissection proceeds.

Closure of the abdomen

At the end of the lymphadenectomy, the pelvis should be checked for haemostasis and any bleeding controlled. In the past, it was felt that drainage of the pelvic space was required to prevent the formation of lymphocysts. However, the editors have shown that, as long as the pelvis is not reperitonized, there is no benefit to drainage. For this reason, a drain should only be inserted if there is any concern regarding haemostasis.

In premenopausal women in whom the ovaries are conserved, consideration should be given to transpose one of the ovaries outside the pelvis in case adjuvant radiotherapy to the pelvis is required. The inferior margins of the ovaries can be marked with metal clips to assist the radiotherapist with planning treatment.

If a suprapubic catheter is to be inserted, this can be inserted by direct vision before the abdomen is closed. The bladder is filled by inserting about 400 mL of saline through the transurethral catheter, facilitating insertion of the suprapubic catheter. The editors have found these to be superior to transurethral catheters in allowing patients to spontaneously initiate passage of urine. They also facilitate bladder training and assessment of residual urine volumes without the need for frequent catheterization with all its attendant risks. Most patients will pass urine spontaneously during the first 10 days postoperatively, but a small percentage will take longer for bladder recovery. In these cases, the women are taught to self-catheterize prior to discharge from the hospital and the suprapubic catheter is removed.

The abdomen is closed by mass closure, as described in Chapter 4.

Complications of radical hysterectomy

Complications may be subdivided into intraoperative, postoperative and long-term (Table 21.1).

Haemorrhage

Haemorrhage during a radical hysterectomy is a significant risk, especially at certain anatomical sites during dissection. Venous bleeding, particularly that arising from injury to the lower vena cava if para-aortic node dissection is performed, requires compression not only inferiorly and superiorly but laterally in order to compress the lumbar perforators. This can best be accomplished using four sponge/swab sticks, thereby collapsing the vein, which allows for primary suture repair while minimizing blood loss. For arterial bleeding or pelvic haemorrhage, in addition to calling for a vascular surgeon, consideration should be given to clamping the aorta below the renal vessels and heparinizing the patient. This is safe if the clamp time is less than 1–2 hours.

Sites associated with a high risk of haemorrhage include:
- ureteric tunnel
- paracolpos and vaginal edge
- external iliac artery and vein
- obturator fossa
- bifurcation of the common iliac artery and vein.

Table 21.1 Complications of radical hysterectomy

Intraoperative	Postoperative	Long term
Haemorrhage and vascular trauma Ureteric, bladder, bowel and nerve trauma	Ileus Infection Thromboembolic disease Ureteric and bladder fistulae Lymphocyst	Bladder dysfunction Ureteric and bladder fistulae Pelvic lymphocyst Leg lymphoedema

Bladder dysfunction

Following radical hysterectomy and node dissection, the commonest complication is bladder dysfunction, manifesting itself as difficulty in initiating micturition and fully emptying the bladder. Catheterization is essential in the postoperative period, but is often unnecessary for a prolonged time.

In attempting to reduce the bladder dysfunction, nerve-sparing techniques have been adopted by some surgeons. As the extent of the soft tissue resection is limited in the nerve-sparing procedures, some have called into question the adequacy of these modifications.

All patients who have had radical hysterectomies should have the urethral catheter removed at 5 days or the suprapubic catheter turned off, and be allowed to initiate spontaneous micturition. If the patient cannot void or can pass only small volumes, catheter drainage should be reinstated for a further 24 hours. When the patient is able to void, the residual urine volume should be assessed on the evening of the first day. If the patient is unable to pass urine spontaneously, or the residual urine volume is greater than 100 mL, at the time of discharge from hospital she should be taught intermittent self-catheterization.

Ureteric dysfunction

Most patients (87%) show ureteric dilatation 48 hours after the operation, usually with complete recovery by 6 weeks. At the end of the first week, 20–30% of postoperative IVUs are abnormal: dilatation of the upper renal tract is seen whereas the distal one-third may be normal or narrowed.

In almost all patients, these changes will have disappeared by the end of the first year after surgery. When irradiation has been used preoperatively, devascularization of the ureter can be critical, result-ing in fistula formation or at least fibrosis, stricture and loss of peristalsis in the affected segment.

The incidence of ureteric fistula appears to be decreasing in the reported literature. It is probably most influenced by the routine use of prophylactic antibiotics, better pelvic drainage and a reduction in the use of preoperative radiotherapy.

Ureteric stricture is very rare following radiotherapy alone, relatively rare following surgery but occurs more commonly after combination surgery and radiotherapy. If there is an obvious external cause for the stricture, such as a lymphocyst or local recurrence of tumour, then appropriate steps must be taken to deal with this problem. If the obstruction does not clear or cannot be simply resolved by the use of stents, then a urinary diversion must be made.

Vesicovaginal fistula

This complication is less common than ureterovaginal fistula in most reported series. It usually follows intraoperative trauma to the bladder, most commonly in the midline and at a high level in the bladder. Consequently, management should be all about masterly inactivity and continuous bladder drainage. Most fistulae heal spontaneously if the bladder is effectively drained, the exceptions being when the patient has had pre- or postoperative radiotherapy.

Urinary tract infection

The most common cause for postoperative febrile morbidity is a urinary tract infection. It is important to use a sterile technique when inserting the urethral catheter and to maintain a high urine output in the postoperative period. In addition, a catheter specimen of urine (CSU) should be collected if there is a pyrexia and at the time of removal of the catheter.

Pelvic lymphocysts

The incidence of lymphocysts detected by ultrasound is approximately 15–20%, with between 1% and 4% being identified clinically. The lymphocyst appears a few days after operation and may grow steadily for the next few months. Thereafter, in most cases, steady resolution occurs as the fluid contained in the cyst is reabsorbed. On rectal examination, they are palpable as a smooth, tense mass attached to the pelvic sidewall and must be distinguished from tumour recurrence and infection. This differentiation is most easily carried out by ultrasonography.

Lymphocysts require active management when they become infected, or produce pain or obstruction. Symptomatic lymphocysts should be drained. This can be performed under scan guidance, but will often recur and may require laparoscopic 'de-roofing', excising a segment of the lymphocyst wall to allow free drainage.

Nerve damage

The nerve damage most likely to occur is to the genitofemoral and the obturator nerves during node dissection on the pelvic sidewall. It is not unusual for the genitofemoral nerve to be present as a number of thin strands rather than a single nerve bundle; these strands may be mistaken for lymphatics and dissected out by the operator. Damage to the nerve results in loss of sensation over a small part of the anterior surface of the upper thigh and the labia of the vulva. The obturator nerve may be damaged when removing the obturator nodes, which lie along the length of the nerve. Damage to this nerve may produce palsy of the adductors of the inner thigh or pain of the muscles or skin in the inner thigh. Should the transection of this nerve be identified during surgery, often it can be repaired with 7-0 Prolene (Ethicon Endo-Surgery Inc.) with excellent functional results.

Prevention is best achieved by carefully identifying the nerves before continuing with the dissection.

Rather less commonly, deep dissection of the pelvis may produce some sciatic nerve damage, usually manifesting itself as sciatica, but it is much more common to have this type of pain following infiltration of the perineural lymphatics by tumour micrometastases.

Peroneal nerve damage is a risk whenever any patient is put into lithotomy poles.

Laparoscopic radical hysterectomy with aortic and pelvic lymphadenectomy

Approach

In this procedure 12-mm ports are placed approximately 3–4 cm above the umbilicus; at or slightly above the iliac crests; and just above the symphysis pubis. If the superior port is placed too close to the umbilicus, the visual field is obstructed by the uterus because it is progressively elevated as the radical hysterectomy proceeds. Occasionally, in the obese patient, a fifth trocar will be placed near the left costal margin in order to insert a fan retractor to keep the bowel out of the operative field. By using 12-mm ports lymph nodes may be grasped with a variety of large graspers allowing for the direct removal of the nodal tissue without the need for changing instruments or inserting an endoscopic bag. This should be reserved for suspicious lymph nodes to try and avoid port site implantation.

Para-aortic lymphadenectomy

If the aortic lymph nodes are to be resected this should be undertaken first as it is the part of the operation most likely to lead to termination of the procedure either because of metastases being identified in the aortic lymph nodes or because of the need to convert to an open procedure owing to vascular complications. This is best accomplished with the camera placed in the suprapubic port with the surgeon operating on the patient's right side, working into the upper abdomen, or between the patient's legs, again working in the same direction as the camera is pointing. To work in the opposite direction of the camera is difficult at best and limits the upward extent of the aortic lymph node dissection. Any number of energy sources and devices have been used and well described to carry out the lymph node dissection, including argon beam coagulation (ABC), the Harmonic Scalpel, Ligasure, the Gyrus PK bipolar device, as well as standard bipolar and monopolar cautery. The editors' preference is to use ABC as it penetrates only 1 mm in depth while providing excellent haemostasis. The peritoneum over the right common iliac artery is incised and the incision extended both superiorly to the level of the duodenum and inferiorly parallel to the rectosigmoid down to the level of the peritoneal reflection.

This is particularly important as it allows for lateral displacement of rectosigmoid later when harvesting the left high common and low aortic lymph nodes. An epinephrine-soaked small-sized swab is inserted into the operative field and the assistant elevates the duodenum by upwardly displacing the grasper inserted through the left lower quadrant trocar. The epinephrine-soaked swab provides a measure of additional haemostasis by causing the constriction of the small vessels in the field of dissection and also provides an interface between the assistant's retracting grasper and the duodenum. Lastly, if irrigation is used, suction applied over the swab minimizes the number of times the intestine will be pulled into the suction device. The skeletonization of the vena cava is then undertaken after instilling saline or water under the node pad. This manoeuvre provides an added margin of safety between the energy source being used and the thin caval wall as well as acting as a dissector. This dissection can then be carried out on the right side to the renal vessels, if so desired. Care should be taken when dissecting near the insertion of the right ovarian vein into the vena cava as undue traction can result in significant haemorrhage. Dissection is then carried out on the left side by removing the intercaval lymph nodes and the nodes between the left ovarian vein and the aorta. On both sides of the dissection the ureters should be identified and mobilized laterally away from the field of dissection. In most cases, the nodal dissection can be carried out inferiorly to the level of the inferior mesenteric artery (IMA). At this point, it is best to replicate the dissection as begun on the right side, starting at the level of the left common iliac artery and moving in the cephalad direction until the IMA is reached. The assistant at this point grasps the mesentery of the rectosigmoid that has been previously freed up and retracts it laterally and superiorly. This provides excellent exposure along the lateral aspect of the aorta. Particular care must be taken in order not to transect the sympathetic nerves lest your patient awakens with a warm foot on this side due to an incidental sympathectomy. Some authors have purposefully transected the IMA, providing the maximum and, in many ways, the easiest exposure to the aortic lymph nodes. There is a 1–2% risk that the marginal artery of Drummond does not provide adequate blood supply to the rectosigmoid, causing a portion of this organ to be compromised. As in all surgical paradigms, the surgeon must decide which risk is greater

to the patient. If macroscopically positive aortic lymph nodes are encountered then the pelvic node dissection would be undertaken only to remove similarly involved lymph nodes. Otherwise, the procedure is terminated and the patient will be treated with chemoradiation using extended field radiotherapy.

Radical hysterectomy and pelvic lymphadenectomy

Once the aortic lymph node dissection is completed, the camera is moved to the supraumbilical port and the operating surgeon now stands on the left side of the patient, working into the pelvis. As in open procedures the paravesical and pararectal spaces are developed and any question of macroscopic involvement of the parametria or lymph nodes by metastatic disease requires biopsy in order to avoid unnecessary surgery in patients requiring chemoradiation regardless of whether the radical surgery is completed. These spaces are easily identified and developed by transecting the round ligament near the point it exits the pelvic sidewall and incising the peritoneum parallel to it and sweeping your dissector medially. This manoeuvre allows for easy displacement of the obliterated hypogastric vessel (superior vesical artery) medially, providing excellent exposure to the obturator space as well as the pelvic floor musculature. Using a similar lateral to medial motion just distal to the bifurcation of the common iliac artery, the ureter along with the rectosigmoid can be swept to the midline, providing an easy way to develop the pararectal space and clearly defining the cardinal ligament. By continuing to mobilize the ureter medially as it passes distally into the pelvis, the point of origin of the uterine artery will become obvious and, by continuing this medial mobilization of the ureter, the lateral cardinal ligament can be secured either with endoscopic staplers or with an energy source of the surgeon's choice. In this area, the argon beam coagulators should not be used as the vessel size can sometimes exceed the limits of its ability to achieve haemostasis. Similarly, at this point, one can choose to resect the superior vesical artery (Piver type IV) for larger lesions. Once the parametrium has been transected, the lymphadenectomy can be easily completed. The skeletonization of the iliac vessels is undertaken in a similar manner using hydrodissection to develop the surgical planes and an energy source to maintain haemostasis and seal the lymphatics.

It helps to mobilize the iliac vessels medial to the psoas muscle with care being taken to leave the genitofemoral nerve intact while securing the small perforators from the psoas to the iliac vessels that can be quite troublesome if transected. Once the vessels are mobilized medially the lymph nodes lateral to the vessels can be easily resected using hydrodissection and haemostatic instruments. The dissection is carried out down to the sciatic nerve then distally to the point the obturator nerve penetrates the obturator muscle as it leaves the pelvis. The medial and anterior aspects of the iliac vessels are then skeletonized and the node dissection completed.

Attention is next turned to completing the radical hysterectomy with or without removal of the adnexa. Regardless of the surgical method used to complete the radical hysterectomy, issues such as ovarian preservation and transposition need to be discussed with the patient and those decisions acted upon. The adnexal blood supply again may be secured by any number of instruments, with the editors' current preference being the Gyrus PK device. This, in combination with hydrodissection, allows for easy development of the rectovaginal septum and the vesicouterine fold. Once the rectum is dissected free of the vagina posteriorly, the uterosacral ligaments can be secured and transected and the cardinal ligament can be further secured. These steps will result in the elevation of the uterus, sometimes limiting the operative field to the point that an additional trocar may need to be placed superior to the initial supraumbilical placement. At this point a disposable Gyne Tube (Fig. 21.12) is inserted, facilitating further distal mobilization of the bladder from the proximal vagina. It is only at this point that the ureters are dissected free from under the uterine arteries and into and through the cervicovesical fascia, the ureteric tunnel. Using hydrodissection with a Stryker irrigation device, the ureter is dissected laterally and posterior within the tunnel and then in the opposite direction. The 'roof' of the tunnel is transected, allowing for the posterior and lateral displacement of the ureters. Once the ureters are displaced, the remaining segment of the cardinal ligament is resected and the vaginal margin identified. As the Gyne Tube is closed distally and sculptured, allowing for the deeper posterior aspect of the vagina, the colpotomy can be performed with ABC without losing the pneumoperitoneum.

Vaginal closure

Once the colpotomy is completed the specimen is removed and the vagina is closed using an Endo Stitch device (Covidien) with a 0 Polysorb suture. The closure begins after securing a looped knot at approximately 2.5 cm. A 'tag' of approximately 4 cm is left distal to the looped knot. The Endostitch is the passed through the suprapubic trocar and suturing of the vagina begins by passing the Endostitch from out to in and then back out in the midpoint of the posterior vagina. The needle of the Endostitch is then passed through the looped knot and tightened. The surgeon follows him- or herself while closing the vagina in a posterior to anterior direction and then back, resulting in a two-layer closure of the vagina. The suture is tied to the tag left distal to the loop as initially described. The Gyne Tube can now be removed. Since beginning to use this technique over 5 years ago the

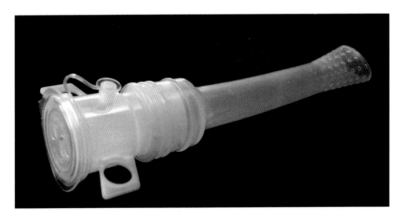

Figure 21.12 The Gyne Tube.

editors have not seen a significant problem with cuff dehiscence or leakage of peritoneal fluid.

Issues

Although there have been no reports of a negative impact on survival with the use of minimally invasive techniques, a few words of caution might be pertinent at this point, particularly regarding the tendency to resect more vagina then necessary and the possibility of devascularizing the distal ureters as the visualization provided with the laparoscope allows for identification and cauterization or clipping smaller ureteral vessels. Some authors have addressed the first potential problem by placing a suture marking the vaginal margin prior to starting the surgical procedure. Many institutions place ureteral stents prior to undertaking the laparoscopic radical hysterectomy and leaving them *in situ* for up to 6 weeks to avoid the problem of possibly compromising the blood supply to the distal ureter and thus to minimize the incidence of ureteral fistula.

Radical vaginal hysterectomy

The vaginal approach for radical hysterectomy was resurrected by Dargent in the 1980s as part of the laparoscopic assisted radical vaginal hysterectomy or coelio-Schauta procedure. When Schauta popularized the radical vaginal operation devised by Pawlik in the early 1900s it met the great need to reduce the significant infective morbidity and sometimes mortality associated with the radical abdominal procedure developed by Wertheim. The operation also met the needs of operating on the very obese and rather unfit patient.

The main failure of the Schauta procedure was that there was no way to deal with the possibility of involved pelvic lymph nodes. As this became an obligatory part of the surgery for cervical cancer, the Schauta operation fell into disuse, excepting when modifications were developed to deal with the need for a lymphadenectomy, such as the Mitra operation, developed to perform an extraperitoneal lymphadenectomy combined with the radical vaginal hysterectomy.

Dargent utilized the modifications of the Schauta technique, together with the modern developments of laparoscopic surgery, to perform a full radical hys-

terectomy vaginally after a minimally invasive laparoscopic procedure, removing the pelvic and, sometimes if appropriate, para-aortic lymph nodes as well.

The radical vaginal hysterectomy described here was developed in Gateshead following the guidance of Dargent and is based on the less radical Schauta–Stoeckel approach. Patient selection is important as performing the procedure in a patient with a narrowed pelvic arch is quite difficult even when using a Schuchardt incision. The procedure as per Dargent's practice is limited to tumours smaller than 2 cm to optimize margins.

The laparoscopic element of lymphadenectomy and ligation of the uterine arteries at source are similar to that described earlier in this chapter.

The principles of the procedure

As with the radical abdominal hysterectomy, the vaginal procedure aims to remove the entire uterus and, if appropriate, the tubes and ovaries, together with an adequate amount of vaginal, paravaginal and parametrial tissues.

Anatomical considerations

When the abdominal approach is used for the radical hysterectomy, the uterine artery crosses medially from its take-off point on the anterior division of the internal iliac artery to cross over the roof of the ureteric tunnel before dividing into an ascending and descending branch to supply the uterus. The ureter runs around the cervix under the uterine artery in a tunnel of loose connective tissue, the upper part of which must be released in order to remove the uterine artery and the lymphatic drainage associated with it. In the vaginal operation, the uterus is drawn downwards into the vagina and the bladder retracted upwards, with the result that the uterine vessels now run downwards and medially while the ureter, because of the tension from the uterine vessels, is caused to also run downwards and then appears to turn upwards to enter the bladder. Thus, a ureteric loop is created, the bend of which is called the ureteric knee by vaginal surgeons with the uterine vessels passing first above and then medial and below the ureter (Fig. 21.13).

It is important to understand the concept that the change in apparent position of the uterine artery from

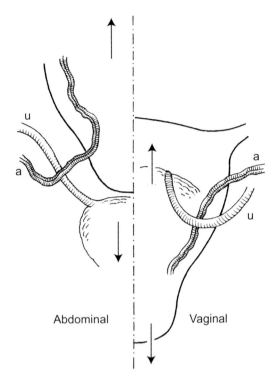

Figure 21.13 Comparison of relative anatomy of ureter and uterine artery between an abdominal and vaginal approach. a, artery; u, ureter.

clearly being above the ureter to appearing to lie below and medial to it is entirely due to tension on the uterus.

Instruments

Similar instruments to those required for the vaginal hysterectomy are necessary. However, it is important to add one or two narrow-bladed Wertheim retractors together with the long-toothed tissue forceps developed by Rudolf Chrobak (Fig. 21.14), a gynaecologist working in Vienna at the same time as Wertheim. These important clamps are used to grasp the vaginal cuff that is developed at the beginning of the procedure. The Schauta element of the laparoscopic lymphadenectomy and radical vaginal hysterectomy (coelio-Schauta) is normally performed after the laparoscopic lymphadenectomy is completed. At the laparoscopic lymphadenectomy, the patient may

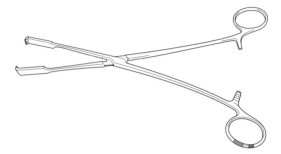

Figure 21.14 Chrobak forceps.

be lying prone, or may already be in the lithotomy position. It is essential for the Schauta procedure for the patient to be in the lithotomy position and, once more, the hips should be flexed as much as possible with the buttocks right on the end of the table.

Anaesthesia

Usually, a general anaesthetic is used, preferably with addition of an epidural or spinal anaesthesia. Blood loss is usually minimal with this operation.

The operation

Preparation of the vagina cuff

As this operation is normally performed for early stage cervical cancer it is common that only a small part of the cervix is infiltrated by the tumour. The cervix should be gently drawn down by grasping a healthy part of the cervix and infiltrating the vaginal tissues above and around it. Using Littlewood or Kocher forceps the vaginal tissue to be removed is defined. This is normally some 2–3 cm of vagina. It is important not to remove too long a length as this can produce debilitating shortening of the vagina. Once the edge of the vagina has been defined and drawn down (Fig. 21.15), infiltration is completed as for a vaginal hysterectomy and, at this point, the vagina is incised just above the position of the Littlewood forceps. As the vagina is incised, the vaginal edge is drawn forwards off the cervix so as to lie in a position to cover over the cervical tissue. The incision is carried circumferentially around the vagina, taking care not to cut too deeply; because of the increased length of vagina being removed, there is a risk to the bladder

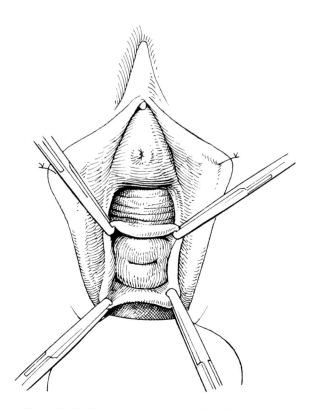

Figure 21.15 Preparation of the vaginal cuff.

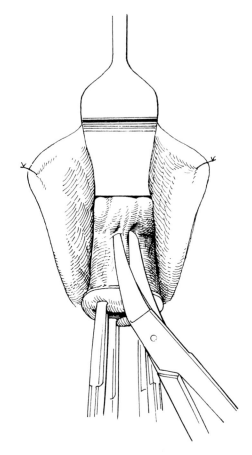

Figure 21.16 Vaginal incision.

anteriorly (Fig. 21.16). Posteriorly, the pouch of Douglas can be simply entered in the upper part of the posterior fornix (Fig. 21.17).

Closure of the cuff of the vagina
It is important to draw the elongated edges of the vagina over the cervix, covering over the carcinoma so that it is completely protected from contact for the remainder of the procedure. Utilizing the Chrobak clamps and beginning at one edge, the anterior and posterior vaginal edges are drawn together over the cervix and the Chrobak clamps applied serially. Normally, four clamps will hold the whole vaginal edge and allow manipulation of the vagina, cervix and uterus, utilizing these four points of attachment (Fig. 21.18).

In the past, other clinicians have sewn the vaginal edges together and maintained a number of threads that can be used to manipulate the cervix and uterus.

The Schuchardt incision
It is the editors' experience that this incision is unnecessary with the laparoscopic approach and can cause significant postoperative discomfort and scarring. The incision, when made, is essentially a large left lateral episiotomy incision extending into the vagina, thereby widening the entrance to the vagina to give greater access.

Elevating the bladder
As the edges of the vagina have been drawn together, the tissues lying immediately above the vaginal cuff can now be gently incised in order to make the bladder as safe as possible. The editors gently dissect downwards rather than upwards on the anterior part of the cervix in order to determine accurately the

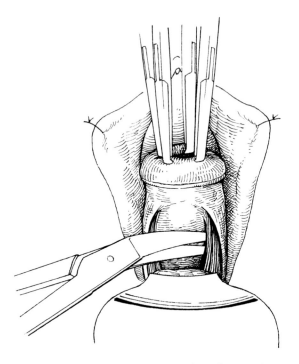

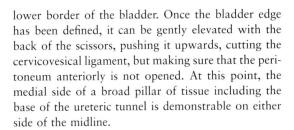

Figure 21.17 Dissection of the rectum from the posterior vaginal wall.

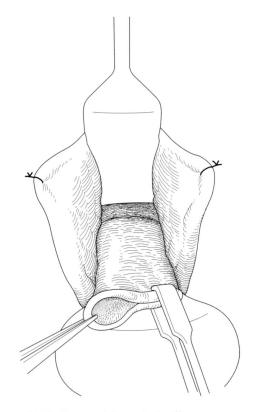

Figure 21.18 Closure of the vaginal cuff.

lower border of the bladder. Once the bladder edge has been defined, it can be gently elevated with the back of the scissors, pushing it upwards, cutting the cervicovesical ligament, but making sure that the peritoneum anteriorly is not opened. At this point, the medial side of a broad pillar of tissue including the base of the ureteric tunnel is demonstrable on either side of the midline.

Opening of the right paravesical fossa
One of the assistants takes the Chrobak clamps and draws the cervix over to one side, and the proximal lateral edge of the cut vagina is grasped with a straight tissue forceps. At this point the Monaghan scissors can be inserted at right angles to the edge of the vaginal skin, upwards and laterally, gently opening the scissors as they advance but taking care not to close them in the space; in this way, each paravesical fossa can be simply and accurately accessed (Fig. 21.19). This space is developed further by placing the narrow curved Wertheim retractor (Fig. 21.20) into

the space. The angled Wertheim retractor fits neatly around the pubic ramus, opening up the space completely. On the medial side of the space that has been so developed lies a pillar of tissue, bordered on its lateral side by the Wertheim retractor and the paravesical space, and on its medial side by the open area which has been separated as the central part of the bladder has been drawn upwards. With the Wertheim retractor in place and the index finger below the bladder lying on the cervix, the ureter can be palpated within the ureteric tunnel and a 'click' can be felt as the firm ureter is rotated against the Wertheim retractor. This gives the surgeon a good idea of the position of the ureter and how far up the pillar it lies. It is now necessary to divide the pillar in order to demonstrate the ureter.

Dissection of the ureters
With one assistant maintaining tension on the Chrobak clamps, the other assistant holding the Wertheim

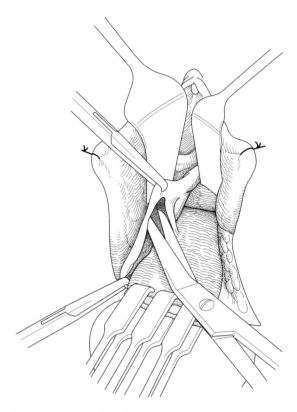

Figure 21.19 Opening of the right paravesical space.

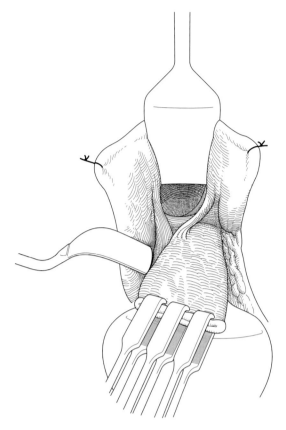

Figure 21.20 Joining the paravesical and pararectal spaces. Horizontal fascia exposed.

retractor in the paravesical space, the surgeon can then gently divide by blunt dissection the lower part of the ureteric pillar. By gently dividing what is in effect the floor of the ureteric tunnel and noting from time to time the position of the ureter knee within the ureteric pillar, the ureter can be identified and gently elevated. As the ureter is elevated (Fig. 21.21), on its medial and inferior side will be seen the descending branch of the uterine artery lying in the soft tissue on the anterolateral part of the uterus. The descending branch of the uterine artery can then be clamped and divided. It is the editors' preference to place a small Navratil right-angled clamp below the uterine artery to elevate it (Fig. 21.22), and following the laparoscopic division of the uterine artery by gently teasing the artery down it will be possible to see the small clip that has been placed on the medial part of the artery where it has been divided close to the internal iliac. In the standard Schauta procedure, which is not combined with the laparoscopic division of the uterine artery, the uterine artery can be divided at a high level by gently drawing it down and then dividing it, having clamped it with the right-angled clamp.

This process of identifying the uterine artery is performed in a gentle and cautious manner, gently teasing it down with a forceps and pushing the ureter away, upwards and laterally.

Dividing the uterosacral ligament and identifying the cardinal ligaments

As the ureter has now been elevated and pushed away and the uterine artery divided, the surgeon can insert his or her finger into the opening in the pouch of Douglas and the uterosacral ligaments can be hooked by the finger. These may be divided and ligated, or in some circumstances may simply require being cut

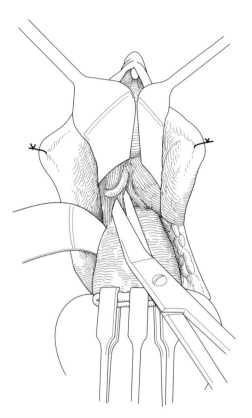

Figure 21.21 Displaying the right ureter.

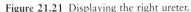

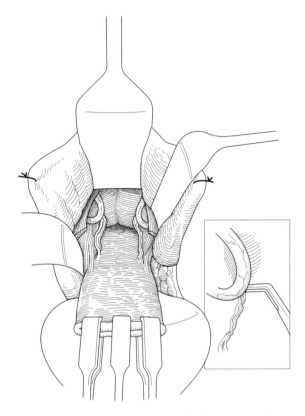

Figure 21.22 Ligation and display of left uterine vessels.

(Fig. 21.23). The next element to be identified is the broad band of the cardinal ligament. This is clearly running at right angles to the cervical tissue and, by placing the index finger around it, the ureter can be elevated well above it and a long length of cardinal ligament identified. These can be grasped with a hysterectomy clamp at a chosen point to include a significant part of the parametrial tissue. The ligament is divided and the lateral ends are sutured and released. At this point, there is nothing holding the uterus into the abdomen apart from the peritoneum which runs across the uterovesical fold, and, unless a pure Schauta procedure is being performed, the round ligaments and uterine pedicles will already have been dealt with laparoscopically. By running the index finger around the side of the uterus, the uterovesical fold can be identified, incised and the entire uterus drawn down simply cutting the remaining peritoneum. At this point, all that is left to be dealt with is the peritoneum of the pelvis if that is to be closed, and the vaginal vault.

Closure of the vault
It is the editors' practice to simply close the vaginal vault, making sure not to foreshorten the vagina too much. Once more a pack is placed into the vagina and a catheter in the bladder, and the procedure is complete. Some authors prefer to close the peritoneum, but this is not essential (Fig. 21.24).

A final laparoscopic check of the intra-abdominal area is made for haemostasis. There are usually minimal problems and the ureters can be observed as they function, and any minor clot removed.

Postoperative care

It has been the editors' experience that the modern variation of the Schauta procedure is significantly

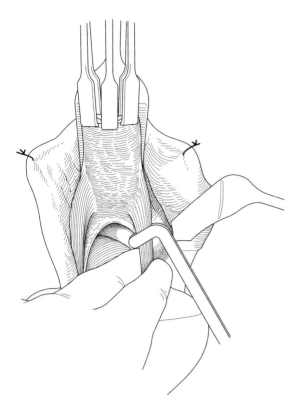

Figure 21.23 Division of uterosacral ligaments.

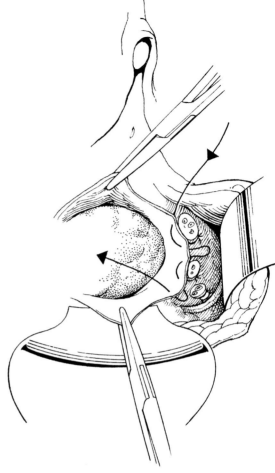

Figure 21.24 Purse-string suture to close the peritoneum.

less damaging to the bladder than has been previously noted. In virtually all patients, the catheter in the bladder can be maintained for 3 days and is then removed and normal function occurs. From time to time more prolonged bladder catheterization may be necessary until normal bladder function resumes. Recovery is rapid. The average time in hospital in the editors' series of patients is just under 5 days. This compares very favourably with the 7 days of the Wertheim procedure.

Radical trachelectomy

In the last 20 years there has been a move to exploring fertility-sparing surgery in young women with small tumours. Dargent performed the first laparoscopic assisted radical vaginal trachelectomy, a radical excision of the cervix and paracolpos in 1987. Ungár

advocated the abdominal approach and has performed the procedure successfully in pregnancy, resulting in a live birth. A total laparoscopic and a robotically assisted approach have also been described with preservation of the uterine arteries.

Vaginal approach

The vaginal radical trachelectomy begins with the laparoscopic pelvic lymph node dissection. Any signs suspicious of metastatic spread demand frozen section analysis or delay of the fertility-sparing procedure until histological confirmation is available. Assuming the pelvic nodes are not involved with disease, the vaginal procedure can then be commenced. The initial steps are as performed in a radical vaginal hysterectomy with incision of the vaginal cuff, protection of the cervix and associated tumour by use of the Chrobak forceps, and opening the pararectal and paravesical spaces. Insertion of a Wertheim retractor into the vesicovaginal space develops the pillars, allowing the ureteric knee and arch of the uterine artery to be dissected and displayed. The cervical branch of the uterine vessels can then be clipped, followed by a gentle push of the ureter towards the more distal structures. The uterosacral ligaments and the transverse cervical ligaments can then be clamped, cut and ligated, mobilizing the uterus into the vagina and allowing access to the uterine corpus. Judgement is then utilized to transect just below the level of the isthmus to release the surgical specimen, which is sent for frozen section analysis to ensure absence of tumour at the surgical margin. A cervical cerclage suture is then placed around the isthmus. The editors' current practice is to use Mersilene (Ethicon Endo-Surgery Inc.) tape and to place the knot posterior to the uterus. A small sound or dilator can be inserted into the os to ensure the suture is not overly tight. The cervical remnant is then sutured to the vaginal cuff using a series of interrupted absorbable sutures. The bladder is catheterized with an indwelling transurethral catheter and a final laparoscopic inspection of the pelvis performed.

Abdominal approach

The radical abdominal trachelectomy is simply a modification of the radical abdominal hysterectomy. The initial clamps alongside the uterus are replaced by clips on the round ligament alone and the ovarian vessels are maintained throughout. The pelvic lymph node dissection is performed as previously described. Dissection and transection of the uterine vessels at source on the pelvic sidewall followed by opening of the ureteric tunnel and entry into the rectovaginal space then allows clamps to be placed on the uterosacral ligaments, transverse cervical ligaments and paracolpos followed by entry into the vagina and dislocation of the uterus from all of its distal attachments. The uterus with cervix, upper vagina and paracolpos with associated uterine vessels and lymphatics are then held in the left hand while the scalpel

is used to cut the cervix just below the isthmus, releasing the surgical specimen, which is sent for frozen section analysis to ensure absence of tumour at the surgical margin. This step is reassuringly associated with blood pulsing out of the parauterine vessels fed solely by the ovarian vessels, evidence that the need to preserve the uterine vessels during the procedure is unnecessary. These parauterine vessels are clipped, followed by insertion of the cervical cerclage at the isthmus. The vaginal cuff is oversewn to deal with any vessels and the cervical remnant is then sutured to the vaginal cuff to seal off the vaginal opening. This step is best performed by inserting a series of suture lengths into the cervix and vagina without tightening and then parachuting the uterus onto the vagina at the end as each suture length is secured and knotted. The clamps are removed from the round ligaments and, at the end of the procedure, the pelvis should be dry and the surgeon should consider the use of adhesion prevention agents.

Further reading

Radical abdominal hysterectomy: history

Bonney V. The treatment of carcinoma of the cervix by Wertheim's operation. *Am J Obstet Gynecol* 1935; 30:815.

Clark JG. A more radical method of performing hysterectomy for cancer of the uterus. *Bull Johns Hopkins Hosp* 1895;6:120.

Freund WA. Method of complete removal of the uterus. *Am J Obstet Gynecol* 1879;7:200.

Monaghan JM. Role of centralization of surgery in stage IB carcinoma of the cervix: a review of 498 cases. *Gynecol Oncol* 1990;37:206–209.

Reis E. Modern treatment of carcinoma of the uterus. *Chicago Med Res* 1895;9:284–289.

Thring ET. On the radical abdominal operation for uterine cancer. *J Obstet Gynaecol Br Emp* 1907;11:239–245.

Wertheim E. Zur Frag der Radikaloperation beim Uteruskrebs. *Arch Gynak* 1900;61:627.

Radical abdominal hysterectomy: classification

Piver MS, Rutledge F, Smith JP. Five classes of extended hysterectomy for women with cervical cancer. *Obstet Gynecol* 1974;44:265–272.

Querleu D, Morrow B. Classification of radical hysterectomy. *Lancet Oncol* 2008;9:297–230.

Laparoscopic radical hysterectomy

Spirtos NM, Eisenkop SM, Schlaerth JB, Ballon SC. Laparoscopic radical hysterectomy (type III) with aortic and pelvic lymphadenectomy in patients with stage I cervical cancer: surgical morbidity and intermediate follow-up. *Am J Obstet Gynecol* 2002;187:340–348.

Laparoscopic assisted radical vaginal hysterectomy

Dargent D, Mathevet P. Schauta's vaginal hysterectomy combined with laparoscopic lymphadenectomy. *Baillieres Clin Obstet Gynaecol* 1995;9:691–705.

Radical trachelectomy

Marchiole P, Benchaib M, Buenerd A, *et al*. Oncological safety of laparoscopic-assisted vaginal radical trachelectomy (LARVT or Dargent's operation): a comparative study with laparoscopic-assisted vaginal radical hysterectomy (LARVH). *Gynecol Oncol* 2007;106:132–141.

Ungár L, Pálfalvi L, Hogg L, *et al*. Abdominal radical trachelectomy: a fertility-preserving option for women with early cervical cancer. *Br J Obstet Gynaecol* 2005;112: 366–369.

22 Uterine cancer

The surgical treatment of uterine cancers is predominantly based upon total removal of the uterus and cervix in conjunction with removal of both fallopian tubes and both ovaries. Peritoneal washings are taken as part of routine staging, usually from the cul-de-sac. Any suspicious nodules or lesions in the pelvic or abdominal peritoneal cavity are biopsied, including removal/biopsy of the omentum if required. Examination of the pelvic and para-aortic lymph nodes is mandatory, followed by removal of any that are suspicious or enlarged. The practice of systematic removal of non-suspicious pelvic or para-aortic lymph nodes varies between continents and centres and is worthy of further discussion.

The great proportion of uterine cancers will be of the endometrioid type. These tumours infiltrate the myometrium and local/nearby tissues and have a tendency to metastasize via the lymphatics. The less common variants of uterine cancer, including uterine papillary serous and clear cell cancers, sarcomas and carcinosarcomas, have a different and more aggressive biology, with uterine papillary serous cancers having a tendency to behave in a similar fashion to ovarian cancers, spreading via the peritoneal cavity, and carcinosarcomas, having a tendency for haematogenous spread. A prior knowledge of the histology and an understanding of the tumour's behaviour are critical when determining the surgical strategy.

It is also important to have an appreciation of the co-morbidities that are often associated with uterine cancers. Endometrioid tumours are commonly associated with the triad of obesity, diabetes and hypertension, and this has to be taken into consideration when determining the surgical approach.

Surgical approach

The procedure can be performed by various routes including an open abdominal using a vertical or transverse incision, a laparoscopic approach either alone or in unison with a vaginal approach, or for seriously debilitated or morbid cases a vaginal approach alone under a spinal or epidural anaesthetic. These procedures are all described in Chapter 11.

The benefits of a laparoscopic approach with the avoidance of a large abdominal incision, especially in the obese, are self-evident. To ensure the approach is acceptable when managing malignant disease of the uterus demands good quality prospective studies, which are currently ongoing. Surgeons skilled in laparoscopic surgery are able to ensure adequate assessment and removal of the other associated tissues including pelvic and para-aortic lymph nodes.

Peritoneal washings

In the 2009 revised FIGO staging for endometrial cancer, positive peritoneal cytology no longer has an impact on the FIGO stage, but the result should continue to be recorded separately.

It is essential that the washings are taken before there has been any significant handling or manipulation of the uterus to ensure that iatrogenic displacement of tumour cells into the peritoneal cavity does not occur. The editors' practice is to apply a straight forceps on either side of the uterus early in the course of the operation to prevent the flow of tumour cells through the lumen of the fallopian tubes. During laparoscopic procedures, some surgeons recommend the application of large Ligaclips (Ethicon Endo-Surgery Inc., Cincinnati, OH, USA) or to apply diathermy to obstruct/fuse the fallopian tubes for the same effect.

Occasionally, there is 20–30 mL of peritoneal fluid already lying within the cul-de-sac and aspiration of this is more than adequate for representative cytology to be obtained. Alternatively, 30–50 mL of saline can be introduced into the pelvis, washing the pelvic structures before it comes to rest in the pouch, from where it can be aspirated and handed to the scrub nurse. Whether further washings taken from the paracolic gutters or upper abdomen provide any additional value is disputable.

Risk of nodal metastases and assessment of nodes

The incidence of lymph node involvement ranges from 3% to 28%, depending on worsening tumour grade, increasing myometrial invasion, presence of high-risk pathological subtypes and when the tumour has already invaded outside the corpus and involves the cervix, vagina, fallopian tubes, ovaries or other pelvic structures. Knowledge of tumour grade and histological subtype is obtained by prior biopsy of the uterine cavity and can be partly used to determine risk of nodal spread. Preoperative MRI scan and, less so, transvaginal ultrasound can give some indication of the degree of myometrial invasion, the benefit of MRI being that it can provide additional information on the possible involvement of nearby structures and lymph nodes. Some surgeons rely on the practice of bisecting the uterus immediately after the hysterectomy so that the degree of myometrial invasion can be visually estimated. The potential value of sentinel

node assessment in the management of uterine cancers is still unclear.

Role of lymphadenectomy

Although there is no disagreement that enlarged or suspicious pelvic or para-aortic nodes should be searched for and removed, the question of whether to systematically remove all pelvic and/or para-aortic lymph nodes in selected or in fact all cases of uterine cancer has been under much debate. Two recent randomized trials were unable to show a survival benefit to performing pelvic lymphadenectomy.

Current practices vary from no lymphadenectomy in any cases, performing pelvic lymphadenectomy in high-risk cases only as a means of determining the need for adjuvant pelvic radiotherapy or chemotherapy, to performing systematic pelvic and para-aortic lymphadenectomy in all cases or in high-risk cases only. It is not the intention of the editors to critique each of the above surgical practices, but to recommend that trainee surgeons make themselves familiar with the surgical procedures, which are described elsewhere in the book, and the associated literature and data.

Radical surgery in advanced disease

Most cases of endometrial cancer will present in the early stages owing to the occurrence of abnormal bleeding during the postmenopausal period resulting in the patient seeking medical advice. Occasionally, however, the warning symptoms arrive later in the course of the disease or do not occur at all, with the patient presenting with signs of more extensive spread, as all too often occurs when associated with the more aggressive histological subtypes.

A thorough history and examination will identify when the surgeon needs to be on guard. The presence of abdominal distension due to the presence of ascites or the palpation of an omental cake, the inspection of tumour involving the lower or upper vagina or cervix, and the palpation of an enlarged, hard, fixed and irregular uterus or additional masses within the pelvis should help avoid any unexpected surprises during the operation. In the presence of such findings, further preoperative investigation, including radiology, is warranted. Occasionally, it will be the isolated finding of a raised CA125 or CEA that will alert the surgeon of impending difficulties.

Several retrospective studies support radical surgical procedures in the management of advanced uterine tumours with outcomes being improved when complete cytoreduction is obtained. There are some early data to suggest that the use of neoadjuvant chemotherapy increases the rate of complete cytoreduction, with a reduction in morbidity related to the surgery. The surgical procedures can be challenging even to the most radical of surgeons as the disease can have a more infiltrative and invasive behaviour than advanced ovarian cancers. Sarcomas and carcinosarcomas can be particularly aggressive and vascular, and it is important to warn the anaesthetist and associated theatre staff of the need for extra vigilance early in the course of the resection if one is to avoid any mishap. Skilful and efficient surgery in conjunction with the use of haemostatic techniques and agents described elsewhere in the text will ensure a satisfactory outcome without excessive blood loss.

Further reading

Randomized studies on lymphadenectomy

ASTEC study group, Kitchener H, Swart AM, Qian Q, et al. Efficacy of systematic pelvic lymphadenectomy in endometrial cancer (MRC ASTEC trial): a randomised study. Lancet 2009;373:125–136.

Benedetti Panici P, Basile S, Maneschi F, et al. Systematic pelvic lymphadenectomy vs no lymphadenectomy in early-stage endometrial carcinoma: randomized clinical trial. J Natl Cancer Inst 2008;100:1707–1716.

Radical surgery for advanced disease

Landrum L, Moore KN, Myers TK, et al. Stage IVB endometrial cancer: does applying an ovarian cancer treatment paradigm result in similar outcomes? A case-control analysis. Gynecol Oncol 2009;112:337–341.

Thomas M, Mariani A, Cliby WA, et al. Role of cytoreduction in stage III and IV uterine papillary serous carcinoma. Gynecol Oncol 2007;107:190–193.

Neoadjuvant chemotherapy in advanced disease

Despierre E, Moerman P, Vergote I, Amant F. Is there a role for neoadjuvant chemotherapy in the treatment of stage IV serous endometrial carcinoma? Int J Gynecol Cancer 2006;16 Suppl. 1:273–277.

23 Ovarian cancer

A systematic approach to achieve optimal cytoreductive status in patients with advanced epithelial cancer of the ovary

The removal of all visible disease in patients with advanced stage epithelial ovarian cancer is associated with prolongation of life, as demonstrated by an increase in median survival when compared with patients left even with 1-cm deposits of visible residual disease and certainly those left with disease deposits measuring more than 1 cm. As it is much more difficult to define the benefit to the patient of aggressive cytoreduction, when more than 1-cm deposits of disease are left behind, it is incumbent upon the surgeon to identify disease that is unresectable as early in the procedure as possible, for this determination should result in the termination of surgery, saving the patient unnecessary morbidity and possible mortality. Undertaking surgical procedures while leaving residual disease of more than 1 cm should be done only to relieve specific symptoms. It is only in this context that such an aggressive surgical approach can be pursued.

Bonney's Gynaecological Surgery, 11th edition.
© Tito Lopes, Nick Spirtos, Raj Naik, John Monaghan.
Published 2011 by Blackwell Publishing Ltd.

The operation

Incision

The surgery requires a midline incision extending from the symphysis pubis to the xiphoid process.

Upper abdomen

As virtually all pelvic disease is resectable, exploration of the upper abdomen and perhaps the thoracic cavity is most critical in determining whether there is unresectable disease. Upon entering the peritoneal cavity, exploration should be done immediately to identify the extent of disease. Once this is accomplished, a complete supra- and infracolic omentectomy should be performed by transecting the short gastric vessels across the greater curvature of the stomach. This can be accomplished with traditional clamps and ties; the LDS (powered single-use stapler with titanium staples) (Covidien Inc., Boulder, CO, USA) stapling device; Endo GIA (Covidien Inc.) stapling devices with vascular loads or any number of bipolar energy devices. The advantage of removing the omentum in this fashion is its removal decreases fluid losses and, more importantly, allows for exploration of the lesser sac and the pancreas. If a primary pancreatic cancer is identified, no further debulking efforts are indicated and surgery should be aborted.

In order to facilitate the complete resection of the omentum and recognizing that 15–20% of patients will require splenectomy to achieve optimal cytoreduction the left colon and splenic flexure should be mobilized. This is best accomplished by incising the left parietal peritoneum from the pelvic brim to the splenic flexure where the phrenicolic ligament can be transected. Hydrodissection in this plane can be used to facilitate the elevation of the parietal peritoneum and descending colon anterior to the left kidney. The distal pancreas and spleen can easily be elevated into the operative field, allowing for complete resection of the omentum and spleen and distal pancreas if necessary. By mobilizing the splenic flexure, mesocolon and descending colon medially the renal vein at the point the ovarian vein drains into it can be easily identified and the lymph nodes in this area can be fully assessed. To assess the lymph nodes involving the coeliac plexus all one must do at this point is transect the lienosplenic and gastrosplenic ligaments and sweep both the spleen and the pancreas over the midline, providing excellent access to this area. By starting the dissection in this manner, not only is the omentum and possibly the spleen easily removed but an evaluation of two areas that might harbour unresectable disease (the pararenal and coeliac lymph nodes) can be evaluated and, if so determined, the need of further debulking can be minimized.

Assuming this portion of the procedure is completed and all disease is determined to be resectable, diaphragmatic disease should be evaluated and removed. In almost all cases, the disease involving the diaphragm can be surgically removed. It is our practice to transect the falciform, right and left triangular ligaments using a Ligasure (Covidien Inc.) device and/or an argon beam coagulator. Similarly, the upper and lower layers of the coronary ligaments are incised using argon beam coagulation; as the dissection proceeds posteriorly, significant care is required to ensure the inferior vena cava is not injured as it penetrates the diaphragm. The liver can now be elevated and mobilized towards the midline, allowing for complete visualization and resection of all diaphragmatic disease or resection of the diaphragm as needed. Special care is also required in mobilizing the liver in this manner as the bare area of the liver is easily fractured, resulting in a significant amount of blood loss. The use of a surgical sponge soaked in a saline and epinephrine 1:100000 dilution can minimize this problem. The surgeon must be prepared to address bleeding caused by this dissection. Techniques used most frequently by the editors include the use of topical haemostatic agents with the application of direct pressure. These agents include Arista (Medafor Inc., USA), Gelfoam (Pfizer Inc., USA) and Surgicel (Johnson and Johnson Inc., USA) soaked in thrombin, or Tisseal (Baxter Inc., USA) applied to the liver surface. In extreme cases, liver sutures are needed to compress large vessels deep to the surface. An alternative to this is using radiofrequency ablation such as the Habib 4X device (AngioDynamics UK Ltd, Cambridge, UK) where a varying length can be inserted into the bleeding site and energy applied until haemostasis is achieved.

Thoracic assessment

A more controversial issue is the appropriateness of addressing disease above the diaphragm. Recent reports suggest that approximately 35–40% of patients with apparent stage IIIC ovarian cancer have subclinical stage IV disease, although in only a few cases was suboptimal disease (greater than 1 cm) found in the thoracic cavity. If identification of this disease influences a surgeon's decision to continue with debulking efforts, or perhaps the decision of whether an intraperitoneal port should be placed for the administration of chemotherapy, there is potential value in opening the diaphragm and placing a 5-mm laparoscope into the right thoracic cavity while the anaesthetist halts ventilation so the parietal and visceral pleurae can be adequately visualized. Small volume disease can be ablated using argon beam coagulation. If disease involves the lung parenchyma and is readily accessible, a TA-60 (Covidien Inc.) stapling device can be used to resect disease on the edges of the lung. Tisseal can be applied after stapling and resecting the involved portion of lung. A chest tube can easily be inserted transdiaphragmatically, although it is not universally agreed that it is necessary to do so. If a chest tube is not inserted, a pursestring suture using a monofilament suture (0-Monocryl or Prolene) should be placed to close the defect in the diaphragm and a large-calibre 'red Robinson' catheter placed into the thoracic cavity. As the anaesthetist hyperinflates the lungs, the catheter, with suction applied, is withdrawn and the purse-string suture secured.

Para-aortic node dissection

In order to complete the resection of all upper abdominal disease, the left and right aortic lymph nodes should be resected. Using an Endo GIA the left ovarian vessels can be transected and resected along with the lymph nodes overlying the anterior and lateral aspect of the aorta down to the level of the bifurcation of the aorta. The dissection should continue across the midline, removing the lymph nodes in the interspace between the aorta and vena cava. If macroscopically involved lymph nodes are encountered posterior to these vessels, the lumbar vessels must be ligated and divided in order to safely resect lymph nodes in this area.

Pelvis

Once the aortic lymph nodes have been removed attention can be turned to the removal of the reproductive organs and the involved pelvic viscera. Typically, 30–40% of patients will require resection of the small intestine or the rectosigmoid en bloc with the reproductive organs. Rarely does complete cytoreduction require partial cystectomy or ureteral resection with ureteroneocystotomy. As small bowel resection is covered in Chapter 27, only the en bloc resection of the rectosigmoid and reproductive organs will be described.

The rectosigmoid should be transected above the level of involvement by metastatic disease using an Endo GIA stapling device. The mesentery should be transected with either Endo GIA staplers or a Ligasure device and the dissection carried out down to the sacrum. The retrorectal space can now be developed either bluntly or with hydrodissection. Both methods are quick, safe and associated with minimal blood loss. Care should be taken to ensure the ureters are safely dissected free laterally and posteriorly, much as is done when performing a radical hysterectomy. The cervicovesical fascia (the ureteric tunnel) can be clamped, cut and ligated in order to facilitate the mobilization of the bladder and the ureters. This is a convenient time to ligate the uterine arteries, which can be clamped at the point they cross over the ureter. Once the ureteral dissection is completed and the uterine arteries ligated, the pararectal and paravaginal tissues can now be divided using an Endo GIA stapler or any preferred energy source, be that the Ligasure, Gyrus PK device (Gyrus ACMI, Southborough, MA, USA) or the Harmonic Scalpel (Ethicon Endo-Surgery Inc.). This dissection and resection is carried out to just below the peritoneal reflection in the posterior cul-de-sac. The vagina can be circumferentially incised with electrocautery or clamped and suture ligated. The rectum can now be transected with a TA-60 stapling device and a primary anastomosis completed using an EEA (Covdien Inc.) stapling device. At this point, issues such as the formation of a 'J' pouch versus a primary end-to-end versus an end-to-side anastomosis must be evaluated on a case-by-case basis. So too, the decision of whether proximal diversion of the gastrointestinal tract is made with either an ileostomy or colostomy.

Closure

At the end of the surgery the incision should be closed, as discussed in Chapter 4.

Further reading

Eisenkop S, Spirtos N, Friedman RL, et al. Relative influences of tumor volume before surgery and the cytoreductive outcome on survival for patients with advanced ovarian cancer: a prospective study. *Gynecol Oncol* 2003;90:390–396.

Eisenkop S, Spirtos N, Lin WM, et al. Regional blood flow occlusion during extensive pelvic procedures for ovarian cancer: a randomized trial. *Int J Gynecol Cancer* 2004;14: 699–705.

Eisenkop S, Spirtos N, Lin WM. 'Optimal' cytoreduction for advanced epithelial ovarian cancer: a commentary. *Gynecol Oncol* 2006;103:329–335.

24 Exenterative surgery

The procedure of pelvic exenteration was first described in its present form by Brunschwig (1948). Over the years, it has been used mainly in the treatment of advanced and recurrent carcinoma of the cervix. Its primary role at the present time is the management of the small number of patients who will develop an isolated central pelvic recurrence of the cervix/vagina following primary chemoradiotherapeutic treatment or after pelvic radiotherapy for recurrent endometrial cancer. However, pelvic exenteration as a therapy for recurrent cancer of the cervix has not been widely accepted, and many patients will succumb to their disease having been through the process of chemoradiation followed by chemotherapy and other experimental therapies without being given the formal opportunity of a curative procedure.

In the early years, high operative mortalities and relatively low overall survival (20% 5-year survival in Brunschwig's series) resulted in few centres taking up the surgery. The more recently published results of exenterative procedures show an acceptable primary mortality of approximately 3–4% and an overall survival/cure rate of between 40% and 60%. The procedures may also be applicable to a wide range of other pelvic cancers, including cancer of the vagina, vulva and rectum, for both primary and secondary disease. It is relatively rarely applicable to ovarian epithelial cancers and melanomas and sarcomas because of their tendency for widespread metastases.

The surgery involved is extensive and postoperative care complex; as a consequence, the operation has become part of the repertoire of the advanced gynaecological oncologist working in a centre with a wide experience of radical surgery. The procedure demands of the surgeon considerable expertise and flexibility, as virtually no two exenterations are identical. Also, considerable judgement and ingenuity is required during the procedure in order to achieve a comprehensive removal of all tumour. A degree of tailoring of surgery can be carried out as it may well be that, with small recurrences, a more limited procedure can be carried out with a degree of conservation of structures in and around the pelvis. Where extensive radiotherapy has been carried out complete clearance of all organs from the pelvis (total exenteration) together with widespread lymphadenectomy may be essential in order to achieve a cure. There is now considerable evidence that, even in those patients with pelvic node metastases at the time of exenteration, a significant salvage rate can be achieved.

Selection of patients for exenterative surgery

Exenterative surgery should be considered for advanced primary pelvic carcinoma as well as recurrent disease. Many patients will be eliminated from the possibility of surgery at an early stage because of

Bonney's Gynaecological Surgery, 11th edition.
© Tito Lopes, Nick Spirtos, Raj Naik, John Monaghan.
Published 2011 by Blackwell Publishing Ltd.

complete fixity of the cancer to the bony structures of the pelvis. The only exception to this rule is the rare circumstance in which a vulval or vaginal cancer is attached to one of the pubic rami, when the ramus can be resected and a clear margin around the cancer obtained.

Palliative exenteration

In general terms, exenterative surgery should not be used as a palliative procedure, except perhaps in the presence of malignant fistulae in the pelvis when it may significantly improve the quality of the patient's life without any significant extension to that life. The patient and her relatives must be made fully aware that the surgery is not being carried out with a curative intent.

Patient assessment

The average age of patients who are subject to exenteration is between 50 and 60 years, but the age range is wide from early childhood through to the eighth or ninth decade. Advanced age is not a bar to success in exenterative surgery.

It is frequently difficult following radiotherapeutic treatment to be certain that the mass palpable in the pelvis is due to recurrent disease and not to radiation reaction or persistent scarring associated with infection or the effects of adhesion of bowel to the irradiated areas.

In recent years, CT scan and MRI have been used extensively in the preoperative assessment of patients for many oncological procedures. The considerable difficulties and uncertainties that are generated for the radiologist assessing the CT or MRI scan where patients have had preceding surgery or radiotherapy is rarely more problematic than when patients are being assessed for exenteration. Some clinicians feel that the scan is an integral part of preoperative assessment, whereas the editors have not found the level of reliability of CT scan in particular to be acceptable, except for the exclusion of chest and abdominal metastases. More recently, with the introduction of PET-CT scans, exclusion of distant disease can be determined more confidently. A tissue diagnosis is essential prior to embarking on exenterative surgery,

and the use of needle biopsy, aspiration cytology or, frequently, open biopsy at laparotomy will need to be performed. As distant metastases tend to occur with recurrent and residual disease, it is sometimes helpful to perform scalene node biopsies and radiological assessments of the pelvic and para-aortic lymph nodes together with fine needle aspiration in order to assist with the assessment. The mental state of the patient is also vital, but should not in itself be a bar to the performance of such surgery.

Absolute contraindications to exenteration

If there are metastases in extrapelvic lymph nodes, upper abdominal viscera, lungs or bones, there appears to be little value in performing such major surgery. However, there is evidence that patients with pelvic lymph node metastases may well survive and have a high quality of life in a small but significant percentage of patients.

Relative contraindications to exenteration

• *Pelvic sidewall spread.* If the tumour has extended to the pelvic sidewall in the form of either direct extension or nodal metastases the prospects of a cure are extremely small and the surgeon must decide whether the procedure will materially improve the patient's quality of life. The triad of unilateral uropathy, renal non-function or ureteric obstruction together with unilateral leg oedema and sciatic leg pain is an ominous sign. The prospects of a cure are poor. Perineural lymphatic spread is not visible on CT and can be a major source of pain and eventual death.
• *Obesity.* This is a problem with all surgical procedures, causing many technical difficulties as well as postoperative respiratory and mobilization problems. The more massive the surgery, the greater are these problems. Barber (1969) noted the very high risk associated with obesity.

Types of exenteration

In North America, the majority of exenterations performed are total (Fig. 24.1b). In the Gateshead series, approximately half of the exenterations have been of the anterior type (Fig. 24. 1a), removing the bladder, uterus, cervix and vagina, but preserving the rectum.

223

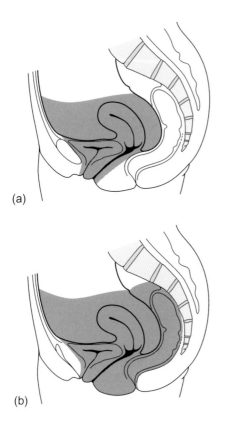

(a)

(b)

Figure 24.1 The limits of resection for (a) an anterior and (b) a total exenteration.

For small, high lesions around the cervix, lower uterus and bladder, it may be possible to carry out a more limited procedure (a supralevator exenteration), retaining considerable parts of the pelvic floor. Posterior exenteration (abdominoperineal procedure) is relatively rarely performed by gynaecological oncologists as these tend to be the areas of activity of the colorectal surgeon. However, a modified posterior exenteration, resecting the sigmoid colon and rectum en bloc with an ovarian tumour, is increasingly performed for maximal cytoreduction in ovarian cancer (see Chapter 23).

Preoperative preparation

It is important that the surgeon and the team of nurses and ancillary workers are confident in their ability to

manage not only the extensive surgery involved but also the difficult, testing and sometimes bizarre complications that can occur after exenteration.

Probably the most important part of the preoperative preparation is the extensive counselling that must be carried out to make certain that the patient and her relatives, particularly her partner, understand fully the extent of the surgery and the marked effect is will have upon normal lifestyle. Of particular importance is discussion about the removal of normal sexual function when the vagina is taken out. It is important to discuss the possibility of reconstructive surgery of the vagina and bladder and the necessary transference of urinary and bowel function to the chosen type of diversionary procedure that will be performed, and to communicate honestly the significant risks of such extensive surgery. During the course of this counselling, the patient should be seen by a stoma therapist. When it is possible, the clinical nurse specialist will arrange for psychosexual counsellors skilled in cancer treatment to make preliminary contact with the patient.

At this very traumatic time, it is important not to completely overwhelm the patient and her family with too much information. A fine judgement has to be made about the pace and volume of information imparted. To aid this communication, the editors find it ideal for the patient to meet with other patients who have had the procedure to discuss on a woman-to-woman basis the real problems and feelings of exenteration.

Most preoperative investigations are now performed in the outpatient setting and will include a full blood analysis, heart and lung assessments, including chest radiograph, and appropriate tests dependent on the patient's fundamental condition.

The patient is usually admitted to hospital the day before the planned procedure in order to obtain high-quality bowel preparation. With the modern alternative liquid diets and antibiotic therapy, complete cleaning of the small and large bowel can be achieved very rapidly. The anaesthetist responsible for the patient's care will see the patient and explain the process of anaesthesia. The editors prefer to carry out all radical surgery under a combination of epidural and general anaesthetic. Although the majority of patients do not require intensive care therapy, its availability must be identified prior to the surgical procedure.

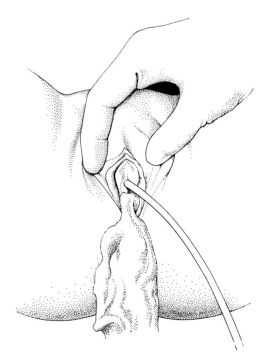

Figure 24.2 Packing the vagina.

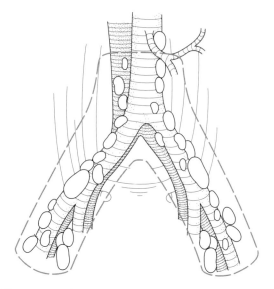

Figure 24.3 Pelvic and para-aortic node assessment.

The operation

The final intraoperative assessment

The final decision to proceed with the exenteration will not be made until the abdomen has been opened and assessment of the pelvic sidewall and posterior abdominal wall has been made utilizing frozen sections when necessary. In the editors' practice, a single team performs the procedure. If the patient has decided that reconstructive surgery such as the formation of a neovagina is to be carried out, usually a second plastic surgical team will carry out any necessary operation.

Once the patient has been anaesthetized and placed in the lithotomy position in the operating theatre the final assessment can begin with pelvic examination followed by catheterization of the bladder with an indwelling urethral catheter. If it is thought likely that an anterior exenteration will be performed, it is useful to pack the vagina firmly with a long gauze roll (Fig. 24.2). The patient is returned to the supine position and the abdomen is opened either utilizing a longitu-

dinal midline incision extending above the umbilicus or a high transverse (Maylard) incision. Exploration of the abdomen will confirm the mobility of the central tumour mass; thereafter, dissection of the para-aortic lymph nodes and pelvic sidewall nodes will be carried out (Fig. 24.3) and sent for frozen section. At the time of this initial intraoperative assessment, the experienced exenterative surgeon will have assessed the pelvic sidewall by dividing the round ligament, drawing back the infundibulopelvic ligament and opening up the pelvic sidewall (Fig. 24.4). This manoeuvre will have opened tissue planes, including the paravesical, pararectal and presacral spaces to a deep level (Fig. 24.5), allowing the surgeon to familiarize him- or herself with the full extent of the tumour. These dissections can be carried out without any significant blood loss. If it is considered not possible to proceed with the operation owing to fixity of the tumour, the abdomen may be closed at this stage as no significant trauma has been carried out by the surgeon. Considerable experience and judgement is required in order to make this decision. It is sometimes helpful to remove any suspicious tissue from the pelvic sidewall and obtain further frozen sections. Time spent here may really mean 'life or death' for the patient. Often, the most difficult decision is to actually stop operating. Very occasionally

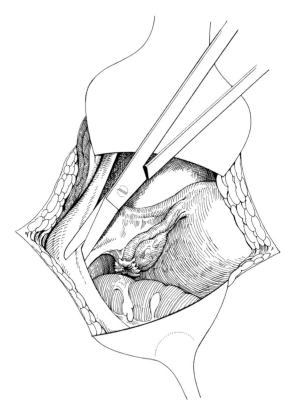

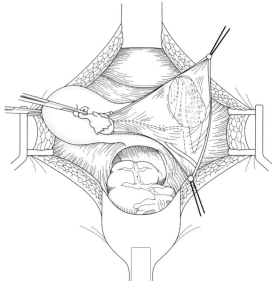

Figure 24.5 Deepening the lateral pelvic dissection to reveal the pelvic spaces.

Figure 24.4 Division of the round and infundibulopelvic ligaments and the beginning of the lateral pelvic dissection.

with some vulval cancers, resection of pubic bones may be necessary, but, in general terms, if there is bony involvement by tumour the procedure should be abandoned.

After the comprehensive manual and visual assessment of the pelvis and abdominal cavity has been made, a line of incision for removal of the entire pelvic organs will begin at the pelvic sidewall, over the internal iliac artery and will pass forward through the peritoneum of the anterior part of the bladder, meeting with the similar lateral pelvic sidewall incision at the opposite side. The peritoneal incision will be carried along around the brim of the pelvis, identifying the ureter as it passes over the common iliac artery and meeting up with the similar incision on the opposite side. Having divided and tied the round ligaments and opened the pelvic sidewall space, the infundibulopelvic ligament can also be identified,

divided and tied. The incision is continued posteriorly and the ureters identified and separated (Fig. 24.6). If an anterior exenteration is to be performed, the peritoneal dissection will be brought down into the pelvis to run across the anterior part of the rectum, just above the pouch of Douglas; this will allow a dissection from the anterior part of the rectum, passing posteriorly around the uterosacral ligaments to the sacrum and releasing the entire anterior contents of the pelvis.

For a total exenteration, the dissection is even simpler, the mesentery of the sigmoid colon is opened and individual vessels clamped, divided and tied. The colon is divided usually utilizing a GIA (Covidien Inc., Boulder, CO, USA) stapling device, which allows the sealed ends of the colon to lie, without interfering with the operation (Fig. 24.7). A dissection posterior to the rectum is then carried out from the sacral promontory, deep behind the pelvis; this dissection is rapid and simple and complete separation of the rectum from the sacrum will be allowed. This enables complete and usually bloodless removal of the rectal mesentery, including lymph nodes. Anteriorly, the bladder is dissected with blunt dissection from the cave of Retzius, resulting in the entire

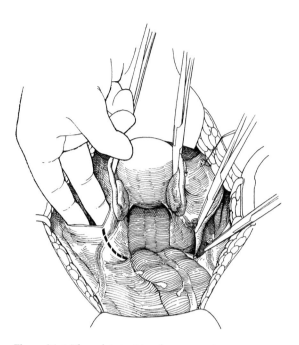

Figure 24.6 The pelvic incision for an anterior exenteration.

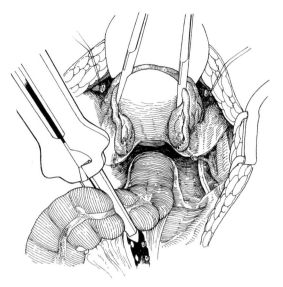

Figure 24.7 Dividing the sigmoid colon with the GIA stapling device.

bladder with its peritoneal covering falling posteriorly. This dissection is carried right down to the pelvic floor, isolating the urethra as it passes through the pelvic floor (perineal diaphragm). As dissection is carried posteriorly into the paravesical spaces, the uterine artery and the terminal part of the internal iliac artery will become clearly visible. By steadily deepening this dissection, the anterior division of the internal iliac will be isolated, the tissues of the lower obturator fossa identified and, at this point, large exenteration clamps or a linear stapling device may be placed over the anterior division of the internal iliac artery and its veins (Fig. 24.8). The ureter, by this time, will have been divided a short distance beyond the pelvic brim. The pelvic phase of the procedure is at this point completed and the perineal phase is now to be carried out.

The patient is placed in the extended lithotomy position and an incision made to remove the lower vagina for an anterior exenteration and the lower vagina and rectum in a total exenteration (Fig. 24.9). Anteriorly, the incision is carried through above the urethra just below the pubic arch to enter the space

of the cave of Retzius, which has been dissected in the pelvic procedure. The dissection is carried laterally and posteriorly, dividing the pelvic floor musculature, and the entire block of tissue is then removed through the inferior pelvic opening. Small amounts of bleeding will occur at this point, usually arising from the edge of the pelvic floor musculature. These can be picked up by either an isolated or running suture that will act as a haemostat.

Once the perineal dissection has been completed and haemostasis achieved, the surgeon has choices available depending on the preoperative arrangements with the patient. If, in the preoperative assessment period, it has been decided by the clinician and the patient that a neovagina should be formed, at this point either the surgeon or a plastic surgery colleague will initiate the development of a neovagina. This may be in the form of a myocutaneous graft using the gracilis muscle, a rectus abdominis graft such as the 'fleur-de-lys' or techniques which revolve around the development of a skin graft placed within an omental pad or the technique of a transposition of a segment of sigmoid colon in order to form a sigmoid neovagina. These individual techniques will not be dealt with in this chapter. For many patients, however, the desire to have a new vagina is a very low priority,

227

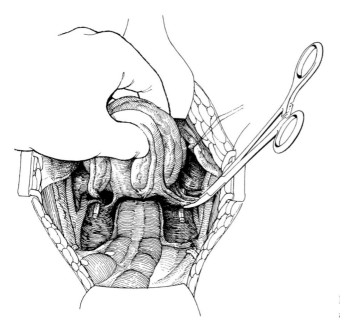

Figure 24.8 Exenteration clamps applied to the anterior division of the internal iliac arteries.

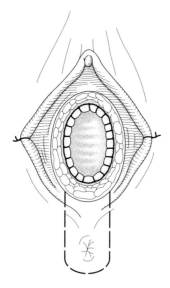

Figure 24.9 The perineal incisions for anterior and total exenterations.

and it is surprising how frequently the patients will put off these decisions until well after the time of exenteration. Survival of the cancer appears to be the uppermost desire that they are determined to achieve. To this end, the careful closure of the posterior parts

of the pelvic musculature, a drawing together of the fat anterior to that and a careful closure of the skin is all that is required. It is usually possible to preserve the clitoris, the clitoral fold and significant proportions of the anterior parts of the labia minora and labia majora so that when recovery is finally made the anterior part of the genitalia has a completely normal appearance. On some occasions, patients will be able to have a neovagina formed some significant period of time following the exenteration. This is now becoming the predominant pattern in the Gateshead experience of over 100 cases.

Once the perineal phase is finished, the legs can be lowered so that the patient is once more lying supine and attention can be addressed to dealing with the pedicles deep in the pelvis. All that remains following a total exenteration will be the two exenteration clamps on either side of the pelvis (unless linear staples have been used) and a completely clean and clear pelvis. The pelvic sidewall dissection of lymph nodes can be completed before dealing with the clamps and any tiny blood vessels that require haemostasis are ligated. As the exenteration clamps are attached to the distal part of the internal iliac arteries, it is important that comprehensive suture fixation is carried out (Fig. 24.10). This is usually readily and easily done, although occasionally the large veins of

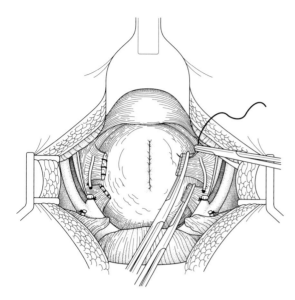

Figure 24.10 Suture of the internal iliac arteries and lateral pelvic pedicle.

the pelvic wall can provide difficulties and the use of mattress sutures may be necessary in order to deal with these complex vascular patterns. Having completed the dissection of the pelvis, the clinician now moves to produce either a continent urinary conduit or a Wallace- or Bricker-type ileal conduit; if the procedure has been a total exenteration, a left iliac fossa stoma will be formed. The individual techniques of these procedures are dealt with in Chapter 27.

Dealing with the empty pelvis

A problem which must be avoided is that of small bowel adhesion to the tissues of a denuded pelvis. This is particularly important when patients have had preceding radiotherapy as the risk of fistula formation in these circumstances is extremely high. There have been a variety of techniques utilized to attempt to deal with this potentially life-threatening complication, including placing in the pelvis artificial materials such as Merselene, Dacron or Gortex sacks, or even using bull's pericardium. Way (1974) described a sac technique in which a bag of peritoneum was manufactured that allowed the entire abdominal contents to be kept above the pelvis. This resulted in an empty pelvis, which from time to time became infected and

generated a new problem – that of the empty pelvis syndrome. Intermittently, over the years, patching with the peritoneum has been used, but the most successful appears to be the mobilization of the omentum from its attachment to the transverse colon, leaving a significant blood supply from the left gastroepiploic artery; this allows the formation of a complete covering of the pelvis, forming a soft 'trampoline of omentum' that will then stretch and completely cover and bring a new blood supply into the pelvis. From time to time, procedures such as bringing gracilis muscle flaps into the empty pelvis have been carried out in an attempt to deal with the difficulty of a devitalized epithelium due to previous radiation.

It is the editors' preference to utilize an omental graft, mobilizing the omentum from the transverse colon using a powered LDS (powered single-use stapler with titanium staples) (Covidien Inc., Boulder, CO, USA) stapling device; this allows a broad pedicle to be left, maintaining an excellent blood supply to the omentum from the left gastroepiploic artery. This is brought down to the right side of the large bowel, dropping into the pelvis immediately to the left side of the ileal conduit, which is anchored just above the sacral promontory. By careful individual suturing around the edge of the pelvis, and sometimes by refolding the peritoneum upon itself, a complete covering of the true pelvis with a soft central trampoline area can be generated (Fig. 24.11). A suction drain is inserted below the omentum that, when activated, will draw the omentum down into soft contact with the pelvic floor. The small bowel can thus come into contact with an area with a good blood supply, obviating the risk of adherence and subsequent fistula formation. At the end of the procedure, the bowel is carefully orientated to make sure that no hernia can develop and the abdomen is closed with a mass closure. The stomas are dressed in theatre and their appliances put in place. The patient leaves the operating theatre and is then transferred back to the ward at the appropriate time.

Postoperative care

The postoperative care of exenterations is straightforward; essentially, it is a matter of maintaining good fluid balance, good haemoglobin levels and, ideally, a significant flow of urine of between 2.5 and 3.5

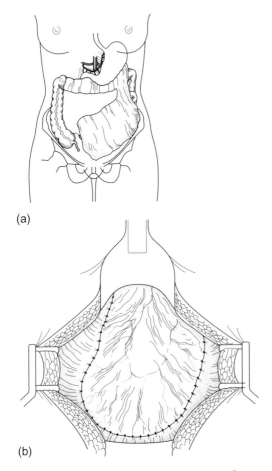

(a)

(b)

Figure 24.11 Development of the 'omental pelvic floor': (a) omental incision; (b) soft trampoline area.

litres per day. Bowel function often returns at the usual time of 2–4 days following the procedure; the nasogastric tube, which is the editors' preference, can be removed on day 3 or 4; and return to oral intake, beginning with simple fluid, is initiated on the third day. During and following the procedure, prophylactic antibiotic cover is maintained, as is thromboembolic prophylaxis.

Mobilization should be rapid, and the patient is most often discharged between 10 and 15 days post-operatively once she is used to dealing with her stomas and the ileal conduit tubes have been removed.

Results of exenteration

Most series show that the 5-year survival following exenteration is of the order of 40–60%; these figures depend very largely upon selection of patients (Robertson *et al.* 1994).

A figure which is rather more difficult to determine is the exact number of patients who have been assessed for exenteration but have then failed at one of the many hurdles that the patient must pass before finally having the procedure carried out. It is, therefore, likely that the final, truly salvageable, figure is an extremely low percentage. In more recent times, the value of carrying out exenterations in patients who have positive lymph nodes has been shown to be low but significant, and it is now many clinicians' practice to carry on with an exenterative procedure even in the circumstances where one or two lymph nodes are involved by tumour.

Further reading

Barber HRK. Relative prognostic significance of preoperative and operative findings in pelvic exenteration. *Surg Clin North Am* 1969;49:431–437.

Brunschwig A. Complete excision of the pelvic viscera for advanced carcinoma. *Cancer* 1948;1:177.

Robertson G, Lopes A, Beynon G, Monaghan JM. Pelvic exenteration: a review of the Gateshead experience 1974–1992. *Br J Obstet Gynaecol* 1994;101:529–531.

Shingleton HM, Orr JWJ. Recurrent cancer: exenterative surgery. In: Shingleton HM, Orr JWJ (eds) *Cancer of the Cervix: Diagnosis and Treatment*. New York: Churchill Livingstone, 1987.

Stanhope CR, Symmonds RE. Palliative exenteration: what, when and why? *Am J Obstet Gynecol* 1985;152:12–16.

Symmonds RE, Webb MJ. Pelvic exenteration. In: Coppleson M (ed.) *Gynecologic Oncology: Fundamental Principles and Clinical Practice*. Edinburgh: Churchill Livingstone, 1992: 1283–1312.

Way S. The use of the sac technique in pelvic exenteration. *Gynecol Oncol* 1974;2:476–481.

Operations on other organs

25 Vascular surgery: applications in gynaecology and gynaecological oncology

Fortunately, vascular injury is rarely encountered in gynaecological surgery, but when injury occurs it takes a calm presence and an understanding of both the anatomy and underlying principles of vascular repair. Vascular injury can occur during minimally invasive as well as during open procedures, and the approaches to repair them differ accordingly.

During minimally invasive surgical procedures, most injuries are associated with initial trocar placement and, to a lesser extent, secondary trocar placement as this is usually done under direct vision. Nevertheless, injuries do occur at this time. It should be noted that there has been no difference noted in the incidence of vascular or visceral injury with initial trocar placement based on whether a closed or open technique is used or whether a Veres needle is inserted to establish a pneumoperitoneum prior to placing the initial trocar. In the editors' opinion, each surgeon should use the technique that he or she is most comfortable with, with one cautionary note: the vast majority of all trocar injuries are due to skin 'dystocia', so every attempt should be made to ensure that the skin incision is adequate to pass the selected trocar and the subcutaneous tissues separated down to the level of the fascia prior to placing the trocars.

Most commonly the vessels injured during minimally invasive surgery are the inferior or superior epigastric vessels. Most of these injuries can be avoided

with transillumination of the abdominal wall prior to inserting the secondary trocars. Alternatively, one can ensure that the secondary trocars are placed sufficiently laterally so that the epigastric vessels can be avoided completely.

In the event that these vessels are injured, a number of techniques have been described to repair them. Some authors have suggested grasping the peritoneum overlying the bleeding vessel with a bipolar forceps inserted through one of the other ports and cauterizing above and below the bleeding site. Others have suggested passing a Foley catheter through the port site, expanding the balloon and leaving the balloon in place so as to compress the vessels between the abdominal wall and the balloon, causing the blood to clot and, thereby, achieving haemostasis. Our preferred method to control bleeding from the epigastric vessels is to pass a Keith needle (triangular pointed straight needle) through the trocar site into the abdomen, grasp the needle laparoscopically and pass it around the vessels and back out through the trocar site. This suture can now be tied down at the level of the fascia and the bleeding controlled. In cases in which this technique is found to be ineffective, the entire abdominal wall can be incorporated in a figure-of-eight fashion, using a Keith needle, and the sutures tied at skin level, to be cut out 1 week later. The Endo Close (Covidien Inc., Boulder, CO, USA) trocar site closure device can be used in a similar fashion and is useful in obese women.

Less commonly, large-calibre vessels are injured during primary trocar placement. When injury to either the vena cava or aorta is identified, it is best for all but the most experienced to undertake immediate

Bonney's Gynaecological Surgery, 11th edition.
© Tito Lopes, Nick Spirtos, Raj Naik, John Monaghan.
Published 2011 by Blackwell Publishing Ltd.

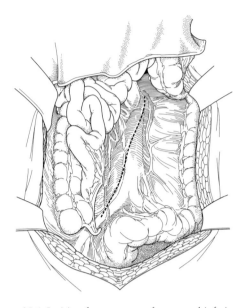

Figure 25.1 Incision for exposure of aorta and inferior vena cava.

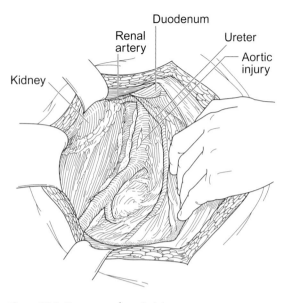

Figure 25.2 Exposure of aortic injury.

laparotomy through a midline incision while calling for the assistance of a vascular surgeon. Injury to both vessels calls for the same basic initial response. Direct pressure applied while the anaesthetist places large-bore intravenous lines either peripherally or centrally, blood products are obtained and, in surgery for benign disease, a cell-saver utilized. A common mistake is attempting to repair the injury without these initial steps having been taken and finding oneself and the patient much worse off.

Aortic injury

Once adequate vascular access and blood products are in place, attempting repair is now a reasonable option. If the injury is arterial, exposure is best obtained by incising the peritoneum over the right common iliac artery and mobilizing the mesentery of the small bowel superiorly and anteriorly (Fig. 25.1). The duodenum is similarly mobilized, providing excellent exposure of both the vena cava and aorta up to and above the level of the inferior mesenteric artery (Fig. 25.2). If necessary the inferior mesenteric artery can be ligated as the blood supply to the distal colon is generally well provided for by the marginal artery. The manual pressure placed on the aorta can be replaced with mechanical compression, using either Satinsky or Fogarty vascular, non-crushing clamps placed above and below the injury site. These clamps have been associated with the least amount of crush injury, which is of particular importance in the elderly or any patient who may have atherosclerosis. Prior to cross-clamping the aorta, most recommend giving heparin at 100 units/kg as a bolus. The defect can now be sutured with small-calibre Prolene suture. There is not usually a need to independently ligate the lumbar arteries to achieve haemostasis in an anterior injury to the aorta. In the rare case of a through and through injury involving the posterior wall then these vessels will need to be individually ligated in order to achieve haemostasis. It is rare in this situation to need protamine (1 mg/kg) to reverse the heparin effect. If cancer primarily or secondarily limits access to the aorta, prohibiting cross-clamping, consideration can be given to balloon occlusion placed via the femoral artery. Although rare when cross-clamping of the aorta is used for less than 1–2 hours, any sign of leg ischaemia requires arterial embolectomy with a Fogarty catheter.

Preemptive clamping of the aorta to limit blood loss during exenterative procedures has been described in the literature.

Iliac artery injury

The same principles as described above of applying non-crushing clamps can be applied to injury to the common and external iliac arteries. Special care should be taken in addressing injuries related to the use of any type of externally applied energy source as the lateral damage caused may mean that primary repair cannot be achieved and a graft will be required to replace the injured segment of artery.

Injury to the internal iliac artery can be repaired or more often its affect alleviated by simply ligating or clipping the vessel and its associated branches, proximally and distally.

Vena caval injury

Injury to the vena cava, whether trocar-related or associated with the dissection of lymph nodes or cancer, should be repaired taking similar precautions as mentioned above before attempting primary repair. It is much more important in repairing the vena cava to compress the vessel both laterally and medially as well as proximally and distally. If the lateral and medial aspects of the cava are not adequately controlled, visualization and repair of the defect will be severely hampered. This four-way compression of the cava can almost always be achieved using four sponges in ring forceps. Once the bleeding is controlled, the wall of the vena cava can be sutured using 4-0 or 5-0 monofilament suture. Although vascular clips may be used, particular care must be used to ensure that these clips do not further the tearing of the vessel wall, which is quite thin. If all else fails, remember the vena cava can be ligated along with the associated lumbar veins. Even if lower extremity oedema develops over the short term, in the vast majority of the cases this will resolve over time as collateralization occurs.

For smaller caval defects any number of fibrin sealants such as Tisseal (Baxter Inc., USA) and Evicel (Johnson and Johnson Inc., USA) are fairly effective. Use of these products as well as other haemostatic agents and products requires a thorough review and understanding of both the intrinsic and extrinsic coagulation pathways (see Chapter 3).

If an attempt at laparoscopically repairing either the vena cava or left common iliac vein is made, the surgeon will be well served to place an additional 12-mm trocar just lateral to the suprapubic trocar and inserting the camera in the suprapubic port and moving the monitors to the head of the table. This will allow the surgeon to grasp the thin-walled vein and apply clips while tenting up the vessel wall. Again, the utility of applying haemostatic agents is left to the individual surgeon.

Presacral bleeding

Occasionally, significant haemorrhage occurs during the undertaking of presacral neurectomy, lymph node dissection or exenterative procedures. Attempts to individually ligate presacral veins most often fail. The most effective measure to control bleeding in this location is the patient application of pressure. Our practice is to ask that someone in the theatre marks the time to ensure that the surgeons do not become impatient, and to keep the pressure applied for at least 20–30 minutes while blood products are made available and proper monitoring instituted. Usually, at this point, fibrin sealants can successfully be applied and the haemorrhage controlled. In rare situations, if the above-mentioned technique fails, sterile thumb-tacks (drawing pins) can be applied directly into the sacrum, thereby compressing the sacral plexus, resulting in control of the bleeding. This is another situation when consideration should be given to clamping the lower aorta to minimize blood loss.

Pelvic packing

When haemorrhage cannot be controlled by the techniques described, packing of the pelvis should be considered. Large packs should be packed into the pelvis to compress the vessels and control the bleeding. The incision can usually be closed, although the sheath can be left open to prevent ventilation difficulties; 24–48 hours later, when the patient is stable and clotting has normalized, the pack should be carefully removed. There is rarely any active bleeding and the abdominal incision can be repaired.

Summary

During minimally invasive procedures, it is often in the patient's best interest to convert to laparotomy without delay; call for a vascular surgeon; initiate proper monitoring; obtain blood products; and apply direct pressure to the injured vessel; and only if comfortable with the steps discussed above proceed with primary repair of the injury.

Further reading

Chapron CM, Pierre F, Lacroix S, *et al*. Major vascular injuries during gynecologic laparoscopy. *J Am Coll Surg* 1997;185:461–465.

Dildy G, Scott JR, Saffer CS, Belfort MA. An effective pressure pack for severe pelvic hemorrhage. *Obstet Gynecol* 2006;108:1222–1226.

26 Urinary tract

The management of injuries to the urinary tract

Urologists joke that gynaecologists perform only three operations: ligating the left ureter, ligating the right ureter and ligating both ureters.

Although injury to the urinary tract is one of the major concerns of the gynaecological surgeon during routine gynaecological procedures, actual injury is rare. The surgeon should know the whereabouts of the ureters and bladder during any procedure to avoid being 'a urinary tract neurotic' and taking ridiculous precautions to avoid the ureters and bladder. These structures should be treated with care but not with the type of respect which results in never handling them.

Anatomical relationship

The source of the gynaecologist's concern is the close relationship of the ureters to the cervix and the uterine arteries, the retroperitoneal course of the ureter in the pelvis and its contiguity with the infundibulopelvic ligament at the pelvic brim. The attachment of the bladder to the anterior part of the uterus and cervix, and the necessity to separate the two structures, often places the bladder in considerable danger of damage.

Bonney's Gynaecological Surgery, 11th edition.
© Tito Lopes, Nick Spirtos, Raj Naik, John Monaghan.
Published 2011 by Blackwell Publishing Ltd.

Predisposing factors

These include:
- congenital anomalies, including duplex ureters and ectopic kidneys
- endometriosis
- chronic pelvic inflammatory disease
- retroperitoneal masses such as broad ligament fibroids and large ovarian cysts
- previous pelvic surgery
- gynaecological malignancy
- radiotherapy with scarring and compromised blood supply.

Preventing injuries

Conditions such as pelvic malignancy, endometriosis, fibroids, radiotherapy and previous surgery can distort the course and position of the ureters and, in particular, cause scarring and constriction of tissues, resulting in approximation of the ureter to the surgical clamps and sutures increasing the risk of injury. Surgical technique, when operating on such conditions, should include a process of 'restoration of anatomy', adequate use of traction and tension by use of retractors and assistants to allow separation of vital structures from the surgical field, an understanding of tissue planes and release of scarred tissues through sharp dissection rather than blunt and forceful manoeuvres. Often, damage is caused through unnecessary trauma to tissues causing irritating vessel injury and bleeding, which is then sutured or clipped prior to obtaining adequate exposure of the surrounding area. An understanding of the retroperitoneal structures and use of the retroperitoneal approach (discussed elsewhere) is essential in reducing the risk of ureteric injury as the ureters can be visualized directly along the majority of their course in the pelvis.

The risk of bladder injury increases during surgery following a previous caesarean section or during cytoreductive surgery for ovarian cancer. Simple tips to avoid such injuries during gynaecological surgery include use of an appropriate retractor such as a Morris retractor and a 'good' second assistant. Proper traction and exposure of the vesicouterine peritoneum allows it to be elevated with the DeBakey forceps or clips and it can be incised safely and the bladder separated from the underlying structures. Alternatively, if the upper area is especially scarred in the midline, a plane in the peritoneum is often found on the right or left lateral aspects of the uterus. Entry and development of this plane should be performed using both blunt and sharp dissection. Another option, especially when the superior aspect of the bladder peritoneum is covered in tumour, which is commonly seen with disseminated ovarian cancer, is that the peritoneal layer and associated tumour are dissected off the anterior surface of the bladder by sharp dissection to the point where the peritoneum becomes densely adherent to the uterus. Separation of the de-peritonealized bladder from the cervix and vagina can then be completed under direct vision.

Injuries to the urinary tract are classified into those recognized at the time of surgery and those which manifest themselves later in the postoperative period.

Damage recognized at the time of operation

Bladder injuries

The most common circumstance for damage to the bladder is when the bladder is being separated from the anterior surface of the lower uterus and cervix during hysterectomy or caesarean section. If the surgeon is unsure about the possibility of an injury he or she should insert diluted methylene blue into the bladder through a urethral catheter and look for any leakage into the peritoneal cavity. Some surgeons use sterile formula milk obtained from the obstetric wards, always available, as this is easily diluted and cleared from the operative field, unlike methylene blue.

Damage to the muscularis If the bladder is not entered but a 'bubble' of mucosa can be seen pushing through from the muscularis, all that is required is that the area should be oversewn with an interrupted or continuous 2-0 Vicryl suture.

Breaching of the bladder wall If the bladder has obviously been entered, the area should be clearly identified by placing Allis tissue forceps or 'stay' sutures on the edge of the defect. The mucosa and muscularis can be sutured in a single layer with a continuous or interrupted layer using a 2-0 Vicryl suture.

It is vital to identify the ureteric orifices if the damage has occurred close to the trigone or the site of entry of the ureters into the bladder wall. In these circumstances, the gynaecologist would do well to call upon the assistance of a urological colleague to perform the repair.

If it is necessary to carry out a repair without assistance, the gynaecologist should open the bladder at its upper part, identify the ureteric orifices, catheterize them with double 'J' stents and proceed with the repair under direct vision. Stenting of the ureters will facilitate identification of the oblique track of the ureter through the bladder wall during repair. Fluoroscopy should be performed to ensure the guidewire has reached the renal pelvis. If not practical, one could use a plain radiograph intraoperatively to ensure proper placement. The stents can be removed 2–6 weeks postoperatively depending on the severity of the injury.

At the end of the repair, an omental flap should be placed between the bladder and the vagina as it increases the vascular supply to the area and adds a layer of separation between the two organs. This is essential when the damage to the bladder has occurred following irradiation, as there is a significant risk of failure of healing and subsequent fistula formation.

Ureteric injuries

When it is suspected that the ureter has been damaged at operation, whether by cutting, crushing or inclusion in a suture, then the ureter should be widely exposed so that a full inspection can be carried out. This is best done by separating the pelvic peritoneum from the pelvic sidewall and exposing the full length of the pelvic part of the ureter. It is not necessary to separate the ureter from the peritoneum for its full length as this would merely jeopardize its blood supply. An immediate repair of the damaged ureter gives a very good prospect of complete recovery without the need for further surgery. A urologist, if available, should be consulted for repair of any ureteric injury.

Injuries to the pelvic ureter

Crushing and thermal injuries These may be caused by crushing or nipping by tissue forceps or by inadvertent ligation. When the injury has resulted from the use of diathermy or other 'energy sources' care must be taken to excise the areas of thermal damage. If the injury is recognized intraoperatively, the surgeon should wait a few minutes before undertaking repair so that the damaged section can be further delineated. The management should be to resect the damaged area and anastomose the two ends.

Incision of the ureter It is rare to partially resect the ureter; more commonly, it is completely resected. In these circumstances, the management is to anastomose the cleanly divided ends of the ureter, having first made the ends spatulate.

The operation

- *Identifying the site of damage.* The area affected is exposed and the damaged area resected.
- *Making the anastomosis.* The clean ends of the ureter are spatulated (Fig. 26.1), and sutured using 4.0 Vicryl over a ureteric stent.
- *Management of the stent.* The commonest stent used is the 'pigtail' Silastic stent (Fig. 26.2), which can remain in the ureter for considerable periods of time. The upper end of the stent is inserted into the renal pelvis and the lower end into the bladder. If a pigtail is used, no fixation is required as the 'memory' of the catheter will unwind the terminal few centimetres and provide adequate fixation.
- *Extraperitoneal drainage.* The operative area should be drained to monitor for leakage of urine during the first few days.

Injuries to the distal ureter

This type of injury tends to occur in association with gynaecological surgery. It differs from injuries higher up the ureter in that it is often difficult to mobilize the ureter sufficiently to anastomose it without tension. In this situation, the method most used to deal with this problem is to produce a new point of

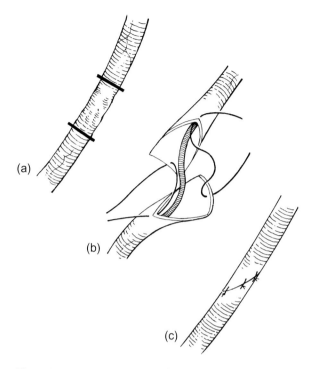

Figure 26.1 (a–c) Anastomosis of the ureter after either transection or resection of a short length of damaged ureter.

entry into the bladder; the damaged distal portion remaining can be either ligated or resected. The ureter should be implanted using an anti-reflux mechanism, which will require the bladder to be opened.

The operation

- *Preparation of the ureter.* The damaged distal end of the ureter must be 'freshened' by removing any necrosed or traumatized tissue. A short length of ureter is mobilized and the distal end drawn towards the bladder.
- *Assessing ureteric tension and bladder mobilization.* If there is any tension, then the bladder should be mobilized by separating it from the symphysis pubis or considering lifting the bladder towards the ureter (the psoas hitch), or developing a 'Boari–Ockerblad flap'.
- *The psoas hitch.* This simple technique involves suturing the bladder wall to the iliopsoas muscle on the pelvic sidewall, thus elevating the bladder and

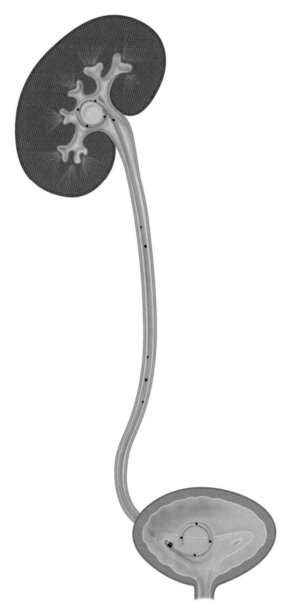

Figure 26.2 A correctly placed double pigtail stent. Drawing kindly provided by Boston Scientific Corporation.

shortening the distance between the bladder and the ureter to be anastomosed (Fig. 26.3).

• *The Boari–Ockerblad flap*. When there has been significant loss of the distal ureter, this technique allows the gap to be bridged by bladder tissue and a

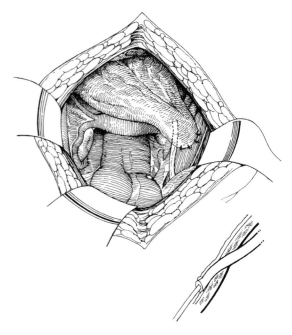

Figure 26.3 The psoas hitch.

satisfactory anastomosis to be achieved without tension. The most important point to be considered when fashioning the flap (Fig. 26.4) is to be careful not to make the flap too narrow. It is extraordinarily easy to forget the relationship between the width of the flap and the tube which it must become. The flap is more readily performed with a full bladder and it may be worth filling the bladder before the incision. An oblique U-shaped incision is then made in the bladder wall, and the distal end of the ureter is either sutured directly to the end or is tunnelled submucosally. Figures 26.4 and 26.5 show the technique for producing a flap with an anti-reflux anastomosis.

• *Direct implantation of the ureter into the bladder*. Once the end of the ureter is clean and it has been decided that it is possible to implant it into the bladder, the first step is to open the bladder and confirm the site of anastomosis. Again, this is more readily performed with a full bladder. An oblique opening is then made in the bladder and the distal end of the ureter is drawn through it using two stay sutures attached to its edges (Fig. 26.6). The edges are then sutured to the mucosa and two further stitches

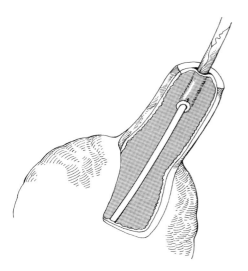

Figure 26.4 The Boari–Ockerblad flap: developing the flap from the bladder wall.

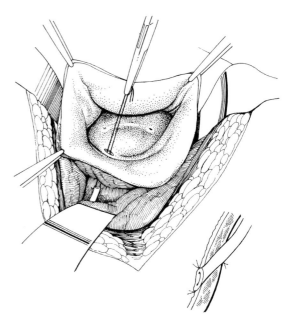

Figure 26.6 Implantation of the ureter into the bladder wall.

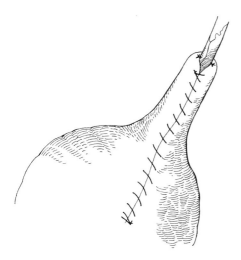

Figure 26.5 The Boari–Ockerblad flap: suturing the flap to form a tube over the antiflux anastomosis.

are placed to fasten the side of the ureter to the outer surface of the bladder in order to anchor it and counter any tendency to retraction. The ureter is stented and the coiled end left to lie in the bladder to be retrieved later using a cystoscope. Another way to reduce the risk of reflux is to directly implant the ureter into the bladder leaving 1–2 cm essentially dangling in the bladder. LaPlace's law provides for the internal pressure in a cylinder (P) to increase as the radius (R) decreases relative to the tension (T) $P = T/R$. The exact calculation of the length of ureter needed to prevent reflux is quite complex as it is influenced by bladder wall tension, which fluctuates as it fills, as well as the pressure within the ureter. As the bladder fills, the rise in the intravesical pressure compresses the ureter, thus preventing reflux. In general, we have found with the bladder filled with approximately 250–300 mL of urine an intravesical ureteral length of 1.5 cm prevents reflux. The ureteric wall is sutured to the bladder mucosa with 3-0 Vicryl and to the serosa with 2-0 Vicryl. This technique potentially reduces the risk of stricture associated with the 'tunnelling of the ureter' meant to reduce reflux. Although the tunnelling of the ureter is commonly discussed as a means to this end, there is little literature describing just how much of the ureter has to be tunnelled to reduce the incidence of reflux.

• *Bladder closure and drainage.* The bladder is drained with an indwelling catheter and the extraperitoneal space is drained with a suction drain.

Postoperative care Prophylactic antibiotics specific for bacteria affecting the urinary tract should be used. The urethral catheter should be maintained for at least 7 days, preferably longer, while the ureteric stents are left in place for 2–6 weeks

An intravenous urogram (IVU) with special views of the lower ureter will confirm the security of the anastomosis.

Less common procedures

• *Transuretero-ureterostomy.* This may be necessary if it is impossible to bridge the gap between the end of the damaged ureter and the bladder. The damaged ureter is cleaned and mobilized; it is then brought across the midline without tension and directly anastomosed into the side of the remaining ureter. Ureteric stents should be used to support the anastomosis until healing has occurred.

Interposition of a segment of small bowel on the left side or the appendix on the right side can also be used to bridge the gap.

• *Bladder augmentation and ileal conduit.* In the rare circumstance when both ureters are damaged and reimplantation into the bladder cannot be achieved, the bladder should be augmented with a segment of small bowel and both ureters implanted into the augmented bladder. This procedure should be considered before creating an ileal conduit, which results in a stoma.

Management of the delayed diagnosis of urinary tract damage

The management of the late diagnosed urinary tract damage is mainly the area of expertise of the experienced urologist; the gynaecologist should not delay in calling for a colleague's advice as further delay will seriously risk the function of the kidney.

The diagnosis of urinary tract damage may be made following the development of symptoms such as urine leakage if a fistula has occurred or loin or ureteric pain when obstruction to the outflow develops.

The management of urinary fistulae is dealt with in Chapter 18.

The management of obstructive damage to the ureters can be divided into the two phases:

• *Drainage* of the obstructed renal tract is best performed by radiologically guided percutaneous nephrostomy. Ureteric catheters can sometimes be passed beyond the point of obstruction, especially when the blockage is due to extrinsic pressure.

• *Repair* of the damage to the ureter needs to be carried out if the obstruction cannot be relieved by a stent. If there is enough ureteric length to obtain a tension-free anastomosis to the bladder, a ureteroneocystotomy can be performed via either laparotomy or laparoscopy.

Laparoscopic ureteroneocystotomy

Two 12-mm trocars are inserted in the midline above the umbilicus as well as approximately 5–6 cm above the pubic symphysis, and two 5-mm trocars are inserted laterally at the iliac crests. The affected ureter is dissected free (Fig. 26.7), maximizing the length to ease the anastomosis. The redundant distal ureteric segment can be clipped or sutured and the proximal end is freshened. The bladder is mobilized off the symphysis pubis and a cystotomy is created anteriorly (Fig. 26.8). After placing a suture (0 Polysorb) through the free end of the ureter, a tract is created through the bladder using a Maryland dissector (Fig. 26.9). At this point, the ureter is sutured to the bladder serosa to maintain its position and a double 'J' stent with a guidewire in place is passed through the urethra, into the bladder and ureter until it reaches the renal pelvis (Fig. 26.10). The guidewire is then withdrawn and the ureter sutured to the bladder mucosa using an Endo Stitch device (Covidien Inc., Boulder, CO, USA) with 3-0 Polysorb. Using the same instrument the ureter can also be further stabilized and tension reduced by suturing its serosal layer to the bladder wall. The bladder wall is then closed using 0 Vicryl in a running fashion either with an Endo Stitch device or using intracorporeal suturing techniques (Fig. 26.11). The procedure can be combined with a laparoscopically created Boari flap if extra length is required.

Other procedures

Frequently it is not possible to bridge the obstructed or damaged length of ureter and more extensive procedures are necessary. These are entirely in the province of the urologist and will be merely listed here.

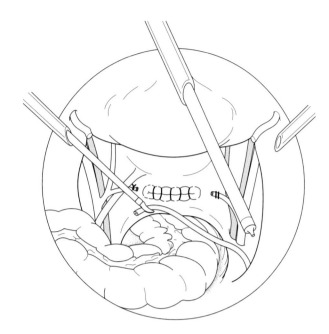

Figure 26.7 The affected ureter is dissected free.

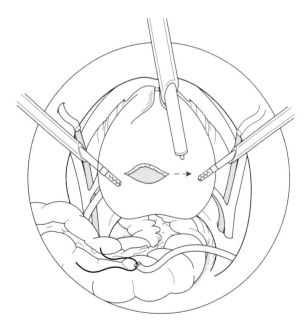

Figure 26.8 A cystotomy is created anteriorly.

• Uretero-ileoneocystostomy, or the use of an isolated segment of ileum to bridge the damaged length of ureter to the bladder.

• Transuretero-ureterostomy may be used if it is not possible to re-anastomose the damaged ureter with the bladder or the urologist feels that the long-term problems of using a segment of intestine are not justified.

• Nephrectomy may be necessary if renal function is markedly impaired.

241

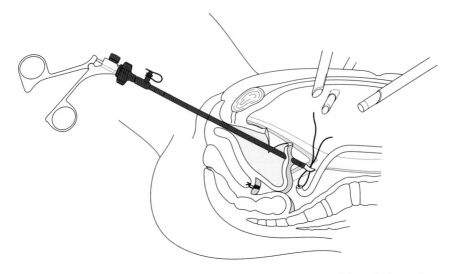

Figure 26.9 Suture connected to the ureter is grasped by a Maryland dissector inserted through the urethra.

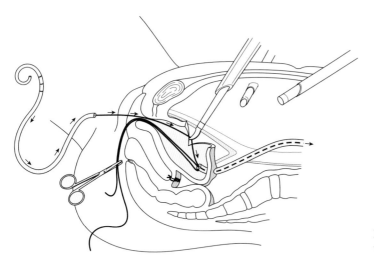

Figure 26.10 Placing of a double 'J' stent through the urethra.

Radiotherapy damage

When the patient has had irradiation to the ureter which is damaged, great care and skill is called for when deciding on the optimal method of repair. It is important to remember that the irradiation may have also compromised the blood supply of organs close to the ureter, particularly bowel; consequently, if conduits are to be produced, a segment of bowel outside the irradiation field should be chosen.

The gynaecologist must not be slow or too proud to ask for advice and assistance from urological col-

leagues; early recognition and management of damage to the urinary tract is in the patient's best interests.

Operations for the formation of a urinary conduit

When it is inevitable that the bladder has to be removed during a surgical procedure, or when the bladder is so badly damaged that it will never function normally again, as occasionally happens after

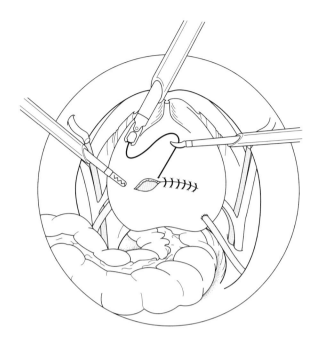

Figure 26.11 Repair of the bladder using an Endo Stitch.

radical radiotherapy, then a urinary diversion must be considered. The production of a urinary conduit may also be part of a larger procedure, such as an exenterative operation.

Various techniques have been used for urinary diversion, including:
• implantation of the ureters into the sigmoid colon (uretero-sigmoidostomy)
• the formation of a wet colostomy, combining bowel and urinary function into one stoma
• the formation of a rectal bladder and a left iliac fossa colostomy
• the production of a nephrostomy or ureterostomy bringing the ureters directly out to the surface, ideally with cannulation.

All these techniques have significant associated problems, especially of infection and electrolyte control in the longer term.

Once Bricker had demonstrated the ease with which an isolated loop of ileum could be used to function as an artificial bladder, variations of his procedure became the preponderant methods of diversion. Many different parts of the bowel may be used, including the ileum, sigmoid colon and, when there has been extensive pelvis and lower abdominal irradiation, the transverse colon.

There are also a variety of ways of joining the ureters to the isolated loop of bowel. In some centres, the Leadbetter technique of implanting the ureters individually into the bowel loop is used; however, the authors prefer the Wallace technique, which is described here.

In more recent years, the development of more complex but aesthetically satisfying procedures, beginning with the Koch pouch and being extended and made more sophisticated by a wide variety of eponymous procedures, have included the Miami pouch, the Mainz pouch and a variety of others, usually taking the name of their originating centre.

All of these continent conduits rely on the use of a low-pressure artificial bladder being generated by denervation and expansion of the small bowel. The stomas are generally brought out through a tiny hole in the abdominal wall, sometimes the umbilicus, which the patient can self-catheterize as and when she wishes to void. These low-pressure systems have many advantages over the relative lack of control of the Wallace diversion; however, they have the major disadvantage of requiring considerable lengths of normal bowel, something which is not always available following extensive irradiation, which is frequently an indicator for this procedure.

Patient preparation

The patient must have the full impact of removal of the bladder explained to her. The advantages and disadvantages must be fairly and honestly explained and the patient and her partner must realize the significance of the permanent alteration in function which will be generated. For many patients, the alteration in voiding habit will bring a definite improvement, especially for those with a post-radiotherapeutic fistula or shrinkage fixity of the bladder. The translation from a complete lack of control of urinary production and the difficulties of maintaining cleanliness when translated into the wearing of a simple ostomy appliance are infinite, and the vast majority of patients have little difficulty in accepting this permanent change.

The patient should be encouraged to meet with other patients who have had diversionary procedures performed and be seen on a number of occasions by the stoma therapist. The surgeon and the stoma therapist should site the stoma and clearly mark the place on the day before operation. The bowel is prepared for resection by giving the patient a low-residue diet for 2–3 days preoperatively. Bowel washouts are unnecessarily debilitating and should be avoided.

Instruments

The instruments required are those in the gynaecological general set described in Chapter 3, augmented with the GIA (Covidien Inc.) stapling devices. If the bowel is to be sutured, soft non-crushing bowel clamps will be needed. A variety of small (no. 6 to no. 10) soft rubber T tubes will be needed, the size depending on the size of the ureters identified at the operation.

Anaesthesia

No special anaesthetic will be required for the conduit to be made; however, an epidural or spinal anaesthetic is of great assistance for any exenterative procedure. Intraoperative prophylactic antibiotics are given.

The operation

The incision

If the conduit is the sole procedure to be performed, a midline or paramedian incision lying alongside the umbilicus will give adequate access.

Opening the abdomen

The incision should be designed so that the lower part of the para-aortic area is accessible at the level of the inferior mesenteric artery. When the operation is performed as part of an exenteration the conduit should lie well above the pelvis out of the irradiated field. Once the abdomen is opened, the bowel is carefully packed away from the operation site aided by a head-down tilt and the ureters are identified and divided.

Identifying and isolating the ureters

It is usually easiest to pick out the ureters as they cross the pelvic brim. They can often be seen shining through the peritoneum, exhibiting movement. The peritoneum close to them is picked up and carefully incised. This incision is extended with scissors and the ureters identified on either side. From time to time one ureter will be found to be disproportionately larger than the other ureter. This is not a contraindication to the use of the Wallace technique, and the ureter should be identified, raised and separated gently from the peritoneum and structures around. The ureters are usually divided at or about the level of the pelvic brim. It is particularly important on the left side not to cut the ureter too high as the ureter has to be drawn across through the mesentery of the large bowel in order to meet with the right-sided ureter over the right side of the aorta and the inferior vena cava. Once the ureters have been identified and divided, the distal ends are tied with Vicryl sutures unless they are to be removed with the pelvic specimen during an exenterative procedure. At this time, the proximal ends of the ureters are allowed to lie free and the relatively small amounts of urine which are exuded can be removed easily at the end of the procedure.

Bringing the ureters to an intraperitoneal position

A point is now chosen on the right side of the posterior abdominal wall approximately 5 cm above the pelvic brim and 5 cm to the right of the midpoint of the aorta. The peritoneum is elevated and incised, usually a continuation of the initial incision for identification of the ureters, and, using a blunt forceps or the index finger, a tunnel is developed so that the divided right ureter can be brought out through the space. The left ureter is a little more difficult to transpose as it has to negotiate the sigmoid colon mesentery. The editors find the easiest way of performing

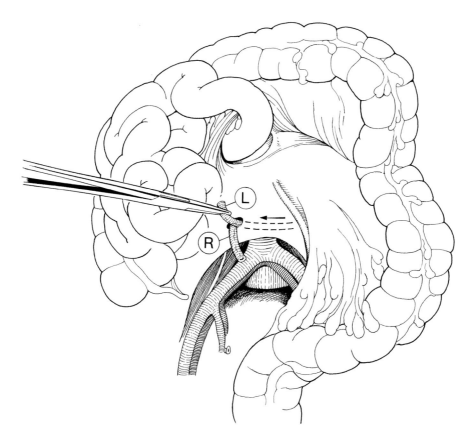

Figure 26.12 Bringing the ureters into an intraperitoneal position.

this transposition is to burrow under the mesentery with the fingers of the left hand, taking care to identify and avoid the inferior mesenteric artery. This gentle burrowing separates the peritoneum, allowing a blunt forceps to be passed from the hole on the right side, across the aorta, through the mesentery, to pick up the ureter on the left and draw it gently out of the hole on the right side of the mesentery (Fig. 26.12).

Preparing the segment of bowel
If the small bowel has not been irradiated then a segment of distal ileum may be chosen for the conduit. If extensive pelvic irradiation has been used, it may be prudent to utilize a more proximal segment of small bowel or a segment of the transverse colon for the conduit as an alternative. The principles involved are identical; therefore, only the ileal segment procedure will be described.

A segment of ileum lying approximately 20–25 cm from the ileal caecal valve is chosen. The bowel is elevated and transilluminated to outline the arterial arcades. Ideally, the segment should contain at least two separate major arcade vessels. It should be approximately 15–20 cm in length depending on the size of the patient, and be fully mobile. The segment is elevated by the surgeon and the assistant and the line of separation identified by incising the two leaves of the mesentery, taking care to either avoid or ligate small vessels which are present (Fig. 26.13). Individual small vessels can be ligated using either clips and ties or small metal clips, which are easy to apply as the dissection develops.

Division of the bowel
This is most elegantly done using the GIA stapling device (Fig. 26.14), producing a sealed isolated

245

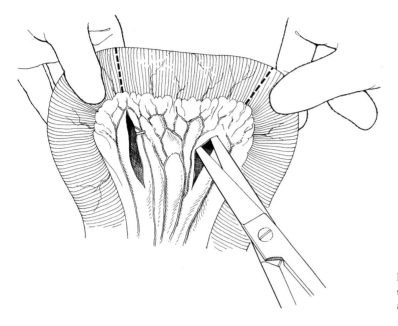

Figure 26.13 Choosing an ileal segment with a broad-based arterial arcade.

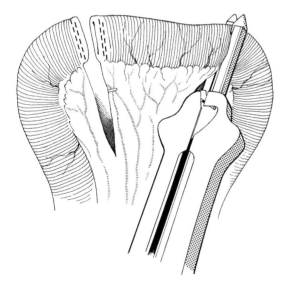

Figure 26.14 Resecting the bowel segment with a GIA stapling device.

segment of ileum. This segment is laid down on a dampened pack below the divided bowel.

In more recent times, the editors have changed their pattern of working to simply divide the bowel using soft crushing clamps so that the bowel is then immediately ready for repair and reconstitution.

Reconstituting the bowel

The two divided ends of the bowel are now elevated so that a functional side-to-side anastomosis can be made. The two ends are held side to side with Babcock tissue forceps so that a small incision can be made alongside each of the staple lines (Fig. 26.15) or, if the open ends of the bowel are present, as is modern practice, the GIA stapler can be introduced down into the bowel lumen and fired. The GIA stapler cuts a communication between the two limbs of the bowel and surrounds this communication with an intact staple line. Thus, a functional side-to-side anastomosis is formed that is completed by repairing the upper part of the anastomosis using a further GIA stapler to close the segment. The space between the mesentery of the small bowel is closed using three or four interrupted fine Vicryl sutures (Fig. 26.16). It is important not to make this repair too tight as it may compromise blood flow to the conduit. It is also important to draw together the individual layers of peritoneum rather than make deep bites into the mesentery and cause injury to the precious vessels feeding the anastomosis.

Formation of the ureteric platform

Having brought the two ureters together intraperitoneally, the terminal 1 cm of each ureter is incised with

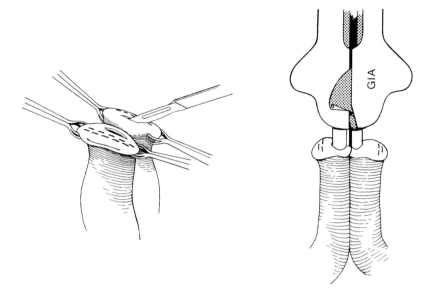

Figure 26.15 Reconstituting bowel continuity using the GIA stapling device.

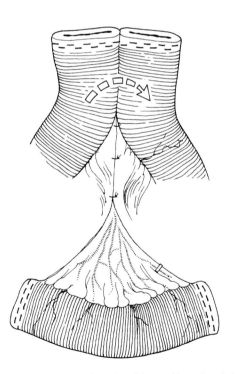

Figure 26.16 Showing the isolated loop of bowel and the completed re-anastomosed small bowel.

scissors so as to splay out the ends. These splayed out ends are then sutured to each other (Fig. 26.17) so as to produce a platform. The central suture is left long so that the T tube, which is now inserted into each ureter, can be anchored onto the base plate. This central stitch is best performed using Vicryl Rapide as, by dissolving quicker, it will allow removal of the anchored T tube sooner during the postoperative period.

Suturing the ileal segment to the ureters

The staples, if used, on each side of the ileal segment are now removed. The long arm of the T tube is threaded through the segment. This is ideally done by passing a soft bowel clamp down the length of the segment, grasping the tube and drawing it gently through. It is important to make sure that the tube passes in the direction of peristaltic flow, and as the T tube is threaded through the segment (Fig. 26.18) the edges of the platform can then be carefully sutured to the edges of the bowel using a series of interrupted Vicryl sutures. The conduit base is attached to the posterior abdominal wall peritoneum with two or three individual sutures of Vicryl. It is important that there is no tension on the ureters themselves, and the conduit does not prolapse into the pelvis.

247

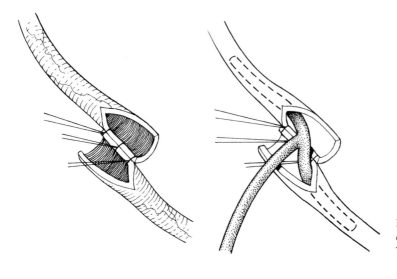

Figure 26.17 Joining the splayed out ends of the ureter and inserting the T tube.

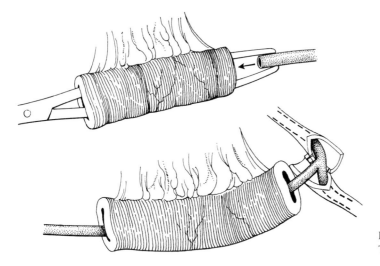

Figure 26.18 Drawing the long arm of the T tube down the segment of the bowel.

Formation of the stoma

A circle is cut in the skin at the site marked by the stoma therapist. This incision is carried down to the aponeurosis, which is cut and the edges clipped. The surgeon now places the left hand in the abdomen and elevates the abdominal wall under this incision. With the right hand the surgeon continues to cut down through the peritoneum, producing a hole through which the index finger can be easily passed.

A Babcock forceps is now passed through the hole and the distal end of the conduit with the T tube is gently drawn through. The conduit should be inspected to ensure that it is lying comfortably without undue tension or torsion. The Babcock forceps is inserted a short distance into the stoma and used to grasp the mucosa (Fig. 26.19). This process everts the end of the bowel, and the edge of the bowel, which is now rolled back on itself, is sutured first to the serosa and then to the skin edge so that a rosebud stoma is formed. The stoma appliance is put in place, feeding the shortened T tube into the back.

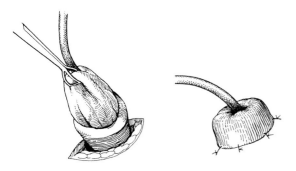

Figure 26.19 Forming the 'rosebud' stoma.

Closing the abdomen
This is carried out as described in Chapter 4. It is prudent to place a suction drain close to the anastomosis site.

Postoperative care
The patient is commenced on fluids soon after surgery and can be converted to a light diet when she is willing and able. The suction drain can be removed a few days after surgery, although this can be left for longer if there is any hesitation relating to the uretero-ileal anastomosis. The T tube is kept in place for approximately 10 days and is then gently pulled to see if it can be removed. If it does not easily release, further attempts should be made on the next 2 days; if it still does not release, the patient can be allowed home with the T tube in place, and it is usually found after a short period of time that the conduit naturally discharges the T tube into the ileostomy bag. The patient will require intensive training in the maintenance of the ileostomy appliance. This is performed by the stoma therapist once the patient is mobile, and confidence is developed at this time. It has been the editors' practice to maintain prophylactic antibiotics, not only during the operation but for some days after the procedure, until good urinary flow is developed, when a lifelong course of low-dose maintenance antibiotic can be commenced.

It is important to maintain good hydration so that a fast flow of urine can be maintained in the postoperative period. This will reduce the risk of clot formation blocking the ureters or the conduit itself.

Further reading

Textbooks

Hinman F. *Atlas of Urologic Surgery*, 2nd edn. Philadelphia: W.B. Saunders, 1998. An excellent book with full descriptions and useful illustrations of the relevant urological procedures.

Historic papers

Bricker EM. Bladder substitution after pelvic evisceration. *Surg Clin North Am* 1950;30:1511.

Kock NG, Nilson AE, Nilsson LO, *et al*. Urinary diversion via a continent ileal reservoir: clinical results in 12 patients. *J Urol* 1982;128:469–475.

Leadbetter WF, Clarke BG. Five years' experience with uretero-enterostomy by the combined technique. *J Urol* 1955;73:67–82.

Penalver MA, Bejany DE, Averette HE, *et al*. Continent urinary diversion in gynecologic oncology. *Gynecol Oncol* 1989;34:274–288.

Wallace DM. Ureteric diversion using a conduit: a simplified technique. *Br J Urol* 1966;38:522–527.

27 Operations on the intestinal tract for the gynaecologist

It is rare for the gynaecological surgeon to be involved with bowel surgery as part of routine gynaecological surgery. However, the gynaecological surgeon should be able to perform an appendicectomy and repair occasional small injuries to the bowel created while separating adhesions. If he or she has any doubt or if the primary pathology is gastrointestinal, the general surgeon should be called.

Appendicectomy

The question of whether to remove the appendix at the time of laparotomy for pelvic disease remains contentious. In the USA, recent studies suggest that incidental appendicectomy at the time of open and laparoscopic hysterectomy is safe. In UK practice, the appendix is not removed, except when it is found to be abnormal on inspection. The appendix should always be removed in cases of pseudomyxoma peritonei as this condition is often associated with tumours of the appendix, including carcinoid tumours. The presence of faecoliths, mucocoeles or any signs of inflammation warrants its removal, provided that the extra operating time does not hazard the patient. The major concern of the surgeon is the risk of contaminating the clean peritoneal cavity with the contents of the appendix. It is

vitally important that a technique should be used which reduces this risk to zero and that the patient is given an appropriate prophylactic antibiotic.

Instruments

The general set described in Chapter 3 will be in use; the only addition which is required is a Babcock soft-tissue forceps and a fine 2-0 Vicryl suture on a round-bodied atraumatic needle.

Patient preparation

No special preoperative preparation is required, although if the appendix is found to be inflamed at laparotomy, or there is evidence of free pus, a Gram-negative-specific antibiotic should be given intravenously during the procedure if not already given.

Anaesthesia

No special requirement is necessary, except for general anaesthesia.

The operation

The incision
The appendix can be reached through most standard gynaecological incisions; therefore, there is no special need to extend or alter the original wound. However, it is important that the edges of the wound should not be soiled by contact with the appendix or the appendix stump when the appendix has been removed.

Bonney's Gynaecological Surgery, 11th edition.
© Tito Lopes, Nick Spirtos, Raj Naik, John Monaghan.
Published 2011 by Blackwell Publishing Ltd.

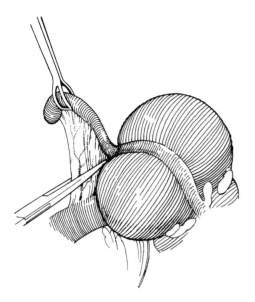

Figure 27.1 Dividing the appendix mesentery.

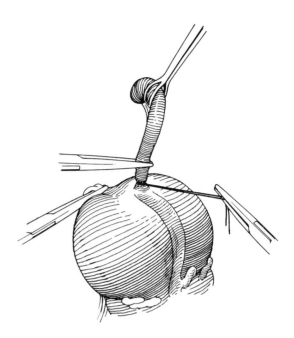

Figure 27.2 Removing the appendix.

Dividing the appendix mesentery
The appendix is elevated using the Babcock forceps, putting the appendiceal mesentery on the stretch. In thin patients, the small appendiceal artery can often be visualized. A short straight tissue clamp is placed across the vessel with its tip close to the wall of the appendix (Fig. 27.1). Using scissors the mesentery is cut, leaving the appendix attached to the caecum solely by its base. When the appendix is long, more than one pedicle may be required.

Placing the purse-string suture
Current practice no longer supports the inversion of the appendix stump with a purse-string suture.

Removing the appendix
The base of the appendix is now crushed using a straight clamp, which is then replaced a short distance down the appendix; a Vicryl tie is placed around the crushed part of the appendix and cut (Fig. 27.2). The surgeon cuts across the appendix below the clamp and places it, and the knife which has been contaminated by the bowel contents, into a dish. (The scrub nurse removes this from the operative field.)

Variations in technique
The appendectomy can be carried out using an Endo GIA (Covidien Inc., Boulder, CO, USA) stapler to secure the mesentery and the appendiceal blood supply as well as the appendix itself at both the open and laparoscopic approach.

Another technique for laparoscopic appendicectomy is to divide the mesentery using any of the energy sources and the appendix base tied using an Endoloop (Ethicon Endo-Surgery Inc., Cincinnati, OH, USA).

Retrograde appendicectomy may be necessary when the tip or part of the length of the organ is involved in adhesions or not readily accessible, such as in the retrocaecal position. The base is cleared around its circumference and clamped, tied and cut as described above. The remainder of the appendix is then dissected free from all adhesions. If the surgeon stays close to the caecum there is a readily found tissue plane which is often very simply separated, reducing the risk of entering either the appendix or the caecum. Rarely, it may be necessary to remove the appendix piecemeal; this should be avoided as the risk of contamination of the abdominal cavity is considerable.

If the appendix is inflamed and pus is present in the peritoneal cavity, the surgeon should carry out peritoneal lavage with an antiseptic solution, having first taken bacteriology swabs for culture and drug sensitivity.

Management of operative injuries of the intestine

The majority of injuries to bowel are avoidable.

One of the commonest circumstances when bowel is damaged is when the peritoneum is opened. This may be due to adhesion of bowel to the parietal peritoneum or simply due to the fact that the surgeon has picked up an edge of bowel in the forceps when elevating the peritoneum prior to incision. The simple safeguard of running the fingers between the forceps will reduce this risk almost to nil.

Other causes include:
• lack of experience in handling bowel, particularly bowel damaged by irradiation or affected by disease such as carcinoma deposits
• an inadequate incision or poor light, which gives poor vision of the operative field and requires assistants to retract unnecessarily forcefully to gain access
• unnecessary haste and carelessness in performing the procedure, resulting in clamps being placed on bowel, or tears produced when adhesions are roughly separated.

The major pathological factors involved in the development of traumatic injuries to the bowel are:
• endometriosis, particularly in the rectovaginal septum
• pelvic inflammatory disease, particularly chronic disease, when multiple adhesions may have developed
• malignant disease, particularly ovarian carcinoma
• infective disease of the bowel, such as acute appendicitis and diverticulitis
• radiotherapy damage and the recently reported adhesive peritonitis, which may develop after the combined use of radiotherapy and some chemotherapeutic agents.

The operation

Closed trauma
If the damage to the bowel has not resulted in opening the lumen but has simply incised the serosa, allowing the mucosa to 'bubble' through, all that is required is for the serosa to be resutured over the defect using a single layer of continuous Vicryl or Monocryl on an atraumatic round-bodied needle.

Open damage
If the lumen has been entered, the surgeon must determine whether the bowel has been devitalized or not.

If the damage is via a clean cut without crushing of the edges of the lesion, it may be possible to perform a primary repair. This should be performed in a single layer apposing the serosa using either a continuous or an interrupted suturing technique with Vicryl or Monocryl. It is important not to narrow the bowel lumen when repairing, so the defect should be repaired transversely and sutures should not be drawn too tightly. The repaired bowel must be examined for patency by grasping the lumen under the repair between finger and thumb, making allowances for the fact that postoperative oedema may further reduce the diameter of the lumen.

Nasogastric tube
If the repair is in the proximal part of the small bowel it is a useful safeguard to ask the anaesthetist to insert a nasogastric tube during the anaesthetic and maintain it until satisfactory bowel action returns in the postoperative period.

Resection of a segment of bowel
If the traumatized length of bowel becomes dark owing to loss of blood supply or when there has been extensive tearing or crushing of the edges, the surgeon must be prepared to resect the segment. This may be performed either in the traditional manner described here or using stapling techniques similar to those described in Chapter 26. The principles are identical.

Identifying the arterial arcade and resecting the affected segment
If the segment of bowel containing the traumatized area is elevated and transilluminated, the arterial arcade can be identified. Soft non-occluding bowel clamps are then applied so that an adequate vascular supply reaches the proposed resection lines (Fig. 27.3). 'Crushing' bowel clamps are placed at either end of the segment to be removed and the segment is resected by cutting along the 'crushing' clamps. The small vessels in the mesentery are tied with 2 or 3-0 Vicryl.

Suturing the bowel
The two ends of the bowel are drawn together and repaired in a single layer, beginning at the posterior layer of serosa (Fig. 27.4) and continuing round (Fig. 27.5) to join the initial suture. The editors use either a continuous suture of 3-0 Monocryl on a round-bodied

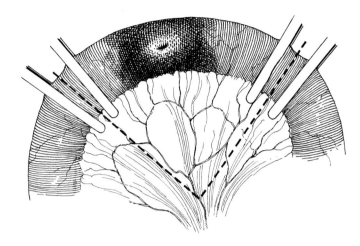

Figure 27.3 Resection of a damaged segment of small bowel.

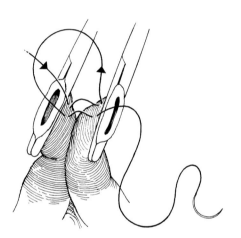

Figure 27.4 Suturing the serosa of the bowel segments.

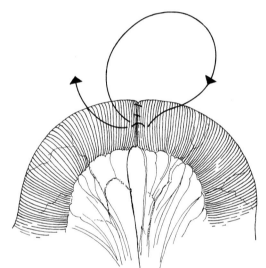

Figure 27.5 Completing the serosal suture.

atraumatic needle or interrupted sutures. Some still recommend repair in two layers.

Suturing the mesentery

The two edges of the mesentery are now apposed using interrupted Vicryl sutures. It is important to pick up the peritoneal edges on both surfaces of the mesentery and not to take bites which are so large as to damage the vasculature (Fig. 27.6).

The mesentery must be handled delicately at all times as it is very easy to traumatize the small vessels, producing a spreading haematoma which may further jeopardize the blood supply to the bowel.

This technique of resection of bowel can be applied to any length of bowel, both large and small.

The formation of a stoma

In current practice it is unnecessary that a gynaecological surgeon should know how to perform a colostomy, but it should be standard practice for a gynaecological oncologist. The indications for this procedure are various and include rectal involvement in ovarian carcinoma, the occurrence of gross radiotherapy damage in the pelvis, as part of the management of

253

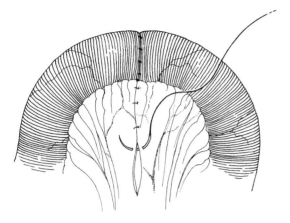

Figure 27.6 Apposing the mesenteric edges.

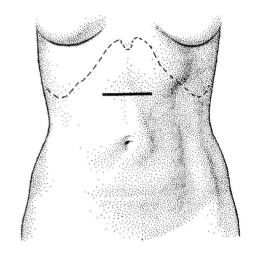

Figure 27.7 The site of incision for a temporary transverse colostomy.

rectovaginal fistulae, certain cases of diverticulitis, and as a preliminary manoeuvre prior to an anovulvectomy. Increasingly, the laparoscopic approach is being used for the formation of stomas.

Siting of the stoma

This is a skill which the gynaecological oncology surgeon should learn, but is normally performed by the stoma therapist, who should visit the patient in the preoperative period if a stoma is planned or likely. For emergency colostomies, the surgeon must rely on his or her own ability to site the stoma correctly.

Patient preparation

If the colostomy is a planned procedure, bowel preparation should be used.

Clearly, when the colostomy has to be made as an emergency procedure, bowel preparation cannot be carried out and the patient should be given intravenous antibiotics during the surgery, if not already administered.

The type of colostomy to be made will depend mainly on whether it is intended to be temporary or permanent.

Temporary loop colostomy

The position of the stoma will depend upon future surgical requirements. The colostomy should be sited away from areas where further intervention is considered. For most purposes, a midline upper abdominal site is suitable, the left iliac fossa site being used for a temporary colostomy only when no further surgery is envisaged in that area. Increasingly, a terminal loop ileostomy is used in preference to a loop colostomy.

The operation

Opening the abdomen
Frequently, the abdomen will be open when the decision to perform a temporary colostomy is made. However, if it is not, the site of choice is usually above the umbilicus in the midline (Fig. 27.7). The incision is made transversely, incising the rectus sheath and separating the muscles so that the peritoneum is entered in the midline.

Forming the loop colostomy
The transverse colon is identified and drawn out of the wound; it is easy to identify the colon because of the taenia running longitudinally. The omentum is seen to extend from the inferior border of the colon and should be dissected from the colon over a distance of about 10 cm; small vessels are easily identified and ligated.

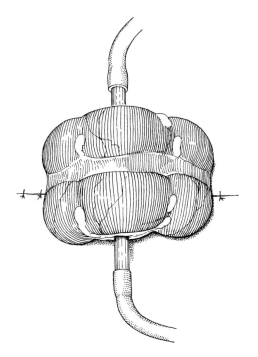

Figure 27.8 Anchoring the loop of large bowel to the surface.

Anchoring the loop
The cleared loop of colon is now drawn out of the wound and a small hole made in the mesentery through which a bridge is passed so as to anchor the loop above the surface (Fig. 27.8).

Closing the abdomen
The fascia is drawn together over the rectus muscles so as not to press too tightly upon the colon and the skin edges are sutured in a similar manner. It is not usually necessary to suture the colon to the edges of the stoma.

Opening the stoma
The bowel is opened along its antemesenteric border through a taenia, as this area is relatively avascular. A stoma bag is immediately applied so that the patient leaves theatre with the colostomy completed and fitted with an appropriate appliance.

Removal of the bridge
The stoma bridge can be removed as soon as serosal adhesions have formed, usually within 4–5 days.

Reversal of the colostomy
The great advantage of the loop colostomy is the ease with which it can be reversed. All that is required is for the adhesions between the bowel wall and the abdominal wall to be carefully dissected free, the bowel closed using a single-layered closure (made transversely so as not to narrow the lumen) and the colon reinserted into the abdomen. The abdominal wall is then closed as described in Chapter 4.

A permanent colostomy

It will be rare for the gynaecologist to have to make a permanent stoma unless he or she is involved in gynaecological oncology. The optimum site for a permanent stoma is in the left iliac fossa, away from bony prominences and fatty folds. The site should be smooth, both when the patient stands and when she sits.

Patient preparation

The bowel should be prepared as per the surgeon's protocol.

The operation

Opening the abdomen
The abdomen is frequently opened for another purpose, but, if not, a lower midline incision will give good access and allow the stoma appliances to be attached without impinging on the wound. Occasionally, it may be adequate to make a small transverse incision at the site for the stoma and pull the sigmoid through it, forming the stoma.

Choosing the bowel segment
The sigmoid colon is usually the site of bowel to be resected; the loop is elevated and transilluminated. If the sigmoid is not mobile, it can be freed further by incising the avascular peritoneum lateral to the colon in the paracolic gutter; this releases and rotates the bowel medially.

Dividing the bowel
The editors use the GIA stapling device at all times for this procedure because of its great accuracy and cleanliness. When a suitable segment has been chosen, the small vessels in the mesentery are divided and

255

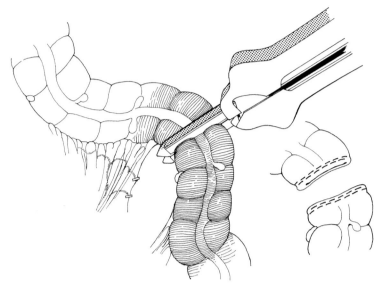

Figure 27.9 Dividing large bowel using the GIA stapling device.

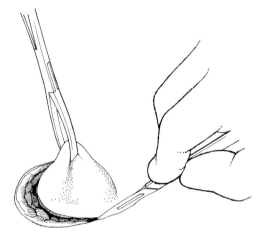

Figure 27.10 Removing the skin disc at the stoma size.

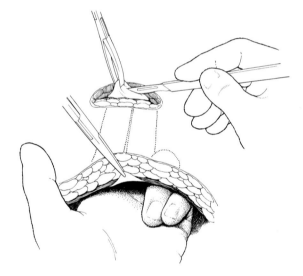

Figure 27.11 Incising the abdominal wall fat, musculature and peritoneum.

ligated so as to release a length of bowel that will reach to the stoma site without tension. The GIA stapling device is placed over the loop at right angles to the lumen and fired (Fig. 27.9). This leaves the distal end of the bowel sealed with the staples which, having been checked for bleeding, is lowered into the pelvis.

Making the stoma

The marked stoma site is now picked up with a Littlewood forceps and, by cutting transversely with the scalpel, a perfect circle of skin is removed, approximately 3 cm in diameter (Fig. 27.10). The peritoneum on the stoma side of the abdominal wound is grasped in a tissue forceps so that it is not drawn towards the stoma and distorts the intra-abdominal opening. The surgeon places the first two fingers of his or her left hand under the stoma site (Fig. 27.11) and elevates the peritoneum and the abdominal aponeurosis,

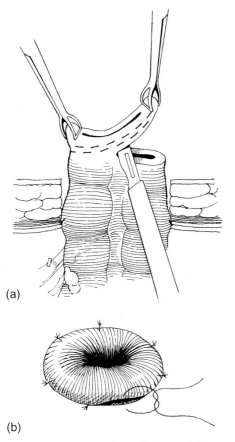

(a)

(b)

Figure 27.12 (a) Removing the staple line and (b) suturing the edge to the skin.

which is incised with a scalpel or diathermy, with the assistant clipping the layers in turn as they are cut. The stoma so produced should comfortably admit the first two fingers of the hand.

Exteriorizing the bowel

By passing a pair of Babcock tissue forceps through the stoma, the stapled proximal end of the sigmoid loop is drawn out of the orifice. The loop is checked for undue tension, and then the line of staples is cut off and the edge of the bowel sutured to the skin (Fig. 27.12). It is unnecessary to suture the edges of the aponeurosis and the peritoneum to the bowel.

Applying the colostomy appliance

The stoma bag is applied in theatre, making sure that it does not impinge on the midline incision.

Closing the abdomen

The abdomen is closed as described in Chapter 4.

The formation of a loop ileostomy

The editors perform a temporary loop ileostomy in preference to a temporary colostomy. The reasons are numerous but include the fact that there is more mobility with the mesentery of the small bowel and the contents are more fluid, reducing the risk of anastomosis breakdown when closed. The procedure is planned as a temporary stoma, but, occasionally, when formed for intestinal obstruction in ovarian cancer, is never reversed. The technique is similar to that for a colostomy.

The operation

Opening the abdomen

The abdomen is usually open when the decision to make an ileostomy is made.

Making the stoma

This is prepared as for the permanent colostomy. Patients with advanced ovarian cancer are often sited preoperatively for both a potential ileostomy and colostomy.

Forming the loop

The intended segment of terminal ileum is pulled through the stoma site using a Babcock tissue forceps. A bridge can be inserted to keep the loop in place but is not routinely used.

Opening the stoma

The bowel is opened transversely at the distal part of the loop and the incision is extended to about half the circumference (Fig. 27.13). The mucosa is inverted and a rosebud is formed, the greater prominence being the proximal segment of the loop (Fig. 27.14).

Removal of the bridge

If used, this can be removed after 4–5 days.

Reversal of the ileostomy

This is similar to that for the temporary colostomy, with the bowel repaired with a single-layer closure.

257

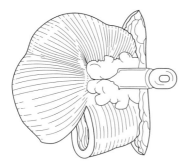

Figure 27.13 Incising the ileum.

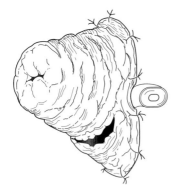

Figure 27.14 Forming a 'rosebud'.

Side-to-side anastomosis procedure

This technique of bypassing a segment of bowel which is obstructed or grossly damaged by tumour or irradiation is a valuable technique to learn.

Preoperative preparation

It may be difficult to achieve perfect preparation of the bowel if there is an element of obstruction. Therefore, the surgeon must be prepared to decompress the bowel if necessary prior to performing the procedure.

The operation

Opening the abdomen

The incision can be any which gives adequate access to the entire abdomen, and is capable of being extended when necessary.

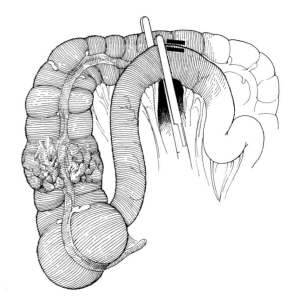

Figure 27.15 Apposing the small and large bowel.

Identifying the site of obstruction

The surgeon must be prepared to spend some time in ascertaining the site of the obstruction and correctly identifying healthy bowel proximal and distal to the obstruction. It is particularly important that the bypass anastomosis should not be performed using irradiated bowel.

Stapling the bowel

One of the commonest techniques necessary is to bypass the distal small bowel and the first part of the large bowel. The healthy ileum is drawn to the transverse colon and laid alongside it. The two lengths of bowel are lightly held using non-crushing clamps proximal to where the anastomosis is to be made (Fig. 27.15). A small opening is made in each segment of bowel and the GIA instrument inserted and fired, producing a stapled communication between the two segments (Fig. 27.16). The device is withdrawn and the two small openings closed with a single-layered closure using a Vicryl or Monocryl suture. The communication between the ileum and transverse colon will be approximately two fingers wide.

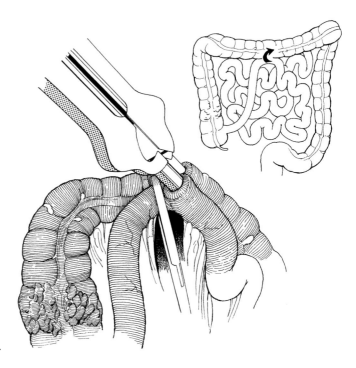

Figure 27.16 Forming a stapled communication between large and small bowel.

Further reading

That one should develop the habit of reading outside the subject is particularly apposite in relationship to this chapter. The gynaecologist must frequently pick up the latest ideas from his or her surgical colleagues and never be too proud to steal an idea or two.

General

Walsh CJ, Jamieson NV, Fazio VW. *Top Tips in Gastrointestinal Surgery*. Oxford: Blackwell Science Ltd, 1999.

Incidental appendicectomy

O'Hanlan K, Fisher DT, O'Holleran MS. 257 incidental appendectomies during total laparoscopic hysterectomy. *JSLS* 2007;11:428–431.

Salom E, Schey D, Peñalver M, *et al*. The safety of incidental appendectomy at the time of abdominal hysterectomy. *Am J Obstet Gynecol* 2003;189:1563–1567.

28 Reconstructive procedures

General comments

The degree to which reconstructive surgery is incorporated directly into one's practice is determined by a number of factors. Most important among them are training and experience. Of lesser importance on a philosophical level, but perhaps of more importance on a practical level, are local hospital politics and standards of practice. The degree to which one involves a plastic surgeon in undertaking these procedures will be influenced by all of the factors. Most importantly, we should never forget that it is the patient who comes first and, whatever combination of surgeons is required to produce optimized care, this is what we should strive for, in whatever hospital or clinical setting in which we practice.

Fortunately, the need to undertake reconstructive surgical procedures in the practice of gynaecology and gynaecological oncology has decreased as the extent of primary radical surgery for vaginal and vulval cancers has been reduced. Over the last 20 years, the use of chemoradiation not only has markedly reduced the need for primary surgery in advanced cases but, when it is required, the extent of it is similarly reduced. A similar trend is noted in the treatment of primary early stage vulval cancer. No longer are many en bloc 'butterfly' incisions used, incorporating large amounts of skin overlying the mons pubis and the skin bridges between the groins and the vulva. Rather, these have been replaced with essentially radical partial vulvectomy and lymph node dissections using sentinel nodes to minimize the need for radical dissection in this area as well. Only in exenterative procedures for locally recurrent gynaecological cancers, generally speaking after chemoradiation failure, are reconstructive procedures commonly undertaken. Once again, as our other treatment modalities have improved, the need for exenteration has also lessened.

Similarly, the need for wide excision of vulval intraepithelial neoplasia (VIN II or III) has been decreased by the use of local ablative therapies, including, but not limited to, the carbon dioxide laser and argon beam coagulation. Despite this, there is still a need for surgeons to be familiar with techniques to close primary vulval defects when primary closure fails.

Vulval reconstruction for localized benign disease, premalignant and early malignant disease

Two commonly used methods to close defects in the areas of the vulva, perineum and vagina involve the use of rotational flaps and Z-plasty. The Lotus petal flap, first described in 1996 by Yii and Niranjan, is being used increasingly to fill vulval defects. These

Bonney's Gynaecological Surgery, 11th edition.
© Tito Lopes, Nick Spirtos, Raj Naik, John Monaghan.
Published 2011 by Blackwell Publishing Ltd.

fasciocutaneous flaps are a versatile alternative to the many flaps available.

Z-plasty (and other variations)

This utilizes the transposition of two or more triangular-shaped flaps of skin in vulval repair to increase the length of an area of tissue which, on a practical level, can be used to cover small defects only; it is not a technique of much practical value in the field of gynaecology. Elongation, once local tissue conditions are taken into account, is somewhat predictable and is based on the angles of the flaps. Flaps of 45° and 60° are most commonly used and provide tissue elongation of 50% and 75%, respectively, without causing significant incisional tension. More complicated techniques of a similar nature include the four- and five-flap plasties (McGregor and McGregor 2000).

Rotational flaps

Rotational flaps, such as the 'lotus petal flaps' are useful for closure of large defects, especially in the posterior aspect of the vulva (Yii and Niranjan 1996).

Full- and split-thickness skin grafts (general considerations)

Full-thickness skin grafts are best used for vaginal reconstruction in women with vaginal agenesis or during vaginal reconstruction following exenterative surgery when the surgeon has chosen to use the omentum along with a skin graft instead of a myocutaneous graft. Full-thickness donor sites should be selected so primary closure can be accomplished without excess tension being placed on the suture line. The inner thigh is ideal for the donor site for this purpose. For split-thickness grafts, donor sites should be smooth and, when possible, the cosmetic aspect given full consideration. Common sites used include the buttocks and the lateral aspect of the thigh. Full-thickness grafts are best harvested freehand using either a no. 10 or a no. 15 Bard Parker blade. All harvested grafts should be placed between saline-soaked gauze.

Split-thickness grafts should be harvested using either a Brown or Zimmer power-driven dermatome. The skin should be cleaned, as should the donor site

for a full-thickness graft, but, in addition, mineral oil should be applied in order to lubricate the skin and facilitate the smooth passage of the dermatome when harvesting the graft. The dermatome should be set at 15/1000 of an inch in thickness. The thickness can be checked by sliding a Bard Parker no. 15 blade between the guard and blade of the dermatome. The donor site should be treated with either epinephrine-soaked sponges or thrombin spray, then covered with either Tegaderm (3M, Loughborough, UK) or gauze permeated with Vaseline. Depending on need, the graft either can be used intact with small periodic incisions made to ensure seromas do not develop or it can be meshed to expand the graft by 1.5–3 times the size, thereby allowing for greater coverage. After either suturing the graft to the host site with 4-0 Monocryl or stapling it in place, it can be covered with bacitracin (1.25 cm in thickness), dressed and left for 4–5 days. Other issues of particular importance include graft contraction and hyperpigmentation, which are more problematic with split-thickness grafts.

It is for this reason that, when undertaking surgery for vaginal agenesis, a full-thickness skin graft should be employed instead of a split-thickness skin graft. Additionally, it should be noted that this surgery can be facilitated by using laparoscopy to help identify and develop the proper space between the rectum and the bladder (see Chapter 8).

Myocutaneous grafts

The vast majority of myocutaneous grafts are used in the repair of pelvic defects related to the treatment or complications of treatment of gynaecological malignancies. Historically, vaginal reconstruction has been accomplished using gracilis myocutaneous or bulbocavernosus grafts and, more recently, the rectus abdominus has become the choice of most gynaecological oncologists. A modification of the standard rectus abdominus graft is the 'fleur-de-lys' flap, as described by McCraw and colleagues, in which the associated defect somewhat resembles the stylized lily of the 'fleur-de-lys'. This defect requires much less tension on the suture or staple lines when reapproximating the subcutaneous tissues and skin. Detailed descriptions of these procedures are beyond the scope of this text and readers are referred to the Further reading section.

Further reading

McCraw JB, Massey FM, Shanklin KD, Horton CE. Vaginal reconstruction with gracilis myocutaneous flaps. *Plast Reconstr Surg* 1976;58:176–183. The definition, history, experimental background, surgical technique, and clinical applications of compound gracilis myocutaneous flaps are presented.

McCraw JB, Arnold PG. *McCraw and Arnold's Atlas of Muscle and Musculocutaneous Flaps*. Cresskill, NJ: Hampton Press Publishing, 1986. See http://www.global-help.org/publications/books/book_mccrawmuscleatlas.html

McGregor AD, McGregor IA. *Fundamental Techniques of Plastic Surgery and Their Surgical Applications*, 10th edn. Edinburgh: Churchill Livingstone, 2000.

Yii NW, Niranjan NS. Lotus petal flaps in vulvo-vaginal reconstruction. *Br J Plast Surg* 1996;49:547–554.

Index

Page numbers in *italics* represent figures, those in **bold** represent tables.

Bonney's Gynaecological Surgery, 11th edition.
© Tito Lopes, Nick Spirtos, Raj Naik, John Monaghan.
Published 2011 by Blackwell Publishing Ltd.